MEDICO-SOCIAL MANAGEMENT OF
INHERITED METABOLIC DISEASE

The Society exists to promote exchanges of ideas between workers in different disciplines who are interested in any aspect of inborn metabolic disorders. Particulars of the Society can be obtained from the Editors of this Symposium.

*Symposia 1–10 published by E. & S. Livingstone

MEDICO-SOCIAL MANAGEMENT OF INHERITED METABOLIC DISEASE

A MONOGRAPH DERIVED FROM
The Proceedings of the Thirteenth Symposium of The Society for the Study of Inborn Errors of Metabolism

EDITED AND ENLARGED BY
D. N. Raine

MTP

Published by
MTP Press Ltd.
PO Box 55, St. Leonards House
St. Leonardgate, Lancaster, England

First published 1977

ISBN 0 85200160 6

MADE AND PRINTED IN GREAT BRITAIN BY
THE GARDEN CITY PRESS LIMITED
LETCHWORTH, HERTFORDSHIRE
SG6 1JS

Contents

ASPECTS OF MANAGEMENT
REQUIRING CENTRAL POLICY

THE FOURTH MILNER LECTURE

Preface

The study of inherited metabolic disease became a subject of more than academic interest in 1953 when Bickel, Gerrard and Hickmans discovered that the totally disabling consequences of phenylketonuria could be prevented if treatment was instituted in the first months of life. This required the widespread screening of all newborn babies and 7 years later this had been successfully achieved in the United Kingdom. The next 10 years was a period of consolidation: screening methods were improved and extended to include other disorders; treatment of phenylketonuria was vastly improved with the stimulus of the increasing numbers of patients being detected, and research into new forms of therapy for some of the other disorders being detected has been initiated. The success of this scheme is illustrated by the remarkable achievement reported by the Phenylketonuria Registry referred to in the present volume.

But at what cost has this progress been made? It is unnecessary to discuss the financial cost for many of the developments would not have been started if their economic value in the system of health care had not been unequivocally established. Many anticipated, and sought to minimize, the anxiety inherent in screening healthy populations; the potential disruption in the family in administering a special diet to one of its members for the first several years of its life; and the immeasurable cost of trials of unestablished forms of treatment before they are perfected—but in retrospect these costs have been greater than some expected. It is towards the solution of these problems and the more controlled development of this aspect of health care that the present book is directed.

That it must develop is without question. In many respects the management of genetic disease is at a stage in its development comparable with that of infective disease about the time of Pasteur. The achievements of the past 25 years are more than could have been expected by those who have lived through them and should more than encourage those new to the subject. No longer is treatment of several inherited metabolic diseases the subject of debate and the present state of the art is described in my *Treatment of Inherited Metabolic Disease* (MTP, Lancaster, 1975). However, genetic disease, more than most aspects of medical care, calls for several services, often simultaneously, and it is essential that these are developed in parallel. Some are proceeding as the result of efforts by individual physicians and medical scientists, but others require the formulation and implementation of policy at a national level.

The present work started as a discussion presented at a symposium of the Royal College of Pathologists in February 1974. This was followed by a decision by the Society for the Study of Inborn Errors of Metabolism to devote its next annual meeting, which all of the present contributors attended, to this subject. Because some of the components of a health care system for inherited metabolic disease are not given the status of chapters in the present work, the original paper is reprinted with the kind permission of the Royal College of Pathologists. Those components that are discussed more fully demonstrate convincingly that a unified service is required and, because of the special nature of some of the problems, the more usual concepts of diagnosis and treatment must be extended and, to be successful, the health care system must be one of total management. If the book helps to achieve this its purpose will have been served.

D. N. Raine

The editor wishes to express the gratitude of all the members of the Society for the generous grants which have been received in support of this symposium from Mr J. Milner of Milner Scientific and Medical Research, Liverpool, and Scientific Hospital Supplies Ltd., Liverpool

Active Participants

CHRISTINE CLOTHIER
Alder Hey Children's Hospital, Eaton Road, Liverpool L12 2AP

CAROL L. CLOW
DeBelle Laboratory for Biochemical Genetics, McGill University—Montreal Children's Hospital Research Institute, 2300 Tupper Street, Montreal 108, Province of Quebec, Canada

VALERIE COWIE
Queen Mary's Hospital for Children, Carshalton, Surrey SM5 4NR

JOAN S. EMMERSON
University Library, University of Newcastle upon Tyne NE1 7RU

P. R. EVANS
Hospital for Sick Children, Great Ormond Street, London W.C.2

JANET HAWCROFT
Phenylketonuria Register Office, Alder Hey Children's Hospital, Eaton Road, Liverpool L12 1AP

A. J. HEDLEY
Department of Community Health, University Hospital and Medical School, Clifton Boulevard, Nottingham NG7 2UH

F. P. HUDSON (DECEASED)
Phenylketonuria Register Office, Alder Hey Children's Hospital, Eaton Road, Liverpool L12 2AP

G. M. KOMROWER
Willink Biochemical Genetics Laboratory, Royal Manchester Children's Hospital, Pendlebury, Manchester M27 1HA

ELSIE D. MAY
Community Health Services Division, Trafalgar House, Paradise Circus, Birmingham B1 2BQ

T. W. MEADE
Epidemiology and Medical Care Unit, Northwick Park Hospital, Watford Road, Harrow HA1 3UJ, Middlesex

D. A. PATRICK

University of London Institute of Child Health, 30 Guildford Street, London WC1N 1EH

T. L. PERRY

Department of Pharmacology, University of British Columbia, Vancouver 8, Canada

D. N. RAINE

Department of Clinical Chemistry, The Children's Hospital, Ladywood Middleway, Birmingham B16 8ET

G. A. RATNER

School of Law, Indiana University, 735 West New York Street, Indianapolis, IN 46202, USA

NANSI G. REES

Department of Clinical Chemistry, The Children's Hospital, Ladywood Middleway, Birmingham B16 8ET

C. R. SCRIVER

DeBelle Laboratory for Biochemical Genetics, McGill University— Montreal Children's Hospital Research Institute, 2300 Tupper Street, Montreal 108, Province of Quebec, Canada

SUSAN H. TERRY

Institute of Mental Subnormality, Lea Castle Hospital, Wolverley, Nr. Kidderminster, Worcestershire

E. WAMBERG

John F. Kennedy Institute, 2600 Glostrup, Denmark

A. WESTWOOD

Institute of Mental Subnormality, Lea Castle Hospital, Wolverley, Nr. Kidderminster, Worcestershire

THE NATURE AND SIZE
OF THE PROBLEM

I

The need for a national policy for the management of inherited metabolic disease

D. N. Raine

Clinical education is based on the apprenticeship system and depends upon the student having personal experience of most of the disorders that he is likely, in the future, to have to deal with. For more unusual or difficult problems, a system of specialist consultants exists and some of these are inclined to specialize even further by seeking out groups of related, but even more unusual, disorders such as muscular dystrophy or childhood celiac disease, and to devise systems of care that would otherwise remain untried and unavailable. For disorders even less common than muscular dystrophy, such as the rare metabolic diseases, the undergraduate educational system breaks down, and unless special attention is drawn to one of these, as with phenylketonuria (because it was one of the first chronic forms of mental subnormality to be treatable), or with galactosaemia (because it often presents with recognizable clinical features and again can be treated) it is likely to pass unrecognized by many medical consultants and to remain unknown to most family doctors (the educational system does not allow it to be otherwise). There are already more than 140 of these rare metabolic disorders inherited by recessive or sex-linked mechanisms for which the precise enzyme deficiency is known: there are altogether 1 200 diseases inherited by similar mechanisms and may soon prove to be metabolic in origin.[1] These diseases collectively constitute a significant part of clinical medicine which the present structure of health care does not allow of satisfactory management.

The present discussion is concerned with the size and nature of this problem and the possible ways in which it can be resolved.

This contribution to the Royal College of Pathologists symposium in February 1974 is reprinted with permission and with minor modifications from *Molecular Variants in Disease*. Ed. D. N. Raine. Symposium organized by the Royal College of Pathologists, February 1974. Published for the Royal College of Pathologists by the Journal of Clinical Pathology, London.

The size of the problem

Many of the inherited metabolic diseases are associated with mental handicap of an order that requires long-term institutional care. Others, which at present are fatal in early life, while they are not an economic burden on the community, are so temptingly near to being treatable that there is a strong human desire to improve the means to do this. Unfortunately, good estimates of the incidence of these diseases are available in very few instances and so the real size of the problem must be approached indirectly. Two approaches are possible: one from the known incidence of known diseases provides a minimum figure; the other, from an estimate of the proportion of paediatric admissions to hospital, paediatric deaths, and patients who are mentally subnormal and have an underlying metabolic disease also provides a useful figure. Estimates by both of these approaches will be made.

INCIDENCE OF SOME SPECIFIC METABOLIC DISORDERS

Surveys of these relatively rare conditions must cover hundreds of thousands of subjects before the number of affected patients is large enough to give a statistically significant assessment of their incidence. The number of satisfactory surveys is regrettably few: the following, however, provide usable data and are summarized in Table 1.1.

World Health Organization (1972)[2]
The source of these data is not stated but the report is prepared by an experienced group of workers in the field of inherited metabolic disease and must have derived from large population screening programmes.

Council of Europe Public Health Committee (1973)[3]
These data derive from centres screening for various combinations of inherited metabolic diseases in the neonatal population in eight countries. The cases discovered and the size of populations screened were: for phenylketonuria, 668 in 5 252 000 (a rate of 12.7×10^{-5}); for histidinaemia 18 in 214 703 (8.4×10^{-5}); and for galactosaemia 21 in 725 857 (2.9×10^{-5}).

Table 1.1 Frequency (per 100 000 births) and rate of occurrence of new cases of specific inherited metabolic diseases

Metabolic disease	WHO[2]	Council of Europe[3]	Frequency used	New cases in UK per year	Estimated life expectancy (years)
Phenylketonuria	7.0	12.7	10	100	50+
Hyperphenylalaninaemia	3.0	—	—	—	—
Histidinaemia	6.0	8.4	7	70	50+
Galactosaemia	3.0	2.9	3	30	20+
Homocystinuria	6.0	—	6	60	20+
Cystinuria	7.0	—	7	70	50+
Tyrosinaemia	0.4	—	0.4	4	5
Maple syrup urine disease	0.3	—	0.3	3	5
Argininosuccinicaciduria	0.5	—	0.5	5	20+
Adrenogenital syndrome	—	—	14.3[4]	143	20+
Cystic fibrosis	50.0	—	50.0	500	20+
Prolinaemia	—	—	10.8[5]	—	50+

Other sources

A careful estimate of the incidence of the adrenogenital syndrome (without considering separately the several different enzyme deficiencies leading to this) was made by Hubble.[4] Data for prolinaemia type 1 were collected for the Council of Europe survey but not published. The incidence from the survey by Raine, Cooke, Andrews and Mahon[5] is included in Table 1.1 and represents six cases in 55 715 babies tested. However, there is an increasing feeling that prolinaemia type 1 may be a biochemical abnormality that is only coincidentally associated with disease symptoms and so this condition has not been included in any of the calculations in the present paper.

Table 1.1 also contains the number of new cases born in the United Kingdom each year assuming 1 million births annually (in 1970 there were 902 500 live births).

The significance of these several diseases, of course, is different. Those so serious as to lead to death in infancy can be largely discounted; others allow the patient to survive childhood with treatment and others do not significantly shorten life. Some of these patients, when well treated, are associated with a normal productive life, but others may need institutional care for many years. It is impossible to be either accurate or even very dogmatic about these factors for a particular disease, but in an attempt to consider one of them, a somewhat subjective assessment of life expectancy is also included in Table 1.1. The life span given is neither the mean nor the maximum age, and the age reached by many patients has been reduced when there is a tendency for death to occur in childhood even though some patients may survive long after this.

Calculating the number of new cases of inherited metabolic disease each year in the United Kingdom on the basis of these 10 diseases the number will be about 985 (say 1000), and most of these will require substantial medical or institutional care for several years if treated satisfactorily. However, if treated inadequately or allowed to remain undiagnosed, many will require treatment or institutional care for much longer, although some would, of course, die.

INCIDENCE BASED ON PAEDIATRIC DEATHS

Two careful studies have been made of the proportion of deaths in children's hospitals that can be attributed to genetic causes. The first,[6] based on 200 deaths, gave a figure of 12%, but did not differentiate single gene defects from chromosome disorders. The second and larger study[7] of 1041 deaths agreed with the earlier that the proportion due to genetic causes was 11%. Of the 2.5% that were chromosomal in origin most were cases of Down's syndrome, but the remaining 8.5% were attributable to recessive or sex-linked disorders, the form of inheritance most likely to be associated with disease of metabolic origin. Indeed 53 of the 88 recessive and sex-linked disorders were certainly metabolic, the precise cause being known.

The number of paediatric deaths in England and Wales can be ascertained from the Registrar General's Statistical Review for 1971[8] as follows: Table 4 of the report shows that there were, in 1971, for children aged 1–14 years, 1.36 deaths per 1000 living children. Table 1 gives 10 894 900 as the population aged 1–14, thus the deaths in this age group were 14 800. For children under 1 year, those who died under 1 month are excluded from the present calculations. The number of deaths of children aged 1 month to 1 year was 4607 (Table 13). The total childhood deaths between 1 month and 14 years was, therefore, 19 407, and the number (8.5% of the total) due to inherited metabolic diseases is 1650. The children dying in less than one month are excluded, not because the illness is less likely to be of genetic origin, but because there is little opportunity to diagnose them and institute effective treatment. This situation could considerably change in the future, in which case the number of deaths under 1 year used in this calculation should be trebled.

INCIDENCE BASED ON PAEDIATRIC ADMISSIONS

In an attempt to determine the frequency of genetic disease the patients admitted to Montreal Children's Hospital in 1969–70 were classified under a number of headings (Ref. 2, Table 1). Of the total admissions, 4.7% had a recessive or sex-linked genetic disorder. Thus, if admissions in the United Kingdom are comparable, this provides another means of assessing the case load of inherited metabolic disease. In 1972 there were 856 670 discharges of children aged 0–14 years in England and Wales (taken from the Report on the Hospital In-patient Enquiry, 1972) and 4.7% of this is 40 260. This should be divided by the average annual discharges for each individual. This figure is not known but is probably between two and five, giving an annual case load between 8052 and 20 130. Dividing these figures by 15 gives an annual occurrence between 537 and 1342.

PREVALENCE OF INHERITED METABOLIC DISEASE
AMONG THE MENTALLY HANDICAPPED

Diagnostic precision in the field of mental handicap is increasing so rapidly that early surveys of the aetiological factors are now of little value. However, Berg[9] found in a survey of 800 consecutive admissions to the Fountain Hospital 22 cases (2.8%) of metabolic disease. In the now classical study in Northern Ireland by Carson and Neill,[10] a survey of 2081 mentally retarded individuals yielded, apart from a number of generalized amino acidurias of unknown significance, 62 (3.0%) cases of specific metabolic disease.

In a later survey by Carson[11] of 5523 mentally retarded subjects and 4126 patients suspected of having an amino acid disorder, 116 patients (1.2%) were found to have an inherited metabolic disease and only 11 of these patients were not mentally retarded. This survey will be affected by the fact that nearly half of those screened did not have mental handicap. The ratio of patients with inherited metabolic disease and mental handicap to the number of mentally handicapped children screened, 105 in 5523, gives an incidence of 1.9%.

A survey of children admitted for assessment or long-term care to Queen Mary's Hospital, Carshalton, showed that of 645 children, 21 (3.3%) had an inherited metabolic disease.[12]

It would seem reasonable to assume that 3% of mental handicap is associated with metabolic diseases that can be recognized by the relatively simple investigations used in most of these surveys and that this is a minimal figure.

INCIDENCE BASED ON PROBABLE PROPORTION OF MENTALLY
SUBNORMAL PATIENTS WITH INHERITED METABOLIC DISEASE

The annual rate of ascertainment of mental handicap can be derived from surveys in Wessex, Newcastle upon Tyne and Camberwell (Ref 13, Table 1). The number of mildly and severely affected individuals, aged 0–14 years, in hospital and at home was 73 per 100 000 total population. Taking the total population of the United Kingdom as 50 million, this gives a total mentally handicapped population of 36 500.

The annual rate of ascertainment will be one-fifteenth of this, 2433, and the number associated with inherited metabolic disease, at the rate of 3.0%, will be 73/year. This is a surprisingly low figure and probably reflects the fact that the surveys are least effective in ascertaining the mild to moderate degrees of mental handicap in individuals living at home. Generally the handicap associated with metabolic disease is of this order rather than the very severe degree of handicap that requires almost all those affected to be cared for in hospitals for the subnormal.

SUMMARY OF ASSESSMENTS OF THE SIZE OF THE PROBLEM

The number of new cases of inherited metabolic disease derived in these various ways is summarized in Table 1.2, and they are all close enough to make them reasonably credible. Although some are for the United Kingdom and others for England and Wales, the difference is scarcely significant considering the error involved in the derivation of the figures.

The annual case load cannot be less than 1000 and it may be as high as 3000. For practical purposes it would be reasonable to assume that at present it is about 2000. It is unlikely that this number will ever be reduced and, as diagnostic skills improve, it can be expected to increase.

Table 1.2   Annual occurrence of cases of inherited metabolic disease in the United Kingdom (UK) or England and Wales assessed by different methods

Sum of known diseases of known incidence	985	(UK)
8.5% Paediatric deaths have a recessive or sex-linked genetic cause	1650	(England & Wales)
4.7% Paediatric hospital admissions are due to recessive and sex-linked genetic disease	537–1342	(England & Wales)
3% Mental subnormality is due to inherited metabolic disease	73	(UK)
For comparison		
Down's syndrome	1312	
Congenital malformations	14 000	

Ideal requirements for satisfactory management

The successful management by family doctors, consultant paediatricians, nurses, social workers, biochemists, obstetricians and geneticists of patients, their parents and prospective parents with some genetic risk involves a number of services, all of which must be readily available and properly coordinated. (1) Accurate information must be assembled and made accessible. (2) Diagnostic services, which may be specialized, should be established. (3) Early detection systems, such as screening for phenylketonuria in the neonatal period, should be instituted in appropriate circumstances. (4) The best information on treatment should be accessible to those concerned with newly diagnosed patients. Existing methods should be improved and new ones devised. (5) Methods of heterozygote detection should be improved and made available. (6) Research into prenatal detection of affected fetuses by amniocentesis should continue until a reliable service can be offered, and the proper place of genetic counselling should continue to be explored. (7) The natural history of the rarer and new diseases needs to be studied in order to ascertain the need for, and the most appropriate form of, management of the condition. (8) A coordinating system for both information and the care of individual patients or subjects at risk, on a national or a supraregional basis, should be designed.

These aspects of the total management of inherited metabolic disease are in different states of development. Thus, while some, such as the Guthrie method of screening for phenylketonuria, and limited extensions of this, are developed to the point where they can be regarded as established forms of service, others, such as prenatal detection by amniocentesis, need further research. Other aspects such as the development of new methods of treatment are still entirely in the research phase. As the different aspects are discussed an indication will be given of their present state of development into those that can usefully provide a service now (S) and those which require further research before their application can be extended beyond a few centres (R).

INFORMATION SYSTEMS

S   *Statements of preferred treatment*

S   *Known patients and their clinicians*

S R Medical literature screen

 R Rapid retrieval from literature file

 R Statement of desirable studies of disease

The value of a continuously revised statement of the treatment of a specific disorder is well illustrated by a patient who suffered a lens dislocation in adult life as a consequence of homocystinuria. Here surgical treatment is moderately urgent but there may be time to treat the patient before the operation in order to minimize the risk of thrombosis. The precise dose of pyridoxine to be given, the optimal frequency of monitoring its effect, the need and extent of reducing the dose after the operation, and the requirements for a low-methionine diet should pyridoxine prove ineffective will rarely be known by the ophthalmologist, and to discover this from the literature would involve unacceptable delays. The information can all be given by telephone and on two occasions recently untreated patients have been improved within two days and rendered safe for surgery within eight days.

For less acute situations, after some initial advice has been given by a reference centre, the clinician will be helped if he can speak directly with those currently treating other patients with a particular metabolic disease. A file of patients and their medical advisers, maintained by the reference centre, would facilitate this.

Keeping abreast of newly published work on all of the inherited metabolic diseases is impossible even for the specialist. It has already been suggested[14] that a population equal to that of the United Kingdom will require five reference centres. Each of these should be able to retrieve from that published sufficient information to deal adequately with about 20 diseases. Having retrieved the information it is necessary to devise means of recovering this from the reference file with the minimum of delay and this will require some experimentation before the best system is established.

As part of the further understanding of a disease and its management it is often necessary to design the care of future patients in a manner that will yield new information. Those treating patients and to whom new ideas occur may wait several years before these can be tested and the reference centre can greatly hasten this process by maintaining statements of desirable new studies. When new cases become available the already planned studies can be proposed and the help of the clinician sought in making them.

DIAGNOSTIC SERVICE

S   Reference laboratories

S R   Selection of crucial diagnostic tests

R   Computer-assisted diagnosis

One of the most inhibiting factors preventing paediatricians taking a greater interest in inherited metabolic disease is the difficulty in making the appropriate investigations. This is illustrated by the fact that histological examination of a liver biopsy is still occasionally the first step in the investigation of glycogen storage disease.

For the more unusual diseases such as the organic acidaemias there may be only one or two laboratories in the country able to perform the appropriate analyses and while they are often willing to do so for clinicians outside their area they have no commitment to do this, or indeed to maintain the diagnostic facility beyond the term of interest of the individual who initiated it. To overcome this, the Department of Health and Social Security has taken the first steps to establish supra-regional reference laboratories, but so far none have been established to cater adequately for the inherited metabolic diseases. Nonetheless, the informal network of interested laboratories has been doing useful service for several years, and will, no doubt, continue to do this within its available resources.

Only if the laboratory or clinician is acquainted with the latest inform-ation will he initiate the most discriminating tests for diagnosis. Thank-fully, the galactose tolerance test is probably never performed now to diagnose galactosaemia, the assay of galactose-1-phosphate uridyl transferase in erythrocytes being more generally available. However, the clinician may not be aware of the extent to which the assay of specific enzymes in leukocytes can effect the diagnosis of several neuronal lipid storage diseases more effectively than the only alternative he may know, namely, histological examination of a brain biopsy. The selection of the most discriminating diagnostic tests needs to be continuously reviewed, and the reference centre should be able to advise on, and undertake, those most useful.

The concept of computer-assisted diagnosis has already been applied to a number of disease areas, and the inherited metabolic diseases would seem to be amenable to similar treatment. A programme for such a system has been written and is currently being examined to discover the extent to which it can reduce the large number of possible diagnoses (many of which will be overlooked during the conventional diagnostic process) given the symptoms and signs of an individual patient with an inherited metabolic disease.

EARLY DETECTION (TOTAL POPULATION SCREENING)

S   *Guthrie testing (phenylketonuria, histidinaemia, methioninaemia, etc.)*

S   *Scriver testing (most amino acid disorders)*

S R   *Limited extensions (e.g., galactosaemia)*

The concept of total population screening for phenylketonuria in the neonatal period is now well established and its effectiveness, in terms of the results of the very early treatment of affected children, that it allows have been most rewarding. The same principle has been applied to the detection of histidinaemia and methioninaemia (for itself and as an indication of homocystinuria). The technique is capable of still further extension, but only testing for phenylketonuria is at present advised by the Department of Health and Social Security (H.M. (69) 72).

An alternative method of screening the total neonatal population is by plasma chromatography. This technique, which can detect in one procedure several amino acid disorders, is used regularly in the Manchester Regional Hospital Board area and in the City of Birmingham. It is reported to detect 3.5 times as many children as a simple Guthrie test[5] but the question of replacing the latter by this test is not a simple one, and this is not the place to discuss the merits or otherwise of the case.

Screening methods suitable for application to the total neonatal population are available for some other diseases, including galactosaemia and, probably in the near future, for cystic fibrosis. However, it is inconceivable that the hundred or so metabolic diseases will be amenable to this form of detection on a total population basis, and any further extensions of this are likely to be limited technically, and will be increasingly difficult to justify in economic terms.

TREATMENT

S   *Treatment centres*

S R   Standardization and improvement of existing methods of treatment

R   Development of new methods of treatment

The Department of Health and Social Security have recommended (H.M. (69) 72) that experience of treating phenylketonuria should be concentrated as much as possible within the limits imposed by the distances that must be travelled by the patients. The same advice must surely be given for all relatively rare diseases if the best results are to be obtained. However, this is not to deprive individual paediatricians or family doctors of the interest and responsibility for their own patients. In practice it is necessary for the treatment centre to have an interested paediatrician and biochemist, and the resources of an expert dietitian, and even a social worker. This team determines the treatment, but once it is established it is usually possible for the supervision to be maintained near the patient's home, and biochemical monitoring can be continued by sending samples to the laboratory, the patient visiting the centre at less frequent intervals as long as metabolic control is maintained.

Centres can maintain a good level of control, even when the patient moves to a different part of the country, and there are considerable advantages in standardizing the treatment of a given condition, provided it does not prevent those centres with a special interest and appropriate facilities from making changes that might result in an improved regime.

There has, in the past, been a rather depressed attitude to the treatment of inherited metabolic disease and, apart from dietary restrictions of the type applied to phenylketonuria, it was believed that there was little to offer. This is no longer so, and a number of diseases are found to respond to various vitamins, some of which act as coenzymes for the defective enzyme, but others are effective by less obvious means. Enzyme replacement has been attempted in various forms, and the results of organ transplants (including bone marrow) justify continuing with these experimental approaches. Treatment of prolinaemia and hydroxyprolinaemia is possible (but as yet of unknown advantage) by blocking renal tubular reabsorption[15] and the treatment of the several glycogenoses is now based on much more rational grounds. These several approaches have been briefly reviewed[14] and more fully by Raine.[16] The scope for further research into new methods of treatment of these disorders is unlimited.

HETEROZYGOTE DETECTION

S R   *Standardization and improvement of existing methods*

S   *Counselling services*

R   *Design of new tests*

R   *Improved methods of reporting*

The assessment of carrier status is often required by the siblings and more distant relatives of an affected patient about the time of their marriage. While many clinicians will arrange such an assessment when requested, it is rarely offered because the conclusion in about one-fifth of subjects is uncertain. While the uncertainty can be reduced by increasing the precision of the test, it is probable that it can never be eliminated. This has led to a change in attitude towards the present methods of testing, whether they are based on direct enzyme assay, in which the heterozygotes have half the normal complement of enzyme activity or on a loading test using the normal substrate of the defective enzyme, in which the heterozygote is less tolerant of the load than a homozygous normal subject. The tests have hitherto been required to give a 'yes' or 'no' answer to whether the subject is heterozygous for the disease in question. By changing this strict requirement and, instead, using the result of the test to calculate the probability that the subject is heterozygous, the accuracy of the conclusion is immediately increased and in certain cases, where a family history is known, an indefinite statement can be made more definite.[17,18]

The value of heterozygote tests will be further improved if different laboratories will agree on standard conditions for such procedures as the phenylalanine tolerance test.

There is still scope for improving tests of heterozygosity, especially those based on enzyme assay. For example, it is better to relate the measured enzyme activity to that of another enzyme, not affected by the disease and of comparable activity, than to such parameters as cell count, protein content, or haemoglobin. Similarly in leukocytes and fibroblasts the use of phytohaemagglutinin to bring the cells into a common growth phase further narrows the range of activity characterizing the heterozygous and homozygous normal populations.

The role of genetic counselling centres is still debated. Edwards[19] believes that for the inherited metabolic diseases at least the genetics are so simple that specialist centres should not be required to give advice which could be given by any family doctor. Nonetheless, many lack the confidence to give this simple advice and until they are able to do so the very real needs[20] of the families at genetic risk should be met—if necessary by specialist counselling centres.

More studies, such as that by Carter, Roberts, Evans and Buck[21] of the effectiveness of such counselling centres will also help to establish their correct place in the management of these disorders.

PRENATAL DETECTION

S R   Counselling

  R   Performance of tests

  R   Design of new tests

The ability to recognize that a fetus is at risk for a genetic disease in time to abort it if this is desired, is an exciting prospect in the management of metabolic disease for which there is no prospect of treatment. Unfortunately, some initial successes have been followed by unbridled enthusiasm and the medical literature already contains reports of mistaken diagnoses and unnecessary abortions and more unpublished cases are known. Much careful work remains to be done before a reliable prenatal detection service can be offered and it is important that this is carried out as quickly as possible in a few centres in order to define safe limits for its more widespread application. Here a nationally organized coordinating system would be of the greatest benefit but none exists and the work is likely to proceed for some time on an *ad hoc* basis.

In this area, too, further research is needed on the emotional, ethical and medical aspects of this form of genetic counselling.[20]

NATURAL HISTORY

  R   Clinico-pathological studies of specific diseases

  R   Recognition of non-diseases

  R   Optimal age for testing and treating

While the better known diseases are receiving more organized and rational attention new diseases will emerge and more cases of hitherto rare conditions will be recognized. Only by knowing the pattern of progress in the untreated disease can the proper treatment or, indeed, the need for treatment, be established. Already there is a growing list of 'diseases' in which an inherited biochemical abnormality was wrongly associated with symptoms and pathology. Cystathioninuria in its inherited form is now known to be a benign biochemical abnormality (there are other serious causes of cystathioninuria but these are not inherited) and Joseph's syndrome, in which proline, hydroxyproline and glycine are excreted in urine in excess, is similarly a benign defect of a renal tubular transport mechanism. By ensuring that healthy relatives of patients are examined for the biochemical abnormality the reference centre can help to reveal further examples of these coincidental associations.

The optimal age of testing for phenylketonuria has been established by the Medical Research Council Working Party on Phenylketonuria[22] as 6–9 days and the optimal age for treating the condition is as soon as possible, but not later than 3 months. However, this information has been obtained by a costly process and it does not exist with anything like the same precision for any other inherited metabolic disease. Thus, while it is suspected that 6 days is too late to screen for galactosaemia, this may be too soon if all cases of homocystinuria are to be recognized. These are further arguments against the extension of total population screening in the neonatal period, but this same information is required for the management of any patient with an inherited disease in which the risk is known and the diagnosis can be established before irreversible damage has occurred.

COORDINATION

S R   *Patient file—computer linked*

  R   *Gene file—computer linked*

S R   *Initial ascertainment*

  R   *Quality control*

  R   *Retrieval conditions—confidentiality*

If the concept is accepted of five reference centres in the United Kingdom, each responsible for keeping itself informed on all aspects of about 20 diseases, so that advice can be given in an immediate fashion on the best methods of diagnosis and treatment, and at the same time offer diagnostic facilities, and be linked with treatment centres using standardized methods, and, where necessary, undertaking the appropriate investigations required for genetic counselling of potential heterozygotes and monitoring pregnancies at risk of genetic disease, then it remains to coordinate this activity and ensure that all centres continue to offer the desired level of service.

Such coordination will be at the national level and details of its structure are open to variation and experiment. It is anticipated that it will require a comprehensive file of affected patients, with or without the aid of a computer. If heterozygote detection develops to the extent some anticipate, a computer-linked file of abnormal genes might also be envisaged, but this will require careful consideration of the conditions for entry into, and retrieval from, the file. The problems of legitimacy and of confidentiality are already being examined by those concerned with computer-linked files of patients.

Testing laboratories now take for granted that their performance will be improved by being subject to a quality control programme and this too should be organized from a national centre.

Finally a system for the initial ascertainment of affected individuals, easy enough for most clinicians to be willing to use, should be devised, and a model for this has already been established by the MRC Phenylketonuria Working Parties, and the MRC/DHSS Phenylketonuria Register in Liverpool.

Discussion

Much of the organizational structure that has been outlined is relevant to the management of many medical conditions that are already being dealt with satisfactorily. The reason for a special case for inherited metabolic disease has already been accepted in Canada where an informal group of investigators and interested parties has formed 'The Committee for the Improvement of Hereditary Disease Management'. Their objectives are stated at the end of a substantial publication[23] aimed at providing a guide to investigators of inherited metabolic disease.

In Britain, responsibility, including finance, for service aspects of health care lies with the Department of Health and Social Security, and is administered via the National Health Service. Research into medical developments, however, is largely undertaken by the Medical Research Council and, hitherto, except for minor departures from these two positions, it has been difficult to support satisfactorily developments of what is essentially a service when the research still needed is only relevant if it is agreed that the service can, and should, be developed. Such situations appear to be provided for by the recommendations of Lord Rothschild[24] but more controversial issues of that report have obscured the need for such customer-contractor-orientated research.

However, regardless of finance, if the need to establish a system of care for inherited metabolic disease could be accepted, the formal coordination of those services that already exist would immediately result in an improvement throughout the country, and a structure would then have been provided within which further developments could take place at whatever rate the national economy will allow.

REFERENCES

1. McKusick, V. A. (1975). *Mendelian Inheritance in Man.* 4th ed. (Baltimore: Johns Hopkins Press)
2. World Health Organization (1972). *Genetic Disorders: Prevention, Treatment and Rehabilitation.* (Geneva: WHO Tecl. Rep. Ser. No. 497)
3. Council of Europe Public Health Committee. (1973). Collective results of mass screening for inborn metabolic errors in eight European countries. *Acta Paediatr. Scand.,* **62,** 413
4. Hubble, D. V. (1966). Congenital adrenal hyperplasia. In K. S. Holt and D. N. Raine (eds.) *Basic Concepts of Inborn Errors and Defects of Steroid Biosynthesis,* pp. 68–74. (Edinburgh: Livingstone)
5. Raine, D. N., Cooke, J. R., Andrews, W. A. and Mahon, D. F. (1972). Screening for inherited metabolic disease by plasma chromatography (Scriver) in a large city. *Br. Med. J.,* **3,** 7
6. Carter, C. O. (1956). Changing patterns in the causes of death at The Hospital for Sick Children. *Grt. Ormond St. J.,* **11,** 65
7. Roberts, D. F., Chavez, J. and Court, S. D. M. (1970). The genetic component in child mortality. *Arch. Dis. Child.,* **45,** 33
8. Office of Population Censuses and Surveys. (1973). *Registrar General's Statistical Review of England and Wales for the year 1971,* Part 1. Tables, Medical. (London: HMSO)
9. Berg, J. M. (1963). Causal factors in severe mental retardation. In *Proceedings of the 2nd International Congress on Mental Retardation, Vienna, 1961.* Part 1, pp. 170–3 (Basle: Karger) (Cited by Crome L. and Stern, J.) (1972), *Pathology of Mental Retardation,* 2nd ed., p. 8. (Edinburgh and London: Churchill Livingstone)
10. Carson, N. A. J. and Neill, D. W. (1962). Metabolic abnormalities detected in a survey of mentally backward individuals in Northern Ireland. *Arch. Dis. Child.,* **37,** 505
11. Carson, N. A. J. (1970). Disorders of amino acid metabolism: results of screening programmes in Northern Ireland. In M. Roth (ed.), *Proceedings of the 7th International Congress of Clinical Chemistry, Geneva/Evian, 1969.* Vol. 3, pp. 320–9. *Hormones, Lipids and Miscellaneous.* (Basle: Karger)
12. Angeli, E. and Kirman, B. H. (1971). Genetic counselling of the family of the mentally retarded child. In *Proceedings of the Second Congress of the International Association for the Scientific Study of Mental Deficiency,* pp. 692–6. (Warsaw: Policy Medical Publishers)

13. Department of Health and Social Security and Welsh Office. (1971). *Better Services for the Mentally Handicapped.* Command 4683. (London: HMSO)
14. RAINE, D. N. (1972). Management of inherited metabolic disease. *Br. Med. J.*, **2**, 329
15. COOKE, J. R. and RAINE, D. N. (1973). Competitive inhibition of renal tubular transport in the treatment of prolinaemia and hydroxyprolinaemia. In J. W. T. Seakins, R. A. Saunders and C. Toothill (eds.), *Treatment of Inborn Errors of Metabolism*, pp. 97–103. (Edinburgh and London: Churchill Livingstone)
16. RAINE, D. N. (1974). *The Treatment of Inherited Metabolic Disease.* (Lancaster: M.T.P.)
17. WESTWOOD, A. and RAINE, D. N. (1973). Some problems of heterozygote recognition in inherited metabolic disease with special reference to phenylketonuria In J. W. T. Seakins, R. A. Saunders and C. Toothill (eds.), *Treatment of Inborn Errors of Metabolism*, pp. 63–77. (Edinburgh: Churchill Livingstone)
18. WESTWOOD, A. and RAINE, D. N. (1975). Heterozygote detection in phenylketonuria: measurement of discriminatory ability and interpretation of the phenylalanine loading test by determination of the heterozygote likihood ratio. *J. Med. Genet.* **12**, 327
19. EDWARDS, J. H. (1972). Genetic counselling. (Letter) *Br. Med.J.*, **2**, 22
20. COWIE, V. (1972). Genetic and social aspects of prenatal and newborn population screening. *Ann. Clin. Biochem.*, **9**, 112
21. CARTER, C. O., ROBERTS, J. A. F., EVANS, K. A. and BUCK, A. R. (1971). Genetic clinic; a follow up. *Lancet*, **i**, 281
22. Medical Research Council Working Party on Phenylketonuria. (1968). Present status of different mass screening procedures for phenylketonuria. *Br. Med. J.*, **4**, 7
23. SCRIVER, C. R., CLOW, C. L. and LAMM, P. (1973). On the screening, diagnosis and investigation of hereditary amino acidopathies. *Clin. Biochem.*, **6**, 142
24. ROTHSCHILD, LORD (1971). *A Framework for Government Research and Development.* (Including Lord Rothschild's Report) Command 4814. (London: HMSO)

2

Genetic screening and allied services: structure, process and objective

C. R. Scriver, C. Laberge and Carol L. Clow

Service programmes formulated under the discipline of medical genetics are designed to reduce the burden of genetic disease among individuals in the community. In this discussion we define, in general terms, the amount and nature of genetic disease in man; then in detail the structures which appear best to serve the processes of patient intake through genetic screening or medical referral; and the processes of diagnosis, counselling and treatment which follow in the application of knowledge to patients with genetic disease.[1] We conclude with comments on an existing programme, the Quebec Network of Genetic Medicine, which articulates all of these principles; their application at the national level is occurring through the accreditation of genetic centres under the newly established Canadian College of Medical Genetics.

Amount of disease due to defective gene expression

The size of the disease burden caused by aberrant gene expression in the fetus and postnatal subject, is revealed in various surveys.

The fourth edition of the catalogue *Mendelian Inheritance in Man*[2] lists 2336 monogenic diseases, of which 1142 are secure in their assigned inheritance patterns (autosomal recessive, autosomal dominant or X linked). The growth rate of enumeration in these catalogues has been exponential through the four editions over the past decade, and is likely to continue at this pace in the near future.

Major malformations arising during the period of intrauterine morphogenesis, often associated with postfertilization chromosomal aberrations, or threshold events in the environment interacting with specific alleles in the fetus, have been identified in a majority of spontaneous abortions.[3,4] Rejection of the deformed products of conceptions is, in fact, a prevalent mechanism for the disposal of 'genetic' errors in the human species.

Multiple-input ascertainment of handicapping disease in a defined population[5] has revised in an upward direction, all previous estimates of the amount of hereditary disease in human populations.[6] The new findings reveal that defective gene expression in liveborn individuals will result in 9.4% of individuals being affected by a handicapping condition. More precisely, the new Canadian data reveal that at least 0.18 individuals per 100 livebirths are born with diseases of single-gene cause. One can expect this frequency to vary under the influence of demography and geography in response to gene segregation and founder effects; accordingly, the figure is likely to be a minimum value. Another 0.16/100 livebirths have chromosomal anomalies. The frequency of this form of genetic disease will also vary among populations as for example in the case of Down's syndrome in relation to the prevailing maternal age. Again, we consider the figure of 0.16/100 to be a minimum value. Congenital malformations of multifactorial origin occur in 3.6/100 livebirths while an estimated further 1.58 persons are born with irregularly inherited disease of multifactorial cause contributing to the illness burden of later life. Trimble and Doughty arrived at an aggregate birth frequency of 9.4% for genetic handicaps by correcting for known causes of underestimation.

The 'fallout' of genetic disease as it is expressed in surviving births, is an important cause of admissions to hospitals. Various studies[7–10] indicate that as many as one-third of paediatric hospital admissions are for various forms of gene-influenced disease, that is: monogenic disease, multigenic and multifactorial illness of imprecise inheritance pattern, chromosomal anomalies, and multifactorial congenital malformations. Genetic disease also accounts for a disproportionately large fraction of the long-term paediatric admissions (those lasting more than 10 days); and of the population of patients with multiple admissions.[8] Data for the adult patient population reveal that single-gene disease and possibly gene-influenced illness consumes 11% of hospital care costs in a large metropolitan hospital.[7] The adult patient data can now almost certainly be revised upward.

Mortality data in the paediatric age group have also been examined.[7,11,12] Deaths accountable to genetic and gene-influenced disease now approach about 40% of the total mortality in childhood. In adult life, diseases with multigenic origins, such as atherosclerosis,[13] now account for a major share of premature mortality.

Whereas the foregoing observations pertain largely to white popula-

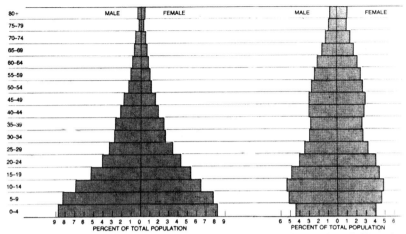

FIGURE 2.1   Age-specific population profiles for a developing nation (left) and a developed country (right). A high birth rate and reduced average life span characterizes the former, where genetic disease is of proportionately less significance than in the latter with a lower birth rate and greater longevity. From Friedman, R. and Berelson, B. *Scientific American*, p.31, vol 231, September 1974 with permission

tions in the relatively affluent societies of the Northern Hemisphere, a burden of genetic disease exists in all races of man throughout the world; therefore the concern for this problem will eventually be global. A mechanism to offset the effects of common, fatal intercurrent illnesses in youth now exists in many populations. Reproductive compensation with high birth rates sustains a pool of genes to pass on to the next generation in these nations (Figure 2.1). The relative importance of genetic disease is of course still small in such countries. However, with the fall in birth rate which occurs in the transition to a post-industrial society and is characteristic of developed nations,[14] the occurrence of genetic disease cannot but achieve a prominence that will demand recognition. In any society where there are few conceptions per parent, each birth is relatively more crucial to the family; accordingly the benefits of genetic knowledge become a matter of the utmost concern. It follows that our own present interest in the structure and the function of genetic services in society is ultimately relevant to other nations and peoples in the forseeable future.

RELEVANCE IN RECOGNITION OF MONOGENIC AND MULTIGENIC DISEASE

The presence of discontinuous variation in the relative frequency distribution with which a particular trait is expressed (Figure 2.2) may

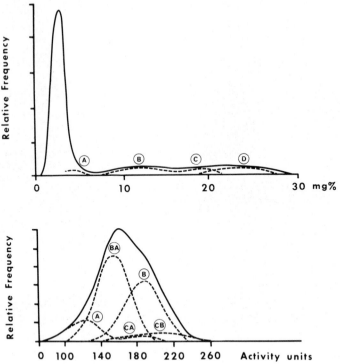

FIGURE 2.2 Relative frequency distribution profiles for a monogenic trait with genetic heterogeneity (top figure) and a polygenic trait (bottom figure). *Top:* The phenomena of normal phenylalanine hydroxylase ontogeny (A) and three different mutant alleles (for example, those for: benign hyperphenylalaninaemia, (B) atypical phenylketonuria, (C) and classical phenylketonuria, (D)) account for the discontinuous variation in plasma phenylalanine in the newborn infant. *Bottom:* Five polymorphic genes account for the quasicontinuous variation in red cell acid phosphatase activity in British Caucasians

permit one to segregate persons who carry a single gene with large effect from those who do not, by means of simple tests and diagnosis.[15-17] Genetic screening and the measurement of metabolite levels or gene product activity are now widely practised modes of generating data for purposes of such classification. On the other hand, quasicontinuous variation[17] in the frequency distribution of a trait is likely to be observed if several alleles account for the trait (Figure 2.2). In this instance, only when we define the way in which each of the genes is expressed does it become possible to interpret the meaning of the variation among individuals.[18,19]

The hyperlipidaemias are a useful model to illustrate the problem of interpreting multigenic origins of disease, and the relevance of this in delineating the structure and function of genetic services. If we consider for example the distributions of blood cholesterol and triglyceride concentrations among individuals in a population, we observe quasicontinuous variation since several genes are responsible for the control of the metabolism of these two types of lipid. Goldstein and colleagues[20-22] adopted the hypothesis that 'hyperlipidaemia' (defined as an outlier value on the respective distribution curves for age-specific fasting lipid levels in serum) is an important predisposing factor to early-onset ischaemic heart disease. They proposed that monogenic forms of hyperlipidaemia occur in 54% of the hyperlipidaemic survivors of myocardial infarction under 60 years of age. These investigators believed they could discern three different mutant alleles by means of genetic studies in the cohort of patients under study, and that each gene was inherited as an autosomal dominant. They further estimated that between 0.6% and 1% of the general population carry these three genes. If we accept their findings, we come to realize that a *small* fraction of the population in the earlier years of life becomes a *large* fraction of those with hyperlipidaemic ischaemic heart disease in their later years. Whereas it has yet to be proven that prospective treatment and change of lifestyle will reduce the risk of heart disease in those at specific risk,[23] it is quite evident that early identification of the owners of the high-risk hyperlipidaemic genes could yield appropriate candidates for research on the specific role of preventive treatment; accordingly conscription of whole populations into such studies and the subsequent dilution of significant findings could be avoided. Furthermore, this genetic approach would rationalize the empiric evidence that the different types of (monogenic) hyperlipidaemia need different forms of treatment.[23]

Let us now examine what might happen in a society when the genetic approach is not utilized by a central agency interested in the prevention of early-onset ischaemic heart disease. In the accompanying diagram (Figure 2.3) simple squares are used to symbolize a cohort of citizens (left side of the diagram) as they might be perceived by the central agency. Each citizen is assumed to be at a similar general risk for susceptibility to the illness; and all are presumed to be equally malleable to a common process of prevention, perhaps a change in lifestyle, indicated as activity A. The agency's approach de-emphasizes the biological diversity among the citizens and produces, as it were, a sociopolitical entropy.

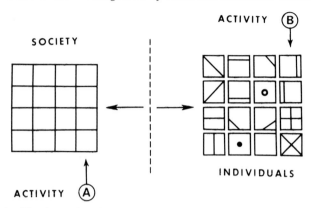

FIGURE 2.3   The 'central authority method' (A) and the 'genetic method' (B) for disease prevention. See text for explanation

On the right side of this same diagram, different symbols are used for different citizens to indicate how they might see themselves, each with his or her own biological identity. The citizens seek an identity in the sociopolitical structure and they invest it with an energy which yields diversity. However, such diversity in the expression of personal identity may be inimical to activity A initiated by the central agency and lead to low compliance with it. Tensions may then arise in the system, symbolized by the arrows pointing in opposite directions.

The 'genetic method' could resolve some of these conflicts between society and the individual, and enhance the efficiency of some of the activities directed at disease prevention. The genetic method does so by recognizing the biological individuality of the citizens. A successful genetic screening activity (indicated as B in the diagram), will identify the individual(s) who are at *specific* risk for developing the illness. In the prevention of ischaemic heart disease, we might choose to find persons bearing alleles causing the autosomal dominant hyperlipidaemias. A preventive action directed at the persons at specific high risk is then likely to yield a better compliance with the preventive measure, be it taking a drug, following a diet or changing lifestyle, than if all citizens were exhorted to comply with a universal regimen.

From this one example, among many, we might choose to illustrate the role of genetic factors in the pathogenesis of common disease, we perceive that if the genetic component of illness in society is as large as we believe it to be, we have good reason to want to know more about the structure and function of those genetic services which can provide specific diagnosis, counselling and treatment. The current programmes which have tended to focus on monogenic disease (and which have endured some criticism for their narrow focus) may indeed be important models for the design of programmes which can effectively serve similar principles of disease prevention in the area of multigenic illness.

Organization of services for management of genetic disease

The aggregate objective of genetic services in their various guises is to reduce the burden and cost of genetic disease in society.[1] A repeating series of structures and processes (Figure 2.4) can be seen to serve the attainment of four major sub-objectives. These may be summarized as follows:

The Process	The Structural Mode
1a Genetic screen	centralized
1b Patient retrieval	regionalized
2 Diagnosis	centralized
3 Counselling and treatment	centralized/regionalized

With respect to the intake of patients, two major points of entry now exist in societies endowed with highly developed health care systems.

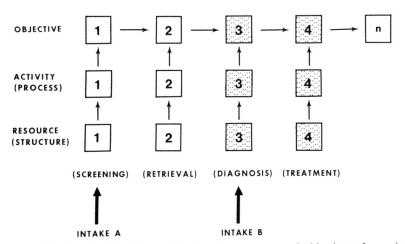

FIGURE 2.4 Organization diagram for structure, process and objectives of genetic services encompassing screening, patient retrieval, diagnosis and follow-up (counselling, treatment, and evaluation). Intake A indicates entry of patients into programme through proband or heterozygote screening; intake B indicates patients entering through referral. The total objective (n) is to reduce the burden of genetic disease

One is through genetic screening programmes (intake A, Figure 2.4); the other is through referral of a proband (or consultand) who seeks diagnosis and the required genetic counselling and/or treatment (intake B, Figure 2.4). Genetic screening has only recently become a major activity; its pitfalls and advantages are the subject of an intense ongoing examination.[24] Specific structures and processes are required to serve this activity and the attendant objective, the discovery of patients discerned to be 'at risk'. If we assume that all homozygotes for the major treatable inborn errors of metabolism could be identified by genetic screening in the newborn, and that all carriers of mutant genes causing hyperlipidaemia leading to ischaemic heart disease, for example, and all heterozygotes for conditions eligible for reproductive counselling and prenatal diagnosis of the fetus at risk could be identified by screening in early adult life, there would be an estimated intake of about 3% of the total population; the fraction would exceed 5% in certain ethnic groups. On the other hand, if the intake were only at the level of diagnosis prior to counselling or treatment for major handicaps with a genetic component, we can anticipate from the studies of Trimble and Doughty[5] that about 10% of all births or about 0.2% of any population base with a birth rate of 2% would require services to meet the demand. Stated another way, the latter would represent the intake of slightly more than one family per day for genetic counselling and workup in a city of 200 000 persons. It is apparent that complete intake through referral of probands and from ascertainment via genetic screening could generate a massive demand for genetic services unlikely to be met by current structures.

STRUCTURE AND PROCESS OF GENETIC SCREENING

The structure supporting the process of screening must facilitate the attainment of high specificity and high sensitivity in the screening activity. Where it is desirable to pursue multiphasic screening, the structure should provide flexibility for the programme, allowing the addition or deletion of tests in accordance with technological developments and experience within the programme. Modifications in the process should incur only marginal costs. A central screening authority (or commission) is likely to be the structure most suitable to provide informed decisions and flexibility in the process.[24]

Definitions and objectives of screening

Screening in the medical context can be defined informally as an investigation which is initiated other than in response to a patient's problem or request for help.[25] The formal definition describes screening as 'the presumptive identification of unrecognized disease or defect by the application of tests, examination or other procedures which can be applied rapidly. Screening tests sort out apparently well persons who probably have a disease from those who probably do not.'[26]

Screening may be large-scale, to encompass a whole population (mass screening); or it may be *selective* and directed at high-risk subgroups. Screening may encompass *case finding* which in contrast to *epidemiological surveys* is a directive form of investigation to detect incipient or established disease and to bring patients to treatment (and counselling in the case of genetic screening). Diagnosis is a specific activity by which the cause for a finding is sought and defined. Screening should be distinguished from traditional *surveillance* activities; screening is usually a short-term cross-sectional activity while surveillance tends to be a long-term vigil on the health of persons and populations. Whitby[27] and Sackett and Holland[28] have recently defined the important facets of medical and public health screening.

Genetic screening may be defined as a search in a population for persons with genotypes (and phenotypes) known to be associated with disease, or which may lead to disease in their descendants; or which may produce initially 'silent' variation and which in a particular environment may incur a specific high risk for the appearance of a disease.[24] Accordingly, the objectives of genetic screening are:

1. to provide opportunities for medical intervention to prevent genetic disease or minimize its effect;

2. to provide opportunities for counselling about reproductive options;

3. to collect data pertinent to public health policy and basic knowledge.

Mass screening of newborn infants for the occurrence of hyperphenylalaninaemia, is a form of case finding, proceeding to specific diagnosis and treatment of probands with phenylketonuria; as such it is an example of the first objective of genetic screening. Selective screening among the Ashkenazim for carriers of the Tay–Sachs gene is an example of the second objective. Prospective screening in order to examine the epidemiological components relevant to persons carrying the genes causing hyperlipidaemia or α_1-antitrypsin deficiency, illustrates the third objective.

Levels of screening

The biological level at which genetic screening could potentially be pursued[15, 29] is an important determinant of the process of screening. The levels are: (a) the gene itself; (b) the gene product which has been modified by mutation; (c) the metabolic function which has been altered because of modification in the gene product; and (d) the clinical phenotype whose signs and symptoms reflect expression of the mutant gene.

(a) Screening at the level of the gene, in the absence of a detailed map of the human genome and knowledge of nucleotide sequences in DNA at specific gene loci, is not yet possible. Only massive abnormalities in the organization of genetic material, as may occur in the chromosomal anomalies, are suitable targets for such screening at the present time. Screening for trisomy-21 in the fetus, under the high-risk circumstance of advanced maternal age, is an example of this form of screening.

(b) Screening for modification of gene product activity, or structure is already well established in several phenotypes. The detection of haemoglobins and modified activity of erythrocyte glucose-6-phosphate dehydrogenase[30] is an example of a widely-practised screen at the level of the mutant gene product.

(c) Screening for abnormalities of metabolite level is the most widely established form of genetic screening.[31] It is well illustrated by mass screening for postnatal hyperphenylalaninaemia. In excess of 25 million liveborn have been screened at this level in the past 15 years.

(d) Clinical examination, of the newborn in particular,[32] will detect many inborn errors of morphogenesis with Mendelian recurrence risks; it may also detect, at an early stage, some inborn errors of metabolism, which confer important clinical signs such as the adrenogenital syndrome; and it will of course discern many of the multifactorial congenital malformations which usually have low but important empiric recurrence risks, or equally important, may not have any genetic component and have, therefore, no recurrence risk to concern the family.

Specificity and sensitivity of the screening test

General issues. The efficiency of the screening test will be determined by its *specificity* (i.e. its ability to exclude those who are normal from detection by the test); and by its *sensitivity*, (i.e. its ability to detect those who are abnormal). Screening tests designed to detect structural variation causing an altered net charge of the protein provide 'binary' answers (change or no change) and consequently they possess high specificity and sensitivity. For example, haemoglobin electrophoresis will detect with simple efficiency the change in electrophoretic mobility of haemoglobin S which accompanies the substitution of valine for glutamate in the sixth position of the β-chain.[31,33] However, screening methods which measure change in gene product activity, or of metabolite concentration, generate data which must be related to a distribution of normal values; the probability that outlier values are normal or abnormal must be defined by the appropriate statistical methods.[16,17,34] Accordingly, any improvement in the accuracy and reproducibility of the method, and any reduction in the standard deviation which defines the normal population, will increase greatly the efficiency with which abnormal signals can be detected under these conditions.[35]

Extensive experience with an inhibition assay for the detection of hyperphenylalaninaemia and with a fluorimetric method for the same purpose, illustrates the impact of specificity and sensitivity on the process of mass screening. The inhibition assay[36] is used to screen about 2 million liveborns per year in North America. A growth zone, the size of which indicates the approximate concentration of phenylalanine in the blood sample placed at the centre of the zone, is used to signal an abnormality. Growth zones equivalent to phenylalanine concentration in excess of about 4 mg/dl are classified as abnormal but the test is often set to a cut-off point of 6 mg/dl. Many laboratories are customarily employed to provide inhibition assay screening within a given population region, and interlaboratory variation in performance of the test must be controlled. On the other hand the automated fluorimetric assay[37,38] determines a specific concentration of phenylalanine in the sample; accordingly values for the mean and standard deviation can be calculated for the screened population and an abnormal value can be given a precise statistical definition (e.g. in excess of $+ 3$ SD). Performance of all analyses at a single laboratory is possible with this method even for a large population base and this structure eliminates interlaboratory variation. The latter method coupled to simultaneous automated tyrosine determination and organisation approach has been employed in the Quebec Network of Genetic Medicine (National Academy of Sciences,[24] Appendix I); the former method and structure has been used in most

Table 2.1 Specificity and sensitivity of newborn screening for 'hyperphenylalaninaemia' and of case detection for phenylketonuria

Country	% Participation (approximate)	Structure	Process	Specificity	Sensitivity
United Kingdom*	90	moderately centralized	bacterial inhibition assay (60%) other tests (40%)	?	1.0
Canada† (Quebec only)	92	highly centralized	automated fluorimetry (Phe + Tyr)	0.999‡	1.0
United States*	89	variably centralized	bacterial inhibition	0.994‡,§	0.917

* Data taken from Starfield and Holtzman[42]—Years covered: UK 1964-1972; USA 1962-1971
† Data provided by Quebec Network of Genetic Medicine—Years covered: 1971-1975
‡ Data from Holtzman and colleagues[62]
§ Mean age at time of screening test, 4 days, in Quebec and the United States. Difference in specificity is therefore not a function of age at testing

state sponsored programmes in the USA. Specificity and sensitivity are high in the Quebec programme and lower in the American programmes (Table 2.1). When translated into practical terms namely the demand for follow-up and repeat testing, the automated process and central structure generates only 2000 call-book requests per 2 million births, while the other process and structure generates 12 000 requests. In addition, the former system misses fewer actual cases of phenylketonuria.

The use of two tests simultaneously, and the application of Bayesian statistics to the findings, enhances case finding.[34,39] For example, with a single venepuncture we obtain a sample which, by the appropriate two-test analysis of phenylalanine and tyrosine[40] allows us to identify in a very efficient manner those who are heterozygous for the gene causing phenylketonuria.[34] We have also performed efficient selective screening for carriers of the Tay–Sachs allele in over 7000 persons and have used Bayesian methods and two-test discrimination to reduce classification error and the need for repeat tests.[31,34] These experiences have convinced us that the efficiency of screening can be improved through the development of a particular structure and process, namely a centralized testing centre where the appropriate technological resources and statistical experience are available.

Recommendation. A *centralized structure* for performance of the screening tests reduces interlaboratory variation in test accuracy. Testing methodology and statistical handling of the screening data should be selected to suit the process of screening.

Screening and process of patient retrieval. When the objective of the screening programme is to initiate medical intervention or to deliver counselling about reproductive options, identification of a positive screening signal initiates the process of patient retrieval. Unfortunately, excellent screening programmes can be lamentably uncoupled from retrieval mechanisms.[24]

A structure providing the appropriate demographic information and the mechanisms for rapid communication is essential to the process of retrieval. Retrieval efficiency is in part related to the basic structure of the medical care system in which the programme is operated.[42] Data on the time elapsed between detection of hyperphenylalaninaemia in the newborn, and retrieval of the subject for confirmatory testing are available for different medical care systems (Table 2.2). The elapsed

Table 2.2 Relevance of structure in process of patient retrieval. Interval between screening test and retrieval of subject for repeat test and diagnosis*

Country	% of cases with interval (in days) of:		Elapsed time (days)	
	<15	>15	mean	SD
United Kingdom†	89.5	10.5	7	7
United States‡	73.5	26.5	12	19

* Data from National Academy of Sciences report[24] and Starfield and Holtzman[42]
† National Health Service with centralized screening laboratories; and regionalized public health system with health visitors available for patient retrieval
‡ No national health system and with less centralization of screening laboratories; no regionalized health visitor programme in most regions

time is considerably shorter under centralized health schemes compared to entrepreneurial systems of medical practice.

A novel tactic has facilitated retrieval in the Quebec Network of Genetic Medicine. In the initial phase of the programme, positive test results were communicated directly to physicians; retrieval rates averaged 50% under these conditions. However, a request for follow-up is merely one of many 'signals' received during the physician's busy day concerning illness in his practice. If the medical significance of the finding is not readily apparent to the physician, the stimulus to respond immediately and to obtain a follow-up test is wanting. On the other hand, the client perceives the screening signal as a very significant and personal event in his life and he is likely to be concerned and will pursue the finding further. Accordingly, the Quebec programme changed the process of retrieval so as to approach the client directly. Approval to do so was readily obtained from the Provincial Corporation of Physicians. Following this simple change in process, follow-up was accelerated and efficiency soon approached 100%. The structure for our follow-up process is the appropriate demographic information which is supplied on the sample collection kits for blood and urine. The appropriate communication methods permit regionalization of the retrieval mechanism from the central screening laboratory to the home of the client.

Recommendation. Establishment of a *regional* authority for rapid communication between the centralized screening agency and the subject at risk encourages rapid and complete retrieval of clients.

Structure and process for diagnosis and follow-up. Classification of a finding in relation to its cause is the third objective of an integrated genetics programme; the action taken thereafter is the fourth objective. The finding may be a positive screening-test result (intake A, Figure 2.4) or it may be a phenomenon bringing the consultand into the programme for information, counselling or treatment (intake B, Figure 2.4). The process of diagnosis, in the case of genetic disease, must take into account genetic heterogeneity and phenocopies.[43,44] The structure which supports diagnosis best at the present time, utilizes centralized expertise whereby special methods of investigation can be pursued; and where experience gained can be rapidly applied to diagnosis in areas where growth of knowledge about genetic disease is taking place at an exponential rate.

Diagnosis applied to screening. The interpretation of a finding such as 'hyperphenylalaninaemia' illustrates the problem of diagnosis when intake occurs through the structure and process of mass screening. Classification of the causes of hyperphenylalaninaemia requires consideration of many factors which include: the rate at which the phenylalanine level in blood rises after birth; the sex of the proband; the absolute concentration of blood phenylalanine in relation to the phenylalanine intake in the diet; the phenylalanine apohydroxylase activity in liver. Hyperphenylalaninaemia may also result from a disorder in the co-factor regeneration system;[45-47] in this form of the trait, treatment by low-phenylalanine diet does not prevent harm to the central nervous system. Accordingly, exact diagnosis of hyperphenylalaninaemia has important, practical significance. The degree of dietary constraint which is to be imposed on the patient with hyperphenylalaninaemia will be determined by the diagnosis.

Prenatal diagnosis related to selective, high-risk screening programmes is another example of a specialized activity which, at present, should again be carried out at centres where the required experience is available. The process of obtaining and handling the sample of amniotic fluid for purposes of chemical investigation or cell culture is in itself a rather specialized procedure and the additional diagnostic methods such as ultrasonic scanning, fetoscopy and placentoscopy require special expertise. Analysis of amniotic fluid samples for purposes of diagnosis also requires delicate procedures, the controls for which must come from data matched for gestational age, among other factors.

Diagnosis applied to referred consultands. The largest intake of patients at the present time, in most genetic programmes occurs through self- or health personnel-generated referrals. The same structure which serves diagnosis for screened probands will support the greater complexity of the diagnostic process in medical genetics. Many genetic subspecialities are required. They include varying degrees of experience in: 'syndromology', and in the use of dermatoglyphics and the various tools of clinical genetics; in biochemical genetics and somatic cell genetics, for delineation of phenotypes; in cytogenetics and in teratology. Familiarity with population genetics, behavioural genetics, developmental genetics, mutagenesis and oncogenesis will further enhance the precision with which knowledge can be applied to the patient with genetic disease.

Responsibility to the patient does not cease with diagnosis. Genetic counselling[48,49] will follow and evaluation of how the counsellor's information is used and interpreted by the client should be an ongoing activity, not only in proband-orientated genetic programmes,[50] but also in non-proband directed activities such as those involving screening for heterozygotes.[51,52] If treatment is required, the quality of supervision and monitoring of the response to treatment will influence the outcome of the medical intervention. Follow-up can be greatly facilitated by allied health personnel.[53] Moreover, a structure which permits patients with genetic disease to be followed and treated in their home can reduce the cost of care and improve the quality of the treatment process.[1]

Recommendations. Diagnosis frequently requires a *centralized* structure at a genetics centre where a team approach can provide expertise for investigation and interpretation of results. Follow-up can be facilitated from a centralized structure by *regionalization* of the relevant processes.

Comment

The development of structures which permit a wide range of processes including screening, retrieval and diagnosis (and prenatal diagnosis), and follow-up genetic counselling, treatment and evaluation is desirable yet difficult.[54] If possible it should occur under a single authority. The Quebec Network of Genetic Medicine illustrates one way in which such an authority may be established.[24,55]

The Quebec Network provides facilities for screening and diagnosis, genetic counselling and treatment of over 30 hereditary conditions. It is operated by four university medical centres in the province on behalf of

the Ministry of Social Affairs. A working committee directs the programme. Its membership includes two representatives from each
university and appropriate representation from the Ministry. A global
budget for the network is provided by the Ministry.

The network observes two working principles: The first is that an
integrated system of communication exists among the four major
regional centres, the central screening laboratories and the patients.
The second is that pilot studies be done before implementation of the
new services.

The committee established a preliminary structure to screen for
post-natal hyperphenylalaninaemia as its initial activity. This demonstration project began in 1969 and was based upon a pilot study[56] which
had demonstrated the feasibility of genetic screening for purposes of
medical intervention in the population to be served. Separate tasks were
later assumed by each of the regional centres after feasibility studies had
been done. The components were then integrated to facilitate retrieval,
diagnosis, counselling and treatment of patients.

Two specific problems were selected for initial research and development. They were: the problem of hereditary tyrosinaemia, an important
autosomal recessive disease of French Canadians;[57] and the evaluation
of ambulatory care of hereditary metabolic disease, by allied health
personnel.[53]

The Quebec Network of Genetic Medicine was formally created in
1972 to encompass the increasing range of inter-related activities, whose
objectives were to provide genetic screening for purposes of medical
intervention, reproductive counselling and enumeration. The responsibility for the operation of the network remains with the universities;
financial support and final approval reside with government. The
ministry agreed early in the development of the network that research
and development for purposes of disease prevention was in its own best
interest; a flexible programme of research and development and service
has remained a cornerstone of the network. At the present time, the
services offered by this network include mass screening of capillary
blood samples collected from the heel at the time of discharge of infants
from newborn nurseries; and of urine, on samples collected in the home
by parents, when the infant has reached 2 weeks of age. Voluntary compliance rates exceed 92% in the former and 85% in the latter. The
blood samples are processed for phenylalanine and tyrosine content and

for thyroxine (T4) levels. Galactose screening was recently discontinued. The urine samples are examined by a variety of chemical tests for reducing substances, cystine and keto acids, and following the elution of the material from the filter paper carrier, by chromatography for amino acids. Estimation of the uric acid:creatinine ratio was recently discontinued.

Several high-risk selective screening programmes are carried out under the network authority. They include: comprehensive prenatal diagnostic programmes at two of the centres, cytogenetic studies of referred patients, Tay–Sachs carrier screening among Ashkenazi Jews and three French-Canadian demes with a high frequency of the Tay–Sachs-like disease. Chemical and chromatographic screening of patients admitted to paediatric wards is routinely performed at the two largest paediatric centres. Selective assays for arylsulphatase, β-galactosidase, sphingomyelinase, and other acid hydrolase enzymes in leukocytes, and techniques for culturing skin fibroblasts and amniotic fluid cells are available in two centres. A two-test discrimination method for classification of carriers of the β-thalassaemia allele has been developed in readiness for the time when prenatal diagnosis of thalassaemia major in the fetus is available.

Retrieval of patients is rapid within the network (see Table 2.2). Confirmatory diagnosis is pursued at the regional centres following referral of the patient. Counselling is provided for all patients with findings identified in the newborn screening programme or who are referred into the programme for other reasons. The counsellors are medical geneticists, paediatricians with genetic expertise and allied health personnel trained for the role. Treatment resources are provided, including diets and medications; continuous monitoring of treatment effects and evaluation of clinical progress is provided. Ambulatory methods have been emphasized, so that care in the home is provided; hospitalization rates have fallen accordingly.

The network also supports two repositories; one is a computer for screening and demographic data, with the appropriate safeguards for confidentiality and privacy,[55] the other is for cultured skin fibroblasts.[58]

The most recent research and development activities within the network have included the development of a blood T4 screening assay for the newborn;[59] the evaluation of advocacy and compliance in genetic screening;[52] and the development of a National 'Food Bank' system for the delivery and supervision of semi-synthetic diets in the treatment of hereditary metabolic disease.[60] Approximately 25 publications have emanated from these and other projects.

The ministry provides a total budget of $425 000 for a programme serving more than 80 000 births per year. The on-going follow-up of approximately 200 families with genetic disease and the various service programmes and the research and development are all included in the budget. Four traineeships are also provided for personnel seeking experience in medical genetics.

The programme is operated on a voluntary basis; the citizen has the right to withdraw from participation should there be an objection to screening, or any medical intervention. The patient's own physician assumes the responsibility for his general care. The regional genetic centres assist the physician with the genetic problem in a consultative capacity; the centre assumes responsibility for genetic care only by agreement with the physicians.

These developments in Quebec have been paralleled by a further innovation in Canada. The establishment of a Canadian College of Medical Geneticists has been enacted[61] and incorporation took place in November 1975. The objective of the college is to ensure that the necessary skills and knowledge of properly trained medical geneticists and allied health personnel can be encompassed by formal programmes; at the same time standardized procedures for ensuring the quality of laboratory and counselling services are to be provided under the auspices of the college. The corporation shall consist of and represent properly qualified Ph.D. and M.D. medical geneticists. The college shall establish and maintain professional standards of health care delivery in the field of medical genetics. Accreditation of medical genetics centres, is to be a function of the college, which shall also inform appropriate levels of government on the role of medical geneticists in health care. The college shall also advise government on the nature and extent of such services and aid in the negotiations with appropriate levels of government upon the methods of funding these services.

It is evident that Canada will have a mechanism whereby there can be a national network of genetic centres and a national cohort of geneticists and allied health personnel who will provide an integrated structure and process for genetic services on behalf of all citizens. We anticipate that our regional, provincial and national experiences will hold some interest to geneticists and health care planners beyond our borders.

The ideas expressed in this essay emanate in part from a long and rewarding association with Barton Childs, chairman of the National Academy of Sciences, Committee for the Study of Inborn Errors of Metabolism. Our own research in the area of genetic services has been funded over the years by grants from the National Institutes of Health (USA), the Dept. of National Health and Welfare (Canada), the Medical Research Council (Canada), the National Genetics Foundation (New York) and the Quebec Network of Genetic Medicine and a donation from Peter and Edward Bronfman.

REFERENCES

1. CLOW, C. L., FRASER, F. C., LABERGE, C. and SCRIVER, C. R. (1973). On the application of knowledge to the patient with genetic disease. In A. C. Steinberg and A. G. Bearn (eds.), *Progress in Medical Genetics*, Vol. 9, p. 159. (New York: Grune and Stratton)

2. McKUSICK, V. A. (1975). Catalogs of autosomal dominant, autosomal recessive and X-linked phenotypes. *Mendelian Inheritance in Man*, 4th ed. (Baltimore: Johns Hopkins Press)

3. CARR, D. M. (1971). Genetic basis of abortion. *Ann. Rev. Genet.* **5**, 65

4. POLAND, J. B. and LOWRY, R. B. (1974). The use of spontaneous abortuses and still births in genetic counselling. *Am. J. Obstet Gynecol.*, **118**, 322

5. TRIMBLE, B. K. and DOUGHTY, J. H. (1974). The amount of hereditary disease in human population. *Ann. Hum. Genet.* (London), **38**, 199

6. World Health Organization. (1972). *Genetic Disorders: Prevention, Treatment and Rehabilitation*, (Geneva: WHO Tech. Rep. Ser. No. 497)

7. CHILDS, B., MILLER, S. M. and BEARN, A. G. (1972). Gene mutation as a cause of human disease. In H. E. Sutton and M. I. Harris (eds.), *Mutagenic Effects of Environmental Contamination*, p. 3. (New York: Academic Press)

8. SCRIVER, C. R., NEAL, J. L., SAGINUR, R. and CLOW, A. (1973). The frequency of genetic disease and congenital malformation among patients in a pediatric hospital. *Can. Med. Ass. J.*, **108**, 1111

9. DAY, N. and HOLMES, L. B. (1973). The incidence of genetic disease in a University Hospital population. *Am. J. Hum. Genet.*, **25**, 237

10. REICH, E., WALLACE, S., BEN-YISHAY, M., SCHLESINGER, S., MARKS, J. and BLOOM, A. D. *Genetic Disease in a Pediatric Hospital.* (In press)

11. CARTER, C. O. (1956). Changing patterns in the causes of death at the Hospital for Sick Children. *Great Ormond Street J.*, No. **11**, 65

12. ROBERTS, D. F., CHAVEZ, J. and COURT, S. D. M. (1970). The genetic component in child mortality. *Arch. Dis. Child.*, **45**, 33

13. MOTULSKY, A. G. and BOMAN, H. (1974). Genetics and atherosclerosis. In G. Schetter (ed.), *Proc. 3rd Int. Symposium on Atherosclerosis*, Oct. 1973 (Berlin: Springer-Verlag)

14. DUMOND, D. E. (1975). The limitation of human population: a natural history. *Science*, **187**, 713

15. SCRIVER, C. R. (1972). Screening and treatment of hereditary (metabolic) disease. In *Human Genetics Symposium, Proc. IV International, Cong. Human Genetics*, p. 10. (Paris: Excerpta Medica Found)

16. WESTWOOD, A. and RAINE, D. N. (1973). Some problems of heterozygote recognition in inherited metabolic disease with special reference to phenylketonuria. In J. W. T. Seakins, R. A. Saunders and C. Toothill (eds.), *Treatment of Inborn Errors of Metabolism*. SSIEM Sympos. No. 10, p. 63. (London: Churchill Livingstone)

17. MURPHY, E. A. and CHASE, G. A. (1975). *Principles of genetic counseling.* (Chicago; Year Book Medical Pub.)

18. HARRIS, H. (1968). Molecular basis of hereditary disease. *Br. Med. J.*, **ii**, 135
19. HARRIS, H. and HOPKINSON, D. A. (1972). Average heterozygosity per locus in man: an estimate based on the incidence of enzyme polymorphism. *Ann. Hum. Genet.*, **36**, 9
20. GOLDSTEIN, J. L., HAZZARD, W. R., SCHROTT, H. G., BIERMAN, E. L. and MOTULSKY, A. G. (1973). Hyperlipidaemia in coronary heart disease. I. Lipid levels in 500 survivors of myocardial infarction. *J. Clin. Invest*,. **52**, 1533
21. GOLDSTEIN, J. L., SCHROTT, H. G., HAZZARD, W. R., BIERMAN, E. L. and MOTULSKY, A. G. (1973). Hyperlipidaemia in coronary heart disease. II. Genetic analysis of lipid levels in 176 families and delineation of a new inherited disorder, combined hyperlipidemia. *J. Clin. Invest.*, **52**, 1544
22. HAZZARD, W. R., GOLDSTEIN, J. L., SCHROTT, H. G., MOTULSKY, A. G. and BIERMAN, E. L. (1973). Hyperlipidaemia in coronary heart disease. III. Evaluation of lipoprotein phenotypes in 156 genetically defined survivors of myocardial infarction. *J. Clin. Invest.*, **52**, 1569
23. LEVY, R. I., MORGANROTH, J. and RIFKIN, B. M. (1974). Drug therapy. Treatment of hyperlipidemia. *N. Engl. J. Med.*, **290**, 1295
24. National Academy of Sciences. (1975). *Genetic Screening. Programs, Principles and Research.* Washington, D. C.
25. NORTH, A. F. Jr. (1975). Personal communication
26. WILSON, J. M. G. and JUNGNER, G. (1968). *Principles and Practice of Screening for Disease.* (Geneva: WHO Public Health Papers No. 34)
27. WHITBY, L. G. (1974). Screening for disease. Definitions and criteria. *Lancet*, **ii**, 819
28. SACKETT, D. L. and HOLLAND, W. W. (1975). Controversy in the detection of disease. *Lancet*, **ii**, 357
29. SCRIVER, C. R. (1965). Screening newborns for hereditary metabolic disease. *Pediatr. Clin. North Am.*, **12**, 807
30. World Health Organization. (1967). *Standardization of Procedures for the study of Glucose-6-phosphate Dehydrogenase.* (Geneva: WHO Tech. Rep. Ser. 366)
31. World Health Organization. (1968). *Screening for Inborn Errors of Metabolism*, (Geneva,: WHO Tech. Rep. Ser. 401)
32. HECHT, F. and Lovrien, E. W. (1970). Genetic diagnosis in the newborn. A part of preventive medicine. *Pediatr. Clin. North Am.*, **17**, 1039
33. World Health Organization. (1966). *Haemoglobinopathies and Allied Disorders.* (Geneva: WHO Tech. Rep. Ser. 338)
34. GOLD, R. J. M., MAAG, U. R., NEAL, J. L. and SCRIVER, C. R. (1974). The use of biochemical data in screening for mutant alleles and in genetic counseling. *Ann. Hum. Genet.*, **37**, 315
35. KIRKMAN, H. N. (1972). Enzyme defects. In A. G. Steinberg and A. G. Bearn (eds.), *Progress in Medical Genetics*, Vol. 8, p. 125. (New York: Grune and Stratton)
36. GUTHRIE, R. and SUSI, A. (1963). A simple phenylalanine method for detecting phenylketonuria in large populations of newborn infants. *Pediatrics.*, **32**, 338
37. McCAMAN, M. W. and ROBINS, E. (1962). Fluorimetric method for the determination of phenylalanine in serum. *J. Lab. Clin. Med.*, **59**, 885
38. HILL, J. B., SUMMER, G. K., PENDER, M. W. and ROSZEL, N. O. (1965). An automated procedure for blood phenylalanine. *Clin. Chem.*, **11**, 541
39. MURPHY, E. A. and MUTALIK, G. S. (1969). The application of Bayesian methods in genetic counseling. *Hum. Hered.*, **19**, 126
40. ROSENBLATT, D. and SCRIVER, C. R. (1968). Heterogeneity in genetic control of phenylalanine metabolism in man. *Nature (London)*, **218**, 677
41. DELVIN, E., POTTIER, A., SCRIVER, C. R. and GOLD, R. J. M. (1974). The application of an automated hexosaminidase assay to genetic screening. *Clin. Chim. Acta*, **53**, 135
42. STARFIELD, B. and HOLTZMAN, N. A. (1975). A comparison of effectiveness of screening for phenylketonuria in the United States, United Kingdom and Ireland. *N. Engl. J. Med.*, **293**, 118
43. CHILDS, B. and DER KALOUSTIAN, M. (1968). Genetic heterogeneity. *N. Engl. J. Med.*, **279**, 1205 and 1267
44. McKUSICK, V. A. (1971). The nosology of genetic disease. *Hosp. Prac.*, **6**, 93
45. Bartholome, K. (1974). A new molecular defect in phenylketonuria. *Lancet*, **ii**, 1580
46. SMITH, I., CLAYTON, B. E. and WOLFF, O. H. (1975). New variant of phenyl-

ketonuria with progressive neurological illness unresponsive to phenylalanine restriction. *Lancet,* **i,** 1108

47. KAUFMAN, S., HOLTZMAN, N. A., MILSTIEN, S., BUTLER, I. J. and KRUMHOLZ, A. (1975). Phenylketonuria due to deficiency of dihydropteridine reductase. *N. Engl. J. Med.* **293,** 785

48. MURPHY, E. A. (1968). The rationale of genetic counseling. *J. Pediatrics,* **72,** 121

49. FRASER, F. C. (1971). Genetic counseling. *Hosp. Pract.,* **6,** 49

50. LEONARD, C. O., CHASE, G. A. and CHILDS, B. (1972). Genetic counseling: A consumer's view. *N. Engl. J. Med.,* **287,** 433

51. KABACK, M. M., BECKER, M. H. and RUTH, M. V. (1974). Sociologic studies in human genetics. 1. Compliance factors in a voluntary heterozygote screening program. *Birth Defects Orig. Article Series.* (Natl Foundation), Vol. X, No. 6, p. 163.

52. BECK, E., BLAICHMAN, S., SCRIVER, C. R. and CLOW, C. L. (1974). Advocacy and compliance in genetic screening. Behaviour of physicians and clients in a voluntary Tay–Sachs testing program. *N. Engl. J. Med.,* **291,** 1166

53. CLOW, C., READE, T. and SCRIVER, C. R. (1971). Management of hereditary metabolic disease. The role of allied health personnel. *N. Engl. J. Med.,* **284,** 1292

54. RAINE, D. N. (1974). Screening for disease: Inherited metabolic disease. *Lancet,* **ii,** 996

55. GRENIER, A. and LABERGE, C. (1974). Depistage des maladies metaboliques hereditaires au Quebec. *Union Med. Can.,* **103,** 453

56. CLOW, C. L., SCRIVER, C. R. and DAVIES, E. (1969). Results of mass screening for hyperaminoacidemias in the newborn infant. *Am. J. Dis. Child.,* **117,** 48

57. LABERGE, C. (1969). Hereditary tyrosinemia in a French Canadian isolate. *Am. J. Hum. Genet.* **21,** 36

58. GOLDMAN, H. (1972). The repository for mutant human cell strains. In L. Dallaire (ed.), *Med. Res. Council (Can.) Prenatal Diagnosis Newsletter,* Vol. 1, No. 2, p. 6

59. DUSSAULT, J. H., COULOMBE, P., LABERGE, C., LETARTE, J., GUYDA, H. and KHOURY K. (1975). Preliminary report on a mass screening program for neonatal hypothyroidism. *J. Pediatr.,* **86,** 670

60. CLOW, C. L., ISHMAEL, H., SCRIVER, C. R., MURRAY, K., CAMPEAU, H., LONG, D. and STEINBERG, H. A. (1975). The national food distribution centre for management of patients with hereditary metabolic disease. *Bull. Genet. Soc. Can.,* **6,** 29

61. MILLER, J. R. (1975). Canadian College of Medical Genetics. *Can. Med. Ass. J.,* **113,** 357

62. HOLTZMAN, N. A., MEEK, A. G. and MELLITS, E. D. (1974). Neonatal screening for phenylketonuria. IV. Factors influencing the occurrence of false positives. *Am. J. Pub. Health,* **64,** 775

PRESENT METHODS OF MANAGEMENT

3

The role of the paediatrician

G. M. Komrower

During the last decade there has been considerable interest in and experience of the management of individuals with an inherited metabolic disorder. These patients usually are long-term responsibilities requiring assistance from several disciplines, some of which, for example dietetics and biochemistry, are of considerable importance. As a result people have questioned the position of the physician in such a team and have suggested that he may not have a principal part to play in the care of these affected individuals.

We must establish a definition of paediatrician, as this will vary from country to country with their differing patterns of health care. In some countries the paediatrician is a general practitioner for children, making house calls, carrying out immunizations and being responsible for the primary care of the children. In the United Kingdom a paediatrician is usually a consultant with a long training in paediatrics. He is responsible for the hospital care of children in his town or district and will receive requests for assistance from the general practitioners around him, as well as being the adviser to a number of local institutions concerned with children. He may have had a special interest within paediatrics, but usually he will not have sufficient time to practise this in depth; as a result groups of specialist consultant paediatricians have emerged throughout the country; these men and women have fewer general paediatric responsibilities and have devoted themselves to the development of a particular aspect of paediatric medicine or surgery. Consequently, the more difficult and special problems tend to be referred to them. The subsequent discussion will be mainly concerned with the two latter categories, that is the general consultant and the specialist consultant paediatrician.

WHAT DO WE MEAN BY MANAGEMENT OF INHERITED DISEASE?

Is this exercise solely concerned with the treatment and support of recognized cases, or does it include detection and accurate diagnosis? If the latter is so, then the management would include population and family screening for designated disorders as well as the study of individual problems. Here the paediatrician would be responsible for the planning of investigations and would be guided by the history and clinical findings as well as any unusual preliminary biochemical result. In those families in which inherited metabolic disease had been detected, he would advise on family planning and future pregnancies and would assist in the detection of heterozygotes. The screening unit would require the paediatrician's help when more than one test was to be carried out due to uncertainty over the diagnosis: this might require the attendance of the child and the family at the hospital for a careful clinical examination by an interested and experienced physician, as well as the carrying out of more sophisticated biochemical tests. Here, the initial contact of the paediatrician with the family, and his careful explanation of the reason for the visit and the nature of the test, would be of inestimable value in restoring family morale and confidence, and would encourage them to stay with the unit while the tests were completed and treatment established, should this prove necessary.

When a diagnosis is confirmed the paediatrician would be required, firstly, to explain the nature of the disorder and the implications for the immediate future, and secondly, together with the dietitian and biochemist, to initiate and then maintain first-class dietary control. As has been indicated earlier these initial interviews are of great psychological importance, and go a long way in establishing a good relationship between the family and the unit concerned with the care of their child. Regular but not frequent visits to the clinic would be needed when, in addition to the clinical and biochemical review, there should be ample opportunity for the parents to talk to the dietitian and the paediatrician, who must be prepared to answer their questions. It is important that they maintain good communication with the general practitioner (family doctor) and health visitor concerned with the case, and spend time giving a full report of the clinical findings and investigations whenever the child visits the clinic. The paediatrician should be capable of interpreting physical and behavioural variations from the normal in order to supervise the emotional and psychological progress of these children, and so explain behavioural upsets to the family. He should watch for any adverse effects of the discipline of the treatment.

Inevitably these exercises include an element of primary care but as far as possible this should rest with the family doctor. As the paediatrician will see the child and the family fairly regularly, the initial genetic counselling should be done by himself and any subsequent back-up should be his responsibility. It is well known that a single consultation is unsatisfactory, as the parents in their distress and anxiety fail to comprehend the full implication of the nature of the disease and the mode of its inheritance, and it is my experience that this exercise must be undertaken at least twice with each family. As counselling is part of family support, the paediatrician should be in a position together with the biochemistry team to assist in respect of heterozygote detection.

EDUCATION

This will be offered to personnel working in, or wishing to work in, the area of inborn errors of metabolism; for example, health visitors, social workers, psychologists and public health doctors. It will be necessary to inform them in general about the screening programme, the methods of diagnosis and the principles of treatment. This will require occasional visits to the areas served by the screening and metabolic unit for lectures and discussions. Here, as well as at lectures and demonstrations in the central unit, there should be ample opportunity for questions and for the clarification of any problems that have arisen, either in the screening programme or with the care of affected cases. There will be some responsibility in respect of the education of undergraduate and postgraduate students. It is unlikely that much time will be allocated to the undergraduates but it is hoped that a small number of postgraduates in training could be attached to the unit for a reasonable period, in order for them to gain experience of the work that is carried out there. The unit must plan long term studies which should contribute to the better understanding and handling of these disorders. This may in part be research, but there is in addition the distillation of good long-term clinical experience which should be available to the people attached to or working in the unit. The paediatrician concerned will have to identify particular areas for study; these may be epidemiological, clinical or psycho-social; they may be related to the special biochemical problems that emerge during the diagnosis and treatment of a case, or possibly during the heterozygote detection tests.

WHAT HELP WILL THE PAEDIATRICIAN REQUIRE?

It is essential that he has a good and interested biochemical team, which has this work as its main responsibility. It should take a real interest in the clinical side of the problem, as it is only in this way that those concerned will offer thoughtful and experienced analysis of the biochemical results, particularly those where the diagnosis has not been confirmed and is still in doubt. The dietitian holds a place of high importance in the team, as apart from the responsibility for the nutritional state of the child, she will be concerned with the production of interesting and palatable diets. In addition, she can give much reassurance to the mothers. Therefore, she will require ample time to devote to the many problems that will arise.

The paediatrician will require help in the community where the primary care of the child is carried out by the general practitioner, assisted by the health visitor concerned with the case. The community physician and senior nursing officer of the area must be involved to ensure that help and advice are given to the school, in particular concerning the diet; and also to support the health visitor, should she run into any administrative difficulties. It is important for the education authorities to be aware of the problem, particularly where the child concerned requires a careful assessment with regard to correct placement in school. In order for this to work efficiently, there must be very good communication between the central unit and the child health services, the general practitioner and health visitor; for this reason an efficient and interested secretary is essential, who will also be responsible for the careful reporting of results in any associated screening programme.

This requires the paediatrician concerned to be a well-informed physician who has had special training in the handling of metabolic and genetic problems, as well as some knowledge of biochemistry. He will work most efficiently in a well-equipped, central clinical investigation area, and as he is required to be a good co-ordinator and communicator, he would seem to be the most suitable person to direct the team.

IMPLEMENTATION OF THESE PRINCIPLES

The principles outlined above have been incorporated in the arrangements for screening and the care of inherited metabolic diseases in the Manchester region. All the activities are contained in the same building which houses the physician's office and consulting rooms, the metabolic ward in which the cases are investigated, and the unit's laboratory which is responsible for the regional screening as well as the back-up services. The dietitian has her room in this building, as does the liaison nurse and unit secretary, who effect the good communication which is essential. The child and her family use one entrance only and are quickly acquainted with the different members of the staff with whom they will come into contact. There is an efficient back-up of the regional screening programme making it possible to check on doubtful cases with considerable speed and to confirm the diagnosis in the cases detected. In addition, there is the prompt handling of the various problems referred to the unit by paediatricians and physicians in the area. Over the years a highly efficient system of communication has been built up between the unit on the one hand, and the parents, the general practitioners concerned and the local authorities on the other. In order to facilitate this the post of liaison nursing sister has been established. This member of the team is an experienced nurse of many years standing who is interested in the problems of long-term treatment and who works in close collaboration with the paediatrician, the dietitian and the ward sister. She attends all the clinics and in this way knows the children and their families, and has time for discussion with them. She is easily available on the telephone and can offer advice directly and also by referring the parent, health visitor, or occasionally the general practitioner concerned to the appropriate unit in the hospital. She has a car allowance and is therefore able to travel to health visitors who have children with metabolic problems in their care; she also visits the school during the child's first term in order to deal with any immediate queries. She is able to make an occasional visit to the home together with the health visitor when the clinical or biochemical checks are unsatisfactory, in order to see whether or not the diet is being taken satisfactorily and to offer appropriate advice. This appointment has been a great success; the liaison sister has been generally welcomed by the health visitors. Her early contact with the family and health visitor allows her to reinforce the advice and explanation given by the dietitian and consultant concerning the nature of the diet, the arrangement for biochemical control and the meaning of the disorder. This has helped to reduce the initial length of stay in hospital, the need to readmit later for restabilization of the diet, and greatly reduced the need to bring children back to the hospital follow up clinics.

There is a close relationship between the laboratory carrying out the biochemical work and the paediatrician concerned with the clinical care of the cases. The latter has his office immediately adjacent to the laboratory so that two-way communication is easy, and apart from spending time in the laboratory, the paediatrician takes part in the weekly laboratory conference and in the reporting session for cases of special interest. He also is present when the reporting on the routine urine screening examinations is made by the laboratory staff. The staff of the laboratory have been encouraged by their close proximity to visit the ward and outpatient clinics and to see the children under investigation and treatment. They explain the nature of the tests to the medical staff and nurses, and they in turn are shown interesting features of the cases they are working on.

Considerable effort has been expended in the education of parents, health visitors, general practitioners and schools; partly by means of the liaison nurse mentioned above, partly at the hospital level where special meetings of health visitors and general practitioners concerned have been held at regular intervals; partly with parent meetings, and finally when the physicians connected with the unit have travelled out into the community to talk to the health visitors, school medical officers and community physicians.

The co-ordinator of all this activity has been the specialist consultant paediatrician who is the director of the Willink Biochemical Genetics Unit: there is no doubt that his responsibilities would have been more difficult had it not been possible to concentrate and integrate the activities of the unit in this way.

4

Management of dietary treatment in the home

Christine Clothier

The ultimate responsibility for the long-term administration of a therapeutic diet to a child rests with the mother in her own home. Her problems include the preparation of special, and often unusual, ingredients; the administration of what may appear to her to be an unpalatable diet to a reluctant child; and last but by no means least in importance, an understanding of the reasons for the treatment and a confidence in the final outcome. Continued education, encouragement and discussion of day-to-day problems are needed by every mother but a busy hospital clinic cannot often provide the quiet intimate and relaxed atmosphere so essential for this work.

Dietary treatment of phenylketonuria

The aim of treatment in phenylketonuria is to reduce the serum phenylalanine to an accepted level which does not lead to brain damage and promotes normal growth and development. This is achieved by giving a diet low in phenylalanine composed almost entirely of an amino acid mixture, with natural fat and carbohydrate and supplementary vitamins. Phenylalanine constitutes 4–6% of all animal and vegetable proteins. The protein-rich foods such as meat, fish, eggs and cheese are, therefore, naturally excluded from the diet, and other foods although containing less protein, for example, bread, cakes and biscuits and pulses are equally unacceptable. Phenylalanine, however, cannot be excluded entirely as it is one of the essential amino acids and a certain amount is required by the body. The requirement varies with age and although in phenylketonuria the tolerance may differ considerably from individual to individual, rarely does it allow the bottle-fed infant more than 6 oz (170 ml) milk or the older child more than a serving of cereal, 3 tablespoons of cooked potato and 2 oz (57 ml) of milk daily. All living matter contains protein and so the list of foods allowed freely is very limited and a mother must draw on all her powers of initiative and imagination to provide palatable and attractive meals. The problem of withholding forbidden foods is equalled by the necessity of administering the protein substitute, the smell and flavour of which is considered by adults at best unusual and at worst unpleasant and revolting. Because of its synthetic nature the low-phenylalanine diet, from the moment it is introduced, is strictly calculated at regular intervals according to body requirements and recommended allowances. The need for adherence to details is one of the early pressures borne by the parents of a phenylketonuric child and because of the strong threat of mental retardation the management of the diet is accompanied by a tense attitude, which at the first signs of difficulty can frequently turn to despair. Problems do not diminish as the infant grows but increase as the child develops his own tastes, character and awareness of the great importance attached to his food.

After the diagnosis has been explained by the physician, the dietitian will need to spend many hours giving individual instruction and support to the new parents. This will be the beginning of a long association. She will need all her resources to advise on this artificial regimen, for it is to her that the mother will turn when she has drained all her own ideas. Constructing a balanced diet, successfully flavouring or disguising the protein substitute and ensuring an adequate calorie intake are just some of the responsibilities of the dietitian. She will learn the theory behind these in her basic training, but only practical experience will enable her to master the art of communicating her ideas to the anxious mother.

THE DIETITIAN'S ROLE

The role of the dietitian in the team is to liaise between patient, biochemist, and physician, and to act as interpreter when explaining the biochemical disorder. The more enlightened parents will soon have a basic understanding of the problem, but others, such as the warm-hearted, football orientated Liverpudlian find it as difficult to grasp as a foreign language. To a person whose medical knowledge is limited, phenylalanine, tyrosine, and amino acids are just words which some even find difficult to pronounce. Once the diagnosis is established, careful dietary treatment is of the utmost importance, and it is therefore essential for parents to be given a simple explanation of the metabolic fault, so that they may understand the treatment and the need for full

cooperation with the team. The dietitian should teach with tact, understanding and sympathy, taking a positive approach to the diet, for any
specific restriction should leave the diet as near to normal as possible, a
very difficult task for the amino acid metabolic disorders.

Large clinics for phenylketonuria and other allied disorders are few
and far between, and naturally draw a number of interested visitors
from the medical and para-medical fields. In the out-patient clinic the
patients and parents are consequently faced with a room full of people,
which disconcerts them and in many cases renders them speechless. It is,
therefore, most important for the dietitian to give continual support to
the parents, in a relaxed atmosphere, encouraging them to contact her
by telephone or in person whenever they feel it is necessary.

The management of special diets in the home is a vast subject, too
large to consider in one chapter, but two points are of particular
significance:

   1. the method and degree of accuracy necessary in the preparation
of an artificial diet,
   2. the psychological effect such a diet has on patients and their
families.

The dietetic therapy for any disorder is calculated mathematically
from food tables, and under ideal and rigid conditions, as in a metabolic
unit, will give perfect control. Food, however, is both physically and
psychologically an essential part of living; meals are a focal part of
family life, food and drink are offered as a sign of hospitality or as a
comfort at moments of great stress, and eating and drinking form the
basis of any celebration or social occasion, from a round in the pub to a
wedding feast.

To interfere with man's natural affinity with food is to meddle with
his whole way of life, and a dietitian or physician who is too rigid in a
patient's treatment will inevitably cause problems, for example, restriction of a child's food intake can lead a mother to over-sympathize and
cause resentment from other siblings. On the other hand if therapy is to
be at all effective it is obvious that some form of control is needed and
successful treatment will largely depend on the parent's ability to strike
a balance between strict limitation and sensible leniency.

Measuring the Diet
It was with the point of exactness in mind that at Alder Hey Hospital

we investigated the need to issue each patient with a small pair of scales for weighing food. Four groups of people were asked to take part, patients' mothers, ward sisters, nurses and hospital cooks. The hospital staff were chosen on their availability at the time. The mothers were the first five who visited the dietitian's office, regardless of whether they had children on a measured diet or not. Each individual in turn was given the same spoon to serve out 3 heaped tablespoons of cornflakes. This is a generally accepted measure equivalent to $\frac{1}{2}$ oz (14 g) of cornflakes or 50 mg of phenylalanine (the standard portion for diet prescription in the United Kingdom). The cornflakes were then weighed on an accurate laboratory balance. Taking all four groups together, the total difference in weight came to 9.8 g, equivalent to 34.0 mg phenylalanine (over half a portion). Table 4.1 shows in detail the variation obtained.

Table 4.1   Test measuring 3 heaped tablespoons cornflakes ($\frac{1}{2}$ oz or 14 g = 50 mg phenylalanine)

	Weight (g)	*Phenylalanine (mg)*
Mothers	17.2–21.9	61–77
Sisters	15.9–21.2	56–75
Nurses	16.4–21.5	58–76
Cooks	16.7–25.7	59–90

The exercise was then repeated with similar groups but different people, only this time the cornflakes were weighed on a small pair of scales of the type often used by diabetics. Each person was first shown how to use the scales, in the same way that mothers are instructed before their children are discharged from hospital. When the portions were re-weighed the variation in weight was 9.2 g or 32 mg phenylalanine (Table 4.2). Interestingly enough in both studies the group showing most consistency were the mothers. The total difference in weight was very similar in both parts of the study due to the very inaccurate weighings of three individuals, however, the rest all showed less variance when weighing the cornflakes than when measuring them with a spoon. Other commodities including milk and cooked potato were then measured and weighed and similar results were obtained. From these studies, and taking into account the wide range in size and shape of household

Table 4.2   Test weighing $\frac{1}{2}$ oz cornflakes for 50 mg phenylalanine

	Weight (g)	*Phenylalanine (mg)*
Mothers	13.3–15.4	47–54
Sisters	12.8–16.4	45–58
Nurses	9.9–14.5	35–51
Cooks	12.2–19.1	43–67

spoons, and the different quantities obtained by people using the same spoon, it was decided that patients would receive a more standard amount of phenylalanine if their food was weighed. The use of scales instead of milk powder scoops also ensured a more accurate intake of protein substitute. These observations emphasize the discrepancy in many diets between that prescribed and that consumed.

PARENTAL UNDERSTANDING AND INVOLVEMENT

A large number of phenylketonuric children are treated at Alder Hey Hospital and the patients in their biochemical and physical progress compare reasonably with other leading clinics. The aim of the medical team has always been to achieve good control without causing the parents and patients too much distress, and each individual member is sympathetic to the difficulties caused by dietary restriction. The majority of parents when seen in the clinic are reserved, and very rarely admit to many problems. To investigate this behaviour of almost complete satisfaction, it was decided that the dietitian should call on a few families in their own home and it was on these, almost social visits, that the parents' true feelings and attitude towards phenylketonuria and their management of the diet was revealed. Everyone was most cooperative and readily answered questions, in fact they welcomed the opportunity for an informal chat in their own surroundings about this disorder which had become part of their lives involving the whole family.

What is phenylketonuria?

I was glad to find that all the parents gave a sensible explanation in reply to this my first question, and some naturally were more detailed than others. For example, one father, a university lecturer, started with an almost textbook reply: 'Phenylketonuria is a rare blood disease caused by a recessive gene, passed on by both parents, who are carriers. The diet will not cure the disease, only control it.' Over half the explanations called it a liver complaint including the simplest; this mother also added, 'There is a lot of protein in the blood and any forbidden food that a child eats causes brain damage, why I've forgotten!' Many of them referred to the fact that only an exact amount of phenylalanine could be taken daily, as the body was unable to dispose of excess, allowing it to build up into a poison causing brain damage. One fact that interested me was the number of times the disorder was said to be caused by an acid, not an enzyme, missing in the liver, and it was not until I was instructing a new mother that I found this misunderstanding must have arisen from my description of protein as a composition of amino acids.

What is the worst factor about phenylketonuria?

My second question released a torrent of repressed feelings and emotions like an explosion from a lighted match dropped into a can of petrol. The parents without exception strongly declared that giving the protein substitute was the most exhausting, time-consuming and disturbing feature of the disorder. All of them felt it was of vital necessity to see that their infant took the complete formula, and one mother even went so far as to say that if her child had vomited she would have had to refeed him; pure fabrication arising from her tense feelings, certainly not a dietetic recommendation. The methods used to accomplish the feeding were ingenious and like the mother who held the child's hands behind his head, occasionally desperate. 'As he grew older', she said, 'it took two of us. He began screaming as soon as he saw me go to the cupboard.' However, Gary's distress was alleviated when protein hydrolysates were replaced by substitutes composed of amino acid mixtures and to his mother's relief and joy he started mixing and flavouring his own substitute and even taking it when he was not required to.

One parent referred to her little boy's infancy, when she finally resorted to an eye dropper to administer the substitute, as a bad period which she had tried to block out of her mind and told of her bitter dislike of the lounge carpet and suite she had at that time. 'Unfortunately,' she told me, 'I still have the carpet but I managed to get rid of the suite.'

A young mother, whose husband left her as soon as he was told of the diagnosis, had with the help of her parents used less drastic, but nevertheless effective, methods: 'You name it and we've done it', she boasted. Her baby had a fascination for clocks so at feeding time all the time pieces in the house were assembled around him to hold his interest. As his mind started to wander they set off the alarm bells at regular intervals, then as his mouth dropped open in surprise they shot into it a spoonful of feed. A similar ruse was used with a little chair swing, the feed being spoon fed to him as he swung happily towards his mother, joining his grandparents in a chorus of Oohs.

To illustrate the depth to which the effect of this disorder can strike, I would like to stress more specifically the case of one particular couple and their little girl. The family have been attending our clinic for over 4 years and during that time the mother has hardly spoken. The father almost entirely dominates the conversation and appears to be in sole control of the child's upbringing. On my visit to their home I discovered that the mother had been so disturbed by the diagnosis of phenylketonuria that she refused to face up to the illness or anything connected with it. For 3 years the father and his mother-in-law had tried daily to explain the disorder to her but she stubbornly ignored them. The father's presence at clinic was, therefore, a necessity to act as spokesman and to learn of any change in treatment. The mother's tense attitude was reflected in the baby's irritable and difficult behaviour and from the little girl's discharge from hospital she refused to be bottle-fed. The mother, who fortunately did look after the child, prised open her mouth with a dummy and poured the feed through a small space between her lips. This lengthy process, the mother herself told me, often resulted in her flinging the child on the bed shouting, 'Do you want to be soft?' Many times she would meet her husband as he came in from work and thrust the child into his arms with a desperate plea, 'You try'. Rows between the couple were frequent and heated and their methods for administering the feed tiring and tedious, and not successful for very long. Solids, and more adult meals were introduced but food never followed the protein substitute as the parents were too exhausted to prepare or serve it. Low phenylalanine biscuits and cakes were not featured in this home, as the little girl took all meals with reluctance and under pressure and the mother was afraid to offer her any dietetically free foods, which would enjoyably satisfy her appetite, in case they aided her continual resistance against being fed.

The mixed acid preparations improved the situation but the child is still obsessed with her diet. At home or at parties she will sit and stare in silence at people eating and whenever food advertisements appear on commercial television she will accompany each one with the comment, 'I can have that', or 'I can't have that'. She refuses to mix with other children, unless they have been personally introduced by her mother, she has become self-centred, continually demanding attention from her parents and giving a first class, dramatic performance at the slightest mishap which befalls her.

What have you explained about phenylketonuria to your child and what effect do you think the disorder has had on the child and you?
Phenylketonuria and its problems are beyond the concept of all children, yet the little ones in the families I visited showed unbelievable self control, accepting the discipline and restrictions made upon them without understanding the necessity for dietary control. Some of the children were satisfied with the misleading explanation that forbidden foods would make them ill, but not sick, others kept to their diet believing any lapse would result in a visit to hospital and more needles, and one mother put the entire blame on the physician. 'I am only carrying out the doctor's orders,' she told her two little boys, 'so if you don't like it don't tell me, tell him.' Three mothers, however, had met the problem head on, using documentary-type programmes on television, showing the mentally handicapped to illustrate their point. The children were told that dietary treatment from birth had saved them from such suffering and enabled them to grow at home normally and attend an ordinary school. 'If you should break diet your brain will be damaged, causing your limbs to relax and you will be unable to walk and talk', was one of the trio's direct approach. Michelle's mother tried another method: she regularly read to her from the diet sheet the list of forbidden foods and told her if she kept to her treatment she would get better. But to the child's frequent appeals; 'When will I get better?' she could only answer, 'soon'. Michelle's grandfather has formally promised that when the doctor allows her to eat normally he will take her to the largest restaurant or cafe and buy her the biggest steak—which she will probably refuse to eat.

In one family where both children, two boys, have phenylketonuria, the mother had striven so hard to make their lives normal that she and her husband were beginning to feel decidedly abnormal. At meal times the children would point to various dishes and ask 'Is that yours or ours?' Although she accepted their handicap the mother was reluctant to discuss it with friends and neighbours and particularly with their school teacher. She felt their development would be critically watched and if they were late walking or slow to read they would be labelled as retarded due to phenylketonuria. This mother has raised two delightful little boys but her rather tense and anxious management of the elder resulted in a number of difficult feeding periods and his serious character contrasts with the easy-going attitude of the younger who has taken everything in his stride, being handled, after experience, in a more relaxed manner. Steven's obsession with his treatment showed as a toddler in his play, when he would force the child from next door to take the role of a patient on a special diet, and numerous spirited calls on his toy telephone to the doctor and dietitian at the hospital always ended in threats and reproofs to his unfortunate playmate. Steven, possibly because of his early discipline accepts 'yes' and 'no' readily and without question in almost all things, a characteristic supported by another child of one of the family's interviewed. One problem that had arisen in two homes was the contradiction in the nutritional education of the phenylketonuric and normal children. Gary has been brought up to believe that if he eats meat he will be ill, but Steven is told 'If you don't eat your meat you won't grow up to be strong and healthy'. Similarly Steven and Michael are asked to eat whatever is put in front of them while Gary is always asked before a meal to select his own menu, because his mother explained, 'He has to eat all of it'.

The years of childhood in any family must produce times of anguish and the parents of these children certainly suffer moments of stress. I sympathized with Michelle's mother when she told me that Michelle, aged 5, shared her parents' anxiety, after the birth of their second child, until the confirmation of the baby's normality was received. Daily she would ask 'Is Paula like me?' and then when her mother told her, 'No, Paula is O.K.' she withdrew into herself, confused by emotions of relief and disappointment. Her classmates too, feel compassion for her, whenever they see her mother they inevitably ask, 'When will Shelly come off the diet?'

The introduction of chocolate sweets as a portion of phenylalanine brought distress to Erica. Having eaten her allowance she would go to the cupboard, and without attempting to touch them, look at the remainder, silent tears rolling down her face.

My interview with one mother revealed the limits to which parents will go to discourage any dietary indiscretions and so ensure satisfactory control of the metabolic fault. To press upon Evelyn the necessity for taking the protein substitute and keeping rigidly to her diet, her mother told her any relaxation in her treatment would be fatal. Not only the child but the entire family, apart from the maternal grandmother who was present at the initial interview with the dietitian, believed this proposition to be a statement of fact. Her 8-year-old brother showed particular concern for her and whenever he saw her taking an interest in food by lifting the lid of a dish on the table, he would smack her hand lightly saying, 'No, Queen, you'll die if you eat that'. To confirm that her methods of teaching were not exaggerated the mother related to me the following incident: An old lady, a neighbour and friend of the family died, and following the custom of many Irish Catholics in Liverpool, the mother took Evelyn to pay her respects to the corpse. Kneeling by the body the child asked, 'What happened to her, Mum?' and making full use of the opportunity the mother instantly replied 'She wouldn't eat her P.K. Aid!' The result of this episode has been that at each meal before drinking the protein substitute Evelyn announces, 'I don't like this, do I, Mum, but I have to take it or I'll be like the old lady in the box'.

Eight families took part in my research, sufficient to show that by talking to parents in their own homes, in the role of their guest rather than as a dietitian, I achieved a relaxed relationship which opened up to me a more complete picture of living with a child on a special diet. My visits enhanced my practical knowledge of the treatment of phenyl-ketonuria by emphasizing the worries not so obvious to the phenyl-ketonuria team, which daily arise and from the parents management of them. I must stress that I have concentrated on the more distressing problems but I have also heard parents describe with pleasure the way they have triumphed over their difficulties by various ingenious methods. I would now consider home visits by the dietitian, particularly during the first year of a family's experience of phenylketonuria, a necessity and of mutual benefit, not only to those parents who are obviously showing signs of stress, but equally to those who give the appearance of being cool, calm and collected. A health visitor specializing in inborn errors of metabolism would also bring help and support to mothers at home, especially to those families who, for geographical reasons, are unable to visit a clinic more than once a year. At Alder Hey Hospital we have already established, through frequent telephone calls, an excellent liaison with a health visitor on the Isle of Man who advises, comforts and encourages our three patients on the island. Until you delve into this subject more deeply you can mistakenly believe that your patients are without problems. I am very grateful to all the parents who helped me with my research and I would like to offer them my sincere thanks.

The tragedy of this inborn error of metabolism is appreciated by both the medical personnel and the families concerned and yet in spite of its heavy burden the attitude of two mothers moved me deeply. Everyone must be aware of the suffering of children who are unwanted and cruelly treated and this fact was underlined one afternoon on two separate occasions when the mothers said, 'If somebody has to have these phenylketonuric children then thank God a family who will love and care for them was chosen'.

5

Residential management

Erik Wamberg

Erik Wamberg

BACKGROUND TO THE KENNEDY INSTITUTE

It is well known and documentated that the results of treatment of metabolic diseases depend upon the earliest possible institution of treatment.[1] Such treatment must continue consistently during childhood with meticulous adherence to the dietary regimen and meticulous biochemical control to maintain constant therapeutic levels.

These requirements are such that children with inherited metabolic diseases are frequently treated by admission or out-patient control in hospitals or institutions, that is environments designed for *sick* children and which, even in the best cases, are unsuitable, expensive and frequently also stressing for otherwise healthy children and their parents.

Another important requirement for good therapeutic results is a multidisciplinary team composed of dietitians, biochemists, psychologists, social workers and paediatricians.[2] The significance of this has frequently been emphasized in the literature but it has become apparent in the course of years that problems connected with dietary treatment and the results obtained also depend to a great extent on well organized cooperation with the *parents*.[3]

In order to fulfil these requirements and to avoid unnecessary hospital admissions, a special treatment home for children with phenylketonuria, the John F. Kennedy Institute, was established in Denmark in 1967. This home serves the entire country and treatment can be carried out in a more home-like atmosphere, if the parents, for one reason or another, cannot manage the task in their own homes.[4,5]

The Kennedy Institute is situated near Copenhagen in the eastern part of the country, which means that parents from western parts of Denmark have a fairly long distance to travel, although the maximum distance is not more than 300 miles. However, equipped with guest rooms the Institute can always offer an overnight stay for parents.

This service is exceptional compared with the situation in the three major general hospitals in which metabolic clinics have been established but without such guest rooms.

Organization of residential management

Screening for phenylketonuria is undertaken in Denmark (population 5 million) by Guthrie's method and now involves approximately 97% of all newly born infants. The annual birth rate is approximately 70 000 and six to eight cases of phenylketonuria are found each year. Cooperation between the screening centre, the family and their general practitioner, and the treatment centre (the Kennedy Institute), is organized in the following manner:

The Guthrie test, which is undertaken on the 5th–7th day of life, is carried out in a central laboratory in Copenhagen for the entire country.[6] If a positive reaction is found, the Kennedy Institute is notified. The general practitioner is contacted by telephone and requested to send control samples both to the screening laboratory *and* to the Kennedy Institute for fluorimetric analysis.

If this second sample shows a positive reaction with a serum phenyl-alanine level of 600 μmol/l (10 mg/dl) or more, the family is notified via their general practitioner or one of the doctors on the staff of the Kennedy Institute and simultaneously arrangements are made for the child to be admitted for a couple of weeks to the Kennedy Institute for further observation and/or treatment. Children from the entire country can be admitted accompanied by their mothers who are offered accommodation in one of the guest rooms for as long a period as they can be away from home. If necessary it is possible for the Institute to offer accommodation also for the father and younger siblings.

In this manner, attempts are made to limit unfortunate psychological problems which may develop following separation of mother and child in the critical weeks immediately after birth. Simultaneously, attempts are made to build up an atmosphere of trust between the mother and the Institute. The mothers are informed about the condition and its treatment by conversation thereby counteracting the effects of the initial shock in the mothers.

UNITS FOR RESIDENTIAL TRAINING

It is our experience that a treatment centre for phenylketonuria, and

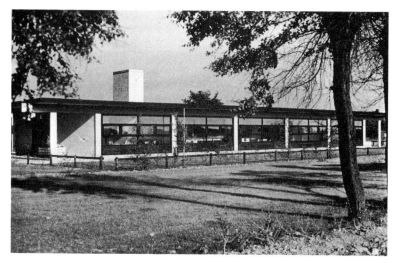

FIGURE 5.1   The front of the John F. Kennedy Institute, a one-storey building with an
internal courtyard

possibly other inborn errors of metabolism, with accommodation for
10–15 children is adequate for a region with a population of 5 million.[5]

A one-storey building with good outdoor space (Figure 5.1) is furn-
ished as a children's home with as home-like an atmosphere as possible
and without hospital or institutional character. A well-equipped diet
kitchen with room for demonstration and teaching the preparation of
diets, adequate laboratory space for routine investigations and research,
and a number of guest rooms are essentials for a treatment centre which
should be attached to a hospital unit with paediatric and neurological
departments and possibly also departments for child psychiatry. The
size and arrangement of the Kennedy Institute are apparent from the
plans shown in Figure 5.2.

The staff consists of a matron and her assistant (both trained nurses),
five nursery nurses, two night nurses, two full-time dietitians, three
laboratory technicians, one part-time psychologist, one full-time paediatrician and two medical consultants in clinical biochemistry and nutritional physiology, respectively.

This treatment home serves the entire country and the treatment of
phenylketonuria is centralized here. This ensures rapid and efficient
service for the families involved. The treatment follows uniform principles and provides experience for the staff and ideal conditions for
clinical and scientific work. Administratively, the Institute is associated

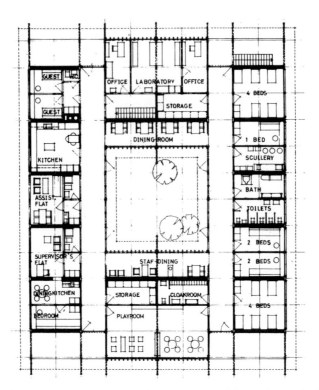

FIGURE 5.2   The John F. Kennedy Institute, ground-floor plan, scale 1 : 200.

with the National Service for the Care of the Mentally Retarded which, in its turn, is under the auspices of the Ministry for Social Affairs.

The Institute offers in-patient and out-patient services and provides an advisory service for the families and general practitioners by telephone or letter. In the case of acute illness in the child, the parents can always obtain advice and directives on contacting the Institute as regards dietary problems. This is a 24-hour service. In addition, the Institute can always admit children for varying periods, should dietary treatment prove difficult or if the parents are ill or on holiday or simply require some relief.

Training of staff

The staff consists mainly of permanent members carefully selected with years of experience in dietary treatment. Changes in the staff are rare, mainly because they prefer the team-work in a small unit with nice working conditions, but also because they become highly involved in every aspect of the treatment. Everybody in this unit knows all the phenylketonuric children and their parents, and this also provides the best possibility for the children to establish the necessary confidence in the staff.

To keep the staff interested in their work all members are invited to the weekly conferences in which they are informed about the therapeutic progress and the total situation regarding individual children.

Lectures (and discussions) given by the consultants and addressed to the nurses as well as to the paramedical staff, are held once a month on current problems connected with the disease and dietary treatment. Subjects could be for instance: composition and advantage of new amino acid preparations, the calculation and the significance of phenylalanine tolerance, different approach of loading-tests, heterozygote detection, problems in connection with the discontinuation of dietary treatment, psychological problems in the phenylketonuric families, etc. The staff are also given opportunity to participate in courses and congresses as circumstances may require.

The dietitians assume a central position among the staff and they are the people with whom the mothers (or possibly both parents) most frequently have contact. In connection with control investigations of the child in the Institute, the mother is taught and advised *personally* by a dietitian during the entire therapeutic period as regards preparation of the diet (formulas, vegetable dishes, special bread, etc.) and calculation of the quantities involved. Small everyday problems involved in the dietetic treatment at home and eating habits or eating problems of the child are frequently elucidated by telephone conversations with one of the dietitians. Successful dietetic treatment demands *inter alia* that sufficient variation in the composition of the diet can be attained and that the individual dishes have an attractive appearance and do not differ greatly from the ordinary diet of the family.

The dietitians must possess considerable imagination and they must always be able to supply recipes for desserts, cakes, biscuits, ice-cream and sweets (to a limited extent) which can provide treats in the child's everyday life. Thanks to the efforts made by our dietitians, it has hitherto not proved necessary to interrupt the diet on practical or psychological grounds in any of the 68 children who receive dietary treatment at present (July 1975) and of whom the oldest is 14 years.

As mentioned previously, cooperation with the parents is an important factor in the complete dietary treatment. In addition to instruction in preparation of the diet, all of the mothers are taught to take blood samples so that they can send these when necessary to the laboratory in the Institute, after which they receive written information concerning the result of the analysis and any necessary alterations in the diet. The mothers (and the family) are thus actively involved in the treatment and kept currently up-to-date concerning the course of the condition. The results of other investigations (EEG, X-rays, psychological investigations, etc.) are, similarly, reported and discussed when suitable opportunities arise.

Practical and psychological problems during treatment are discussed in connection with the regular control visits to the Institute and family advice is given as considered necessary. Similarly, parents are informed about results of recent research at home and abroad. During these visits, the mothers will also meet other mothers with whom they can exchange experience.

PRINCIPLES OF TREATMENT

In principle, dietary treatment of phenylketonuria in our Institute is carried out on an *out-patient* basis but treatment is invariably commenced with a stay of approximately 3–4 weeks as soon as possible after birth.[7] During this period, the diagnosis is verified and decisions are made concerning treatment or continued observation.

By means of a diet low in phenylalanine, the serum phenylalanine in the child is adjusted to a therapeutic level of 180–425 μmol/l (3–7 mg/dl) which has been found by experience to be possible in the course of 1–2 weeks. During the subsequent period, the child's eating habits are observed and the number of meals and their size are adjusted. Once the child is thriving and the mother feels capable of undertaking dietary treatment and has done so for several days under supervision, mother and child can be discharged. Simultaneously, the mother is instructed in the technique of taking blood in capillary tubes so that she can take samples *every week* throughout the first year and every second week in the following years. These blood samples are sent to the laboratory in the Institute as a link in the continuous biochemical control of the treatment.

During the first year of life, the child is investigated clinically every third month with 1 or 2 days admission to the Institute. During the second year of life, the child is seen every 6 months and once annually thereafter provided that treatment and the child's progress are satisfactory. In connection with the investigation at 6 or 12 months, a phenylalanine-loading test is undertaken in order to classify the type of the child's phenylketonuria.[8] This investigation requires admission for 3 days. Simultaneously, tolerance tests are undertaken on both parents and possibly also the siblings. In this connection, it should be pointed out that the principles outlined here concern infants in whom treatment has commenced within the first months of life. In older children, the task is more difficult and the sojourn in the Institute is correspondingly longer.

In addition to the routine visits, it is always possible to undertake extra investigations or arrange brief periods of admission should the diet involve problems in the child's home or if there is a tendency not to adhere to the diet, refusal to eat, failure to thrive or other conditions which necessitate observation. Many parents make use of our offers to admit their children in the course of the year, for example should one of the parents take ill at home or be admitted to hospital, during week-ends, holidays or other reasons requiring relief. In occasional cases, unstable social and/or family conditions have necessitated admission of the child to the Kennedy Institute for more prolonged periods (months to years) and, similarly, in a number of cases, day-care of the child during normal working hours has proved necessary. It will be apparent that there is a certain, although limited, need for beds for treatment of children with phenylketonuria during the initial phase of the treatment but beds should always be available for observation, to relieve the parents or in the case of unstable conditions in the home. In addition, two or more guest-rooms are essential (Table 5.1).

It is our opinion that treatment should be continued as long as possible, that is as long as the children are willing to adhere to the diet and the parents are willing to continue the regimen. In practice this means that we try to keep the boys on the diet at least until puberty. Girls should never be taken off the diet completely, but after puberty a less restricted diet is recommended. It is pointed out to the parents, that their girls must take up a fully restricted diet before and during pregnancy in order to avoid the hazards to the fetus from maternal phenylketonuria.

The oldest child in this study is 14 years and we have not yet been

Table 5.1   Number of occupied beds for children per year and per day together with number of parent/guest days and bed-nights per year

Year	Children		Adults	
	Bed-days per year	Average no. per day	Parent/guest days per year	Bed-nights per year
1968	1821	4.9	224	95
1969	2700	7.3	184	111
1970	2357	6.4	334	219
1971	2475	6.7	295	190
1972	2160	5.9	328	214
1973	1499	4.1	389	250
1974	1046	2.8	330	219
1975	1460	4.0	423	296

forced to abandon treatment in any case. The diet is maintained rigidly until the age of 8 years after which some modifications are introduced, including more milk, free amounts of fruits and bread, and a therapeutic level of about 610 μmol/l (10 mg/dl) of phenylalanine in the serum is permitted. During subsequent years, the diet is less restricted and serum phenylalanine levels of up to 910 μmol/l (15 mg/dl) are permitted provided no striking changes in the child's behaviour occur. In many treatment centres, the dietary treatment is withdrawn at about the age of 6–8 years, and, in some centres even earlier [9-12]. It is not, however, yet certain that this early withdrawl can be undertaken without detriment to the intellectual functions of the child and his scholastic achievements.

Results of treatment

It is outside the scope of this discussion to present a detailed account of the results obtained by the treatment outlined here for children with phenylketonuria but it should be noted that physical growth has been normal in practically all of the cases and the height and weight curves of the children have been within normal limits. The therapeutic level of serum phenylalanine has been satisfactory in the majority of the fasting blood samples: 62% were within the therapeutic level of 180–425

Table 5.2 Percentage of the total number of fasting serum phenylalanine determinations falling within certain ranges. (Desirable therapeutic level, 3–7 mg/dl)

Range (mg/dl)	Samples (%)
3–7	62.3
2–9	95.2
< 2 and > 9	4.8

μmol/l (3–7 mg/dl) and 95% were between 120 and 550 μmol/l (2–9 mg/dl) (Table 5.2).

The intellectual development depends upon the time at which treatment is instituted. In infants in whom treatment is commenced in the course of the first month of life, we have demonstrated entirely normal mental development while the children in whom diet is not instituted until the second or third months of life attain mental development at the lower limit of normal or at the borderline with the educationally subnormal[5] (Table 5.3). In three cases, in whom dietary treatment was started in the third month of life, symptoms of 'minimal brain damage' were noted, that is hyperactivity, restlessness, distractibility, short attention span, rapid changes in mood, etc. in addition to their educationally subnormal development. If treatment is commenced at a later date there is danger of mental retardation.

Table 5.3 Median IQ related to age of starting dietary treatment for 50 children with classical phenylketonuria

Age diet started (weeks)	Number	Age at last test (years and months) Median	Range	IQ Median	Range	P*
< 4	24	2 y 1 m	(1 – 6 y 4 m)	106	(94 – 123)	0.01
5–13	7	6 y 6 m	(1 y 1 m–9 y 1 m)	94	(82 – 110)	
14–52	10	8 y 6 m	(2–11 y 6 m)	90	(40 – 115)	0.05
52	9	8 y 10 m	(5 y 2 m–13 y 3 m)	65	(30 – 87)	

*The Mann–Whitney Rank test

The family situation during treatment

Dietary treatment at home of children with metabolic diseases makes great demands on the parents. These conditions are only scantily illustrated in the literature but the few studies available agree on the problems of treatment and their influence upon family life.[13-15]

By means of a questionnaire sent to 34 families from our group all of whom had children who had received dietary treatment for at least 6 months, we attempted to obtain an impression of the effect of treatment on the psycho-social climate in the family.[16]

Questions were grouped in order to illustrate the following problems:

1. Parents reaction to the diagnosis: phenylketonuria
2. Problems concerning the diet (preparation and management)
3. Practical and psychological influence on family conditions by dietary treatment
4. Assessment of the assistance from the Institute
5. Suggestions made by parents

In more than 90% of the cases, the parents' reaction to the diagnosis of phenylketonuria is more or less one of shock. This can, however, be overcome by means of *repeated* conversation with information concerning the cause of the disease, its course and treatment and by meticulous answers to all questions regarding the prognosis and the mode of inheritance. Nevertheless, our investigations have revealed that one-third of the parents are worried because they are carriers of the condition and more than half of them do not wish to have more children.

Preparation of the diet has not caused difficulties in any of the families and could be successfully continued for up to 10 years, although occasional breaches of the dietary regimen occurred in approximately one-third of the cases. The eating habits of the families were not particularly influenced as, in 30 of the 34 families questioned, the phenylketonuric child ate his meals with other members of the family. This is probably because three-quarters of the children had commenced dietary treatment prior to the age of 6 months.

The every-day life is of course influenced in various ways by the presence of the phenylketonuric child, particularly where social activity is concerned. Thus nearly half of the families had cut down on visits to restaurants or visits to relatives and friends and holiday visits and other

Table 5.4   Changes in some social activities for 34 families with phenylketonuric children

| Social activities | Number of families (%) | | | |
	Unchanged	Reduced	Increased	Don't know
Visit to restaurants	18 (52)	15 (45)		1 (3)
Visit to family friends	23 (67)	11 (33)		
Holidays	16 (46)	14 (42)	1 (3)	3 (9)
Other activity	17 (49)	15 (45)	1 (3)	1 (3)

leisure activities had to be restricted. It is worth noting, however, that 16 families went on holiday as usual. This was possible, among other reasons, because the phenylketonuric child in these cases could have a sojourn in the Kennedy Institute (Table 5.4).

Although we have attempted to support and help these families as much as possible, dietary treatment will, of course, complicate family life. Both fathers and mothers describe themselves as more unstable mentally compared with their situation before the phenylketonuric child entered the family, although without actual conflict situations developing between the parents on this account. Dissolution of the marriage on account of the phenylketonuric child has not been demonstrated. In a number of cases, the parents are exposed to influences from relatives and friends who do not consider it necessary that the dietary regimen is strictly adhered to, but, in the present material, influences of this type have not resulted in breaches of the diet.

In summing up, it may be concluded that by employing advice and support from a multidisciplinary team with good routine and well-developed cooperation with the parents we feel that we have created the necessary requirements for out-patient management of the demanding and prolonged diet in the great majority of cases and without serious disturbances of family life. Parents, to a great extent, are spared from financial problems resulting from treatment—a fact which is of undoubted significance for the results obtained. According to the Danish Health Scheme, treatment and stays in the Kennedy Institute are free of charge. The cost of the diet powder is defrayed by the Ministry for Social Affairs and local authorities can refund the expenses involved for travelling to the Institute and may, further, provide financial support for the expenses incurred in the child's diet at home.

COST–BENEFIT ANALYSIS

Priorities given for tasks and investment of funds and working power in health care services have been in the limelight in recent years and have frequently been the subject of debate. However, when·prevention of mental retardation is concerned, deliberations of this nature must be omitted in lands with social welfare systems.

A working party in the Council of Europe has, however, worked with the problem. They compared the expenses involved in tracing and providing dietary treatment of children with phenylketonuria with the cost of institutional care for the entire lives of untreated children. Although calculations of this type are associated with considerable uncertainty and completely unjustifiable from an ethical point of view, these figures give grounds for reflection and justify the efforts made to trace the threatened children and institute treatment in time. The expenses for each child receiving dietary treatment for phenylketonuria consist of three main elements: (1) tracing of the disease (screening), (2) dietary treatment at home, and (3) share of the running expenses of the treatment institution.

During the financial year 1971/72, we have carried out calculations of the individual items in Denmark, presuming that seven cases of phenylketonuria are demonstrated annually and that dietary treatment is maintained for 10 years and that the Kennedy Institute has an average of 50 children under control and supervision. Employing a socio-economic method of calculation in which future expenses involved in the treatment of the disease are related to the time of birth and are compared with the similarly classified alternative expense of institutional care for life (average duration of life 67 years) for the untreated patient, the following figures are found *per child*:

1. *Early detection and treatment*	Danish crowns
Screening	17 143
Extra cost of dietary treatment	105 584
Share of expenses of Kennedy Institute	153 616
Total	276 343

2. *Institutional care*
    Cost of care from 3 to 67 years   822 571

Net gain (2 — 1)   546 228

These expenses are calculated as follows:

Screening: 80 000 Guthrie-tests are performed each year with an average cost of 1.50 Danish crowns per test. Assuming that seven phenylketonuric children are found per year the cost per case detected will be 17 143 Danish crowns.

Extra expense for dietary treatment: this amount is calculated as the total cost for 10 years of dietary treatment for a given phenylketonuric child, minus expenses for ordinary food in the same period to a normal child. Thus the costs for hydrolysates, special low-phenylalanine bread, extra fruits and vegetables, etc. are included in these calculations.

Share of running expenses of Kennedy Institute: in the fiscal year 1971/72 the total running expenses for this residential unit was 985 383 Danish crowns—covering staff salaries, laboratory costs, heating, food and medicaments during admission. 6% of this sum represents payment of interest and amortization of the capital invested in buildings and equipment. Assuming 50 children are under treatment and supervision per year the share in running expenses for a given child through 10 years of dietary treatment has been calculated to 153 616 Danish crowns.

It may thus be established that, for every child with phenylketonuria in whom dietary treatment is instituted, at least half a million Danish crowns are saved. This example illustrates the great socio-economical aspects involved in prophylaxis of mental retardation.

For the sake of completion, it may be recorded that, in these calculations, the social product of the normally developed individual has not been taken into account. On the other hand, however, the value of the resources of which the normal individual can take advantage has not been taken into account either.

Suggestions for future units

On the basis of 7 years' experience with a treatment home for phenylketonuria, we can now establish that the expectations have been fulfilled. The results of treatment are satisfactory and cooperation with parents has been such that dietary treatment could be carried out in the children's homes for the period required without noteworthy complications.

In addition to phenylketonuria, we have had the opportunity of treating a few children with other inborn errors such as tyrosinaemia and homocystinuria and there are good reasons to presume that a residential unit for the treatment of phenylketonuria as described here could also be used for diseases such as histidinaemia, galactosaemia, argininosuccinicaciduria, prolinaemia and cystathioninuria. On the other hand, other congenital metabolic diseases which are amenable to dietary treatment are frequently so severe that treatment can only be instituted and controlled in a paediatric department, for example maple syrup urine disease, hyperammonaemia, methylmalonicaciduria, cystinosis, hydroxyprolinaemia, isovalericacidaemia, propionic-acidaemia, Lowe's syndrome, Mencke's syndrome, etc. These conditions require intensive clinical observation and supplementary laboratory investigations to an extent which cannot be attained in a treatment home of the type described here.

We have, however, frequently felt the lack of more numerous and more extensive laboratory facilities with the possibility of examining blood amino acids and urine metabolites by column chromatography and gas chromatography respectively and we have still too little accommodation for intensifying the research projects on heterozygote detection which are at present in progress.

PROBLEMS CONNECTED WITH RESIDENTIAL TRAINING UNITS

It has been pointed out previously[5] that centralization of treatment of phenylketonuria in an institution designed for the purpose and with the character of a children's home and calculated for a population of 5 million with an annual birthrate of 80 000 has many advantages of which the following may be noted:

1. Early diagnosis of new cases in cooperation with the screening centre and immediate start of treatment, often within the first 2 or 3 weeks of life.

2. More experience and better research possibilities are obtained when the comparatively few cases available receive treatment and follow-up in one place.

3. It is easier to set up a multidisciplinary team and an experienced nursing staff in one place.

4. The parents will show more confidence in, and cooperate better with, the permanent staff who are familiar with the children.

5. A regional treatment centre will grant the parents a better service, for instance if the child gets fever or anorexia. Staff familiar with the child will always be ready to instruct the parents when they phone or write.

6. In case of illness, holidays or unsettled social conditions in the home the child can be admitted to the Institute so that the dietary treatment and control is maintained.

These advantages of centralization far outweigh the few disadvantages, as for instance in Denmark:

1. Our Institute is situated in the most eastern part, near Copenhagen, involving fairly long journeys. The well-developed system of local airlines, however, makes travelling easier.

2. The university clinics in the rest of the country are deprived of cases for education of students.

3. Doctors in paediatric training at provincial departments will not be acquainted with the treatment of phenylketonuria.

4. The present situation of the Kennedy Institute is too isolated. Preferably it should form a special department at a major regional hospital or a university clinic in close connection with other special departments, but without losing its character of a treatment home.

REFERENCES

1. HUDSON, F. P., MORDAUNT, V. L., and LEAKY, I. (1970). Evaluation of treatment begun in first three months of life in 184 cases of phenylketonuria. *Arch. Dis. Child.*, **45**, 5
2. CLAYTON, B. (1971). Phenylketonuria. *J. Med. Genet.*, **8**, 37
3. SCHILD, S. (July, 1972). Parents of children with PKU. *Child. Today*, **20**
4. WAMBERG, E. (1969). The background and aims of the Kennedy Institute. *Acta Paediatr. Scand.*, **58**, 544
5. WAMBERG, E. (1973). A survey of centralised treatment of phenylketonuria in Denmark. In J. W. T. Seakins, R. A. Saunders, and C. Toothill, (eds.), *Treatment of Inborn Errors of Metabolism.* p. 35. (Edinburgh and London: Churchill Livingstone)
6. LUND, E. and WAMBERG, E. (1971). Screening for phenylketonuria and other inborn errors of metabolism in Denmark. 1962–1970. *Scand. J. Clin. Lab. Invest.*, **118**, (Suppl.) 47
7. WAMBERG, E. (1969). The principles and experience in dietary treatment of phenylketonuria. *Acta Paediatr. Scand.*, **58**, 547
8. GÜTTLER, F. and WAMBERG, E. (1972). Persistent hyperphenylalaninemia. *Acta Paediatr. Scand.*, **61**, 321

9. HANLEY, W. B. and LINSAO, L. (1973). Termination of PKU dietary treatment in 62 patients. *Pediatr. Res.*, **7**, 383
10. HUDSON, F. P. and HAWCROFT, J. (1973). Duration of treatment in phenylketonuria. In J. W. T. Seakins, R. A. Saunders, and C. Toothill, (eds.), *Treatment of Inborn Errors of Metabolism*, p. 51. (Edinburgh and London: Churchill Livingstone)
11. KANG, E. S., SOLLEE, N. D. and GERALD, P. S. (1970). Results of treatment and terminations of the diet in phenylketonuria. *Pediatrics*, **46**, 881
12. MURPHY, D. (1969). Termination of dietary treatment of phenylketonuria. *Irish J. Med. Sci.*, **2**, 177
13. McBEAN, M. S. (1971). The problems of parents of children with phenylketonuria. In Bickel, Hudson and Woolf (eds,). *Phenykletonuria*, p. 280. (Stuttgart: Georg Thieme Verlag)
14. KELESKE, L., SALOMONS, G. and OPITZ, E. (1967). Parental reactions to phenylketonuria in the family. *J. Pediatr.*, **70**, 793
15. WOOD, A. C., FRIEDMAN, C. J. and STEISEL, J. M. (1967). Psychosocial factors in phenylketonuria. *Am. J. Orthopsychiatry*, **37**, 671
16. MIKKELSEN, I., SCHARLING, E., SVENDSEN, F. U. and WAMBERG, E. (1974). The influence of dietary treatment on the psychosocial conditions in families with phenylketonuric children. *Näringsforskning*, **18**, 78 (Engl. summary)

COMMUNITY REACTION
TO PRESENT PRACTICE

6

Parent reaction to medical care and screening

Elsie D. May

The 'good press' accorded various diseases and their treatment by the medical correspondents of newspapers, magazines, radio and television has increased the awareness, knowledge and, partially, the understanding of medicine by the general public. Whilst raising the level of public acceptance of investigation and treatment, the media have raised the level of public expectation and the need for clear information from hospital and community medical services where illness or disorder affects themselves or their families. The scientific, social, ethical and legal implications of the rapid advances in the fields of genetics and biology have stimulated considerable discussion in the medical and lay press about hereditary disorders and screening procedures.[1]

Screening tests are not intended to be diagnostic but to sort out apparently well persons who have a disease or defect, from those who probably do not.[2] While these developments increase knowledge which may improve the quality of life, scientific results are not always applied to ends which most people consider desirable, and with increasing knowledge and understanding of defects and disorders, the old standards of morality and ethics may not be inalienable in the midst of all this change.[3] Knowledge is power and enables society to improve the quality of future generations by advising present and future parents about the nature and nurture of their children. Cowie has stated that it is the right of all parents of reproductive age to have the benefit of genetic counselling in terms that they can understand.[4]

Although all of the measures in the management of inherited metabolic disease have been introduced with good intention, and could not have found such extensive application without both professional and public support, it was considered desirable to investigate the experience of parents to this aspect of health care.

This was done by inviting from three different cities, parents whose experience varied widely and covered as many aspects of this area of paediatrics as possible, to report confidentially on anything they wished to describe, whether helpful or otherwise. Before reporting the results in detail, it is necessary to consider the types of interference, from the point of view of those who offered it, in the three cities studied.

Whole-population screening—the initial test

For one inherited metabolic disorder only, phenylketonuria, a screening test between the 6th and 14th day of life is recommended for all infants born in Britain. Hospitals are responsible for testing infants still in their care on the 6th day, those discharged sooner or born at home or in nursing homes are the responsibility of the Medical Officer of Health and his staff,[5] now the Area Health Authority of the reorganized National Health Service.

Phenylketonuria an inherited deficiency of liver phenylalanine hydroxylase activity, results in accumulation of phenylalanine which affects mental development, often resulting in severe handicaps associated with epilepsy, behaviour disorder and eczema. Its incidence in Caucasians is 1 : 10 000 live births.[6]

The recommended screening tests involve a heel prick to collect either on paper or in a heparinized tube, a sample of capillary blood from the baby. This procedure is carried out by a midwife or health visitor at home or in hospital and the blood sample forwarded to a central hospital laboratory. The tests used are either the Guthrie test, a microbiological assay of phenylalanine,[7] or the Scriver test, analysis of plasma by paper chromatography.[8] The latter procedure can detect, in addition to phenylketonuria, about 20 amino acidopathies[9] and so exceeds the official recommendation for screening. Parental cooperation in screening of infants in England and Wales is 99%[10] which appears to denote satisfaction with the method, the service received, and parents' willingness to cooperate with professional advisors in caring for their children. But all screening procedures involve intrusion into the privacy of the individual and no one should be expected to submit to the inconvenience and anxiety this may involve without the prospect of treatment or benefit.[11]

Before the screening programme was started in Birmingham, the press, radio and television were utilized to inform the public of the tests and the reasons for doing them. Educational programmes for midwives and health visitors were set up, and hospital staff and Medical Officers of Health cooperated in offering training and refresher courses which were usually repeated annually. Thus the staff became both competent and confident and in Birmingham, as elsewhere, it was noted that after the first year of screening there was a diminution in technical errors.

REPEATED SCREENING TESTS

Repeat tests are especially necessary with the Scriver test since several of the amino acids other than phenylalanine show abnormalities, most of which are transient, but any one of which might indicate a specific metabolic disorder. These account for 80% of the repeats in Birmingham,[9] the remainder being for administrative or technical reasons such as testing before the 6th day of life, haemolysis or tube breakage. In Manchester,[12] repeat tests were necessary in 9% of cases in an initial series of 6901 births, although in a later series involving 87 982 infants the repeat rate fell to just over 6%,[13] similar to the Birmingham rate on 55 715 babies of 6.5%.[9] About 10 parents per year refuse repeat tests in Birmingham[9] but in Manchester up to 9% refusals are reported.[13]

Where an abnormal plasma pattern requires a third and subsequent test, these are combined in both Birmingham and Manchester with an out-patient appointment when the parents are seen by a member of the specialist team at the regional hospital. After examination of the baby, the nature of the chemical abnormalities is discussed and the need to follow all chemical abnormalities until they either resolve or there is more positive indication that treatment is required, is explained. Since almost all chemical abnormalities prove to be transient, a generally reassuring approach is adopted.

OBSERVATION OF PATIENTS WITH UNTREATED DISORDERS

The natural history of a number of specific metabolic disorders is still unknown and there is ample precedent for believing that present opinions on others may need revision. This has lead to a cautious approach to treatment, and even a few years ago when management policies in relation to screening for metabolic disease were being formulated the evidence that patients with type 1 prolinaemia should be subjected to a proline restricted diet was considered inadequate, and in neither Birmingham nor Manchester was such treatment instituted. None the less, it was essential that infants with the biochemical disorder should be watched closely for any symptoms or signs that might cause this policy to be reversed and parents were required to attend clinics every few months with their apparently well baby who, they were told, was suffering from a somewhat abstract 'disorder' they found difficult to believe in or understand.

TREATMENT OF SPECIFIC METABOLIC DISORDERS

Approximately 50 cases of phenylketonuria per year are discovered in England and Wales, and if treated with a low phenylalanine diet within the first 6 weeks of life mental retardation can be avoided. The diet must be regulated by laboratory analysis of the blood level of phenylalanine to prevent over- or under-treatment—both equally dangerous.[14] Female patients so treated will need to re-embark on a low phenylalanine diet when pregnant—how soon in pregnancy is not yet known but the diet may have to be initiated prior to pregnancy[15] for normal fetal development.

When hyperphenylalaninaemia is found on first testing, an indication that this may be due to phenylketonuria, the child's family doctor is contacted by the hospital and immediate arrangements made for introduction and establishment of a low phenylalanine diet. Usually this involves further investigation, and if necessary, the baby's admission to the regional hospital. The parents, especially mother, are encouraged to take an active part in the feeding and management of the baby in hospital under the supervision of the ward staff and the dietitian. The period of admission is kept as short as possible, and when problems occur following the baby's discharge from hospital, the parents are encouraged to get in touch with the staff they know, often the dietitian, between out-patient follow-up visits. Careful follow-up is necessary for the first 2–3 years, as some cases of hyperphenylalaninaemia resolve spontaneously. Treatment is available for tyrosinaemia, branched-chain amino aciduria, homocystinuria and histidinaemia,[13] as well as phenylketonuria. The need to treat histidinaemia is still not finally resolved.

The study

To investigate the care, management and information offered to parents by the hospital and community medical and nursing services involved, a small number of parents in Birmingham, Manchester and Liverpool were invited to report their reaction to screening and medical care. In Birmingham, those who did not reply were visited at home and this either stimulated a written reply or, in a few cases, the health visitors report was used.

These selected parents were divided into four groups on the basis of the experience to which they had been exposed:

    1. Routine screening only with a normal result, hence no further involvement

    2. Children having repeat tests but soon found to be normal

    3. Children with abnormal plasma patterns requiring follow up in the clinic but for which no treatment was offered

    4. Infants and children found to have phenylketonuria who were then treated in the usual way

The number of families contacted and the number of replies, both spontaneous and requiring home visits are shown in Table 6.1. The first

Table 6.1 The number of families invited to report, and the number who replied spontaneously, and in parentheses, the additional number who only replied after a home visit

Group	Birmingham Invited	Responded		Manchester Invited	Responded	Liverpool Invited	Responded
1	20	12	(8)	25	5	5	0
2	20	9	(5)	25	8	5	0
3	19	10		25	4	5	0
4	16	11	(4)	25	11	5	3
Total	75	58		100	28	20	3

group were selected from those born in the preceding 3 months to ensure that the parents would be able to recollect the occasion and their reactions.

Few parents (15) commented on the test as part of a national screening programme, and six of those who did so had children with phenylketonuria. They were all favourable to national screening programmes of infants and to their own babies being tested in the first instance. Fifty-nine parents indicated that the test carried out on their babies was acceptable as part of the routine post-partum management: however three mothers requested pre-natal information, and one father thought: 'The screening test should be made compulsory as a right of the child to prove his or her well being'—an interesting comment in the light of the possibility that future legislation may relate to the rights of the unborn infant.[16] Parents would like to know the result of the test even when negative—this, whilst not routinely given, happened in two cases and was greatly appreciated.

Health visitors and midwives as the initial contact with parents and the new baby have enormous potential for relieving or creating anxiety, and as they are involved in all the four groups studied, they elicited comment from the majority of parents (56). The health visitors' and midwives' aptitude for relieving or creating anxiety is most marked with repeat tests, especially where either pregnancy, labour, or both have been difficult or there is a history of previous miscarriage or stillbirth, or a family history of handicap. Parents remarked how happy they were with: a midwife or health visitor who explained, 'why the test was done and what would happen if they found some abnormality', reassurance and explanation from the midwife and family doctor, 'who made a point of calling to see the baby to explain the purpose of the test and assured me that there was no cause for worry at this point', and a midwife's management, 'very confident, extremely reassuring and very gentle with the baby'. Contrast this with the unhappiness of parents unable to obtain what they considered a full explanation and reassurance: 'It was the most nerve wracking experience I have ever been through. I let her go, not believing a word she said,' and, 'Neither the midwife who took the blood, nor our family doctor knew anything about it (or would not tell us)'. One can almost feel the suspicion arising from the brackets enclosing those words. Relations with hospital out-patient staff also pose problems in the field of communication. It is interesting that an equal number of parents of group 3 infants expressed their feelings (good or ill), about hospital and community staff, and were often angry and confused.

It is hoped that hospital medical staff spend time explaining in a simple manner, and giving written information, so that parents feel they are being considered. Many parents complained of their dismissal without information. 'What really upset us was the lack of communication', 'The results of the tests were given to us only because *we asked* for the results', 'We were told to go back for the results of it 2 weeks later. At this stage no one told us what "it" was'. Parents also commented on the good doctors. 'Information given to us was explained clearly and adequately', 'The doctor went to great lengths to explain to me just what he had done and I came away from the hospital with my mind a lot easier'.

Better facilities in out-patients for coping with hungry, crying, naked infants would improve parental morale, as would consideration of the timing of blood tests, especially with older children. Most parents wished to be present when the blood sample was taken and requested that the sample be obtained as soon as possible after arrival in the out-patient department to relieve the children's fear—a lesson in compassion that no children's hospital should need.

As it seems reasonable to concentrate facilities for these children in a laboratory that can cope with the analysis of the more unusual diseases such as the organic acidaemias[17] consideration must be given to the cost and time spent by parents and children in travelling. With increasing specialization in medicine there is a multiplicity of hospitals to attend, and in our group 3, parents with two sets of twins were attending both the maternity and the children's hospital.

All the parents whose children were diagnosed as having phenylketonuria were delighted that their children had started treatment early enough to benefit from dietary management. Rapid admission to hospital, although frightening at the time, was offset by the immediate advice about the disorder and its treatment from the consultant concerned, and all parents found in-patient care, attention to themselves and management of their babies from all the staff, medical, nursing and dietitians exceptionally good. The dietitian, probably one of the most important people involved in the management of phenylketonuria, is offering an excellent service to out-patients as well. However, the diet at home causes fearful problems '3 to 4 hours to feed her' or, 'To try to feed him was a dreadful process'. Two families noticed a change in their babies' temperament when on the diet, from being grizzly miserable infants they became contented ones who would sleep through the night.

There were occasional problems with local pharmacists (6) who would not stock the specialist foods and parents had to shop around.

Mothers with a first baby affected felt diffident and unsure about weaning, and reassurance of their child's future only came for two mothers when they 'saw an older child with the same complaint and my mind was at rest', despite excellent hospital and general practitioner advice and reassurance. The parents of four phenylketonuric children, all of whom were first babies, mentioned their thoughts on whether or not to have other children, and appeared to have received genetic guidance. One family had two further unaffected children and showed some resentment of the advice given after diagnosis of their first child as this had made them fearful of the result of further pregnancies. Of the other three families, one thought they would quite happily encounter further pregnancies whether or not affected; the other two had serious doubts not only about the problems of managing another affected child but also their ability to cope with a normal baby as well as their phenyl-ketonuric child—which concurs with Dr Lorber's statement that a handicapped child in a family often prevents the birth of a normal one. The opportunity to meet other parents was requested by many parents with phenylketonuric children.

Discussion

This small study shows that the initial heel prick test to obtain blood in early infancy is an acceptable procedure to parents and confirms the findings of an earlier survey in Liverpool.[18] The requested information about the screening procedure in the pre-natal clinic might usefully be incorporated into a talk on maternal and infant diets. Difficulties arise in communication between parents and medical and nursing personnel as soon as there is deviation from the normal pattern. Despite articles in the mass media, continuing education of midwives and health visitors and the availability of specialist hospital staff, many mothers at this early stage in the post-partum period will over-react to the request for a repeat test. The Manchester paediatricians produced an excellent typewritten summary of the test procedure and reasons for repeat testing which is issued to the community health staff involved in the screening programme and they, as do most other centres, have recurrent lectures by the hospital staff.

Parents should be able to receive the results of the screening test from their health visitor when this is issued to them by the Area Health Authorities, and may be given to the mothers either at the health visitor's primary visit (14th day) or, where routine developmental screening is established, at the baby's 6th week screening.

Improved facilities in out-patient departments for dressing and feed-ing babies requires thought and reorganization. For example, mothers should be offered facilities for warming feeds on arrival and should not have to ask for them—a not insuperable or expensive service which could easily be made a routine in specialist clinics.

The Area Pharmaceutical Officer could supply parents, on discharge from hospital, with a list of pharmacists prepared to stock the special foods for phenylketonuric children.

An excellent booklet by Holten and Tyfield is available for parents with phenylketonuric children.[19] Another pamphlet for parents whose children have other amino acidopathies would be useful as an adjunct to out-patient follow-up. Both community and hospital staff need to allow more time to answer parents queries and provide early follow-up to make sure that explanations have been absorbed and understood. Pamphlets and written material supplied must satisfy parents and will need careful monitoring to make sure they answer the real needs of parents and not just those anticipated by medical and nursing staff. Any written material given to parents does not reduce the responsibility of the doctor to explain his advice to the parents of affected children.[20]

Discussion with the parents about the future of their affected children does appear to be taking place, and four parents of phenylketonuric children had specifically raised the question of having further children and had found the discussion helpful. They will need to be educated to understand the ethical problems their children may face in the future— mass screening for diagnosis, counselling and treatment has widened the horizons of persons exposed to major genetic illness.[21] Every family should have received sufficient information and guidance to enable them to discuss amongst themselves, at home, the implications of any disorder or handicap affecting one of its members. Failure on our part to assist this debate is a serious disservice to our patients.

Thoughtful consideration must be given in the future to the possible effects of counselling and education. The cost of screening mothers-to-be for evidence of a phenylketonuric gene followed by amniocentesis and possible abortion may be less than the cost of screening all newborn children and give parents the choice of abortion or bringing up a child with phenylketonuria.[1]

Another face to this genetic coin, first recognised by Munro[22] in 1947, and supported by more recent work, namely that siblings of patients with phenylketonuria appear to have superior intelligence five times in excess of expectation suggests that genetic recessive diseases whose carriers are at an intellectual disadvantage acquire compensatory genetic mechanisms,—a gene for superior intelligence giving a positive advantage to the normal siblings.[23] These findings should be included in decisions on future policy.

Diligent follow-up of all affected children into adult life and, if possible, their children as well, may help us to answer some of the ethical problems posed as a result of the present state of progress and treatment. The need for sympathetic understanding of the problems imposed upon parents supports the need for a system of centres with highly skilled staff able to cope with the problems of management and counselling. Continuity of care, and the building up of a relationship with the children concerned as they grow into adulthood could hold the key to many future problems and help to allay the anxieties of parents and their children. Screening for phenylketonuria is accepted as ful-filling all the criteria laid down by Wilson and Junger[24] and is considered the only screening test for whole populations to be at present justified.[25] It would appear to hold exciting keys to the future management of inherited genetic disease.

We warmly appreciate the help, and commend the courage of the paedia-tricians in Liverpool and Manchester, Drs F. P. Hudson, G. Komrower and I. B. Sardharwalla and their colleagues for allowing us to make this a multicentre study thereby sharing the opprobrium (and some praise) that would otherwise have centred on those in Birmingham represented by Drs B. S. B. Wood and M. Addy, from whom we enjoy continuous support, and my personal thanks to Dr D. N. Raine for his help and encouragement.

REFERENCES

1. JONES, A. and BODMER, W. F. (1974). *Our Future Inheritance: Choice or Chance.* (London: Oxford University Press)
2. WHITY, L. G. (1974). Screening for disease: definitions and criteria. *Lancet*, **ii**, 819
3. SMITH, A. (1975). *The Human Pedigree.* (London: George Allen and Unwin)
4. COWIE, V. (1972). Genetic counselling and social aspects of prenatal and new born screening. *Ann. Clin. Biochem.*, **9**, 112
5. Department of Health and Social Security. (1969). *Screening for early detection of phenylketonuria.* HMSO (69) 72
6. RAINE, D. N. (1974). Screening for disease: inherited metabolic disease *Lancet*, **ii**, 996
7. GUTHRIE, R. and SUSI, A. (1963). A simple phenylalanine method for detecting phenylketonuria in large populations of newborn infants. *Pediatrics*, **32**, 338
8. SCRIVER, C. R., DAVIES, E. and CULLEN, A. M. (1964). Application of a simple micromethod to the screening of plasma for a variety of amino acidopathies. *Lancet*, **ii**, 230
9. RAINE, D. N., COOKE, J. R., ANDREWS, W. A. and MAHON, D. F. (1972). Screening for inherited metabolic disease by plasma chromatography (Scriver) in a large city. *Br. Med. J.*, **3**, 7

10. HUDSON, F. P. and HAWCROFT, J. (1975). M.R.C.—D.H.S.S. Phenylketonuria Newsletter No. 3
11. Nuffield Provincial Hospitals Trust. (1968). *Screening in Medical Care*. (London: Oxford University Press)
12. KOMROWER, G. M., FOWLER, B., GRIFFITHS, M. J. and LAMBERT, A. M. (1968). A prospective community survey for aminoacidaemias. *Proc. R. Soc. Med.* **61**, 294
13. SARDHARWALLA, I. B., KOMROWER, G. M., BRIDGE, C. and GORDON, D. B. (1972). One-dimensional chromatography of plasma in Manchester. *Ann. Clin. Biochem.*, **9**, 126
14. World Health Organization Scientific Group. (1968). *Screening for Inborn Errors of Metabolism*. WHO Tech. Rep. Ser., No. 401
15. Committee for the study of Inborn Errors of Metabolism. (1975). *Genetic Screening Programs, Principles and Research*. (Washington: National Academy of Sciences)
16. RATNER, G. (1976). The coming of the second genetic code: eugenic abortion in the United Kingdom. This volume, p 119
17. RAINE, D. N. (1974). The need for a national policy for the management of inherited metabolic disease. In Raine, D. N. (ed.), *Molecular Variants in Disease. J. Clin. Pathol.*, **27**, (Suppl.) (Roy. Coll. Path.) **8**
18. HUDSON, F. P. and MORDAUNT, V. L. (1968). Opinions of health visitors and mother on screening for phenylketonuria. *Med. Off.* **120**, 205
19. HOLTON, J. and TYFIELD, L. (1974) *The Child with Phenylketonuria*. (London: National Society for Mentally Handicapped Children)
20. STEELE, S. J. and GOODWIN, M. F. (1975). A pamphlet to answer patient's questions. *Lancet*, **ii**, 822
21. SCRIVER, C. R., CLOW, C. L. and LAMM, P. (1973). On the screening diagnosis and investigation of hereditary amino acidopathies. *Clin. Biochem.*, **6**, 142
22. MUNRO, T. A. (1947). Phenylketonuria: data on 47 British families. *Ann. Eugenics*, **14**, 60
23. FULLER, R. N. and SHUMAN, J. B. (1974). Genetic divergence in relatives of PKU's: low I.Q. correlation among normal siblings. *Dev. Psychobiol.*, **7**, 323
24. WILSON, J. M. G. and JUNGER, G. (1968). *Principles and Practice of Screening for Disease*. (Geneva: World Health Organization)
25. HOLLAND, W. W. (1974). Screening for disease: taking stock. *Lancet*, **ii**, 1494

7

Screening for Tay–Sachs Disease

P. R. Evans

Tay–Sachs disease is a rare but invariably fatal malady affecting babies. It is transmitted as an autosomal recessive condition and 'screening,' in the sense used here, involves finding the healthy carriers in order to give them a chance to avoid having children who will suffer the disease itself.

The pathological process involves accumulation of lipid in the central nervous system and the retina, producing the cerebromacular degeneration known as GM2 gangliosidosis. There are three clinical forms, the infantile which runs its course in 3 or 4 years, and the much more uncommon and slower late infantile and juvenile forms. The infantile form may be subdivided according to differences in the amounts of hexosaminidase isoenzymes, the most important being the A fraction. In the commonest form (infantile type I), which is the only one considered here, patients have almost no hexosaminidase A, while their parents' blood serum contains moderate amounts which are nevertheless smaller than those present in noncarriers. This is the basis for detection of heterozygotes in screening programmes for this disorder. The amounts are expressed in terms of the percentage activity of heat-labile hexosaminidase A in relation to total hexosaminidase activity. Figures differ in different laboratories, especially when different temperatures and times of heat-inactivation are used. Those of O'Brien[1] and Kaback and colleagues[2] are very similar but differ from those of Ellis and Masson[3] (Table 7.1).

Table 7.1   Hexosaminidase A as % of total hexosaminidase
(Ellis)

	Serum	*Leukocytes*
Control	67 ± 5	61 ± 5
Parents	45 ± 5	43 ± 6

A few equivocal results are obtained, and in such cases the estimations are repeated using leukocytes instead of serum. (Serum is generally preferred because of ease of handling, especially with automated apparatus.) Leukocytes are also used in women more than 4 months pregnant, and in patients with diabetes mellitus or debilitating disease, who may have misleadingly low values in serum. So may some women taking contraceptive pills.[2]

Those tested are told of the result, in writing, with a caveat, 'I am glad to tell you that you are not a carrier of the gene for Tay–Sachs disease, within the limits of accuracy of the test'. Carriers are encouraged to telephone for further discussion or for an appointment, but in our experience few do. The mere fact of knowing that you carry this gene does not appear to be hurtful or usually a matter for secrecy.[4] This is not the case in all genetic diseases.[5]

When a married couple both turn out to be heterozygotes, explanation and discussion must be undertaken promptly, but without hurry, and repeatedly. Husband and wife should, if possible, agree on their choice of doing without children, of adoption, or of monitored pregnancy with prenatal diagnosis and abortion if the fetus is affected.

Prenatal diagnosis involves obtaining 10–20 ml of amniotic fluid by abdominal puncture. This cannot be done until the uterus has risen out of the pelvis in the twelfth week, and in practice it is better deferred until the fourteenth or fifteenth when the volume of fluid is greater. It should not be done after the seventeenth week as cultured cells are required for reliable results and it may take up to 3 weeks for sufficient to grow for analysis. Abortion after the twentieth week is inadvisable particularly if the mother has already felt fetal movements, although amniocentesis for Tay–Sachs diagnosis has been done as late as the twenty-eighth week.[6]

Racial selection for screening

To screen all fertile women for Tay–Sachs heterozygosity would hardly be possible, but to screen a group which is particularly at risk is another matter. In 1887 Sachs noted that in New York the afflicted children were mostly Jewish and it has been found that the disease occurs particularly in the Ashkenazim, a group of Jews descended from those who fled to the north when Titus destroyed Jerusalem in AD 70. Many ended up in the Eastern European regions of Lithuania, Poland and

Russia. (Sheba[7] gives an exposition of Jewish groups). At the end of the nineteenth and the beginning of the twentieth century thousands emigrated to America, some dropping off in Western Europe, so that it is not surprising that Tay–Sachs disease was first described in London and, not long afterwards, in New York. More than half of the world's population of Ashkenazi Jews are in the USA and it has been calculated that the incidence of the disease is a hundred times as great in the Ashkenazim as in other Jews or other races.

It follows that the higher the proportion of Ashkenazi Jews in a population, the greater will be the number of patients with Tay–Sachs disease who are Jewish (Figure 7.1). Examples are given in Table 7.2,

Table 7.2　Proportion of Jews among Tay–Sachs patients

Britain	1974	*ca.* 33%
USA	1957	67%
New York City	1945	95%
Israel	1952	100%

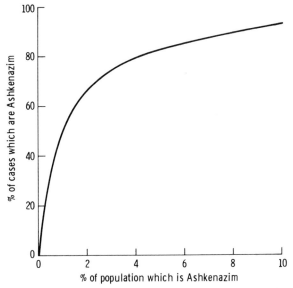

FIGURE 7.1　Theoretical curve relating the % of all cases of Tay–Sachs disease that are Ashkenazi Jews to the % of Ashkenazim in the total population. This assumes that the gene frequency in the population is stable and that the frequency is 1 in 30 for the Ashkenazim and 1 in 300 for non-Jews

which shows that in Britain Jewish patients form a minority, for Jews comprise only 0.7% of the whole population, whereas in the USA, where Jews form 3% of the population, Jewish patients exceed others. (In either country, the other major Jewish group, the Sephardim, form only a small proportion of the total.) There is no census of religious or racial groups in Britain but Table 7.3 shows the estimated population, of whom perhaps 70 000 might be taken to be of progenitive age.

Table 7.3   Jewish population in the United Kingdom[13]

London	280 000
Rest of UK	130 000
Total	410 000

A genetic approach to public health

Thus we have a fairly well defined group with a special risk of having children doomed to die miserably. We also have a chemical method of finding which married couples among them have a 1 in 4 chance of this happening, compared with a 1 in 3600 liability in the Ashkenazi group as a whole, or 1 in 360 000 in the rest of the world.

Dr Michael Kaback had the imagination to see this eugenic opportunity and the energy to organize it, as well as having other advantages—theatrical experience, training as an enzyme chemist and as a paediatrician. His medical school was Johns Hopkins and the neighbourhood of Baltimore and Washington contained nearly as many Jewish people as there were in the whole of Britain.

Kaback aimed at young married couples; he would not test children, or women who were already pregnant beyond the fourth month or pregnant women whose husbands had negative tests. He tried to reach people, after discussion with each rabbi, by engaging the active interest of the leaders of the sisterhoods of each community. They were able and influential in its social pursuits—in that neighbourhood it is customary for people to drop in at the community hall at the synagogue for coffee and conversation on Friday evenings. It was also to be the community leaders upon whom he would eventually rely to organize the actual sessions when specimens of blood were taken for testing, they were his 'volunteer task force'. Once they were fully au fait with his intentions, publicity was increased through dispersal of brochures and use of the press. These, with word of mouth communication in the community and 'public forums' were his chief means. Local television and radio, and encouragement of obstetricians and paediatricians were widely used but were less influential.

He spent 14 months in this way, and in perfecting his methods, with his staff which consisted of only one technician and a secretary, before holding his first bleeding session. It was amazingly successful. More than 1000 people turned up; he engaged students and interns, some paid and some not, some Jewish and some not, to take the 5 ml venous specimens. Logistically and chemically, arrangements were admirable. Within a year he had tested 6938 people and identified 315 carriers, among whom were 11 at-risk couples. Initially 5% of the serological tests were inconclusive. Four of the 280 inconclusives remained persistently in the inconclusive range after retesting, using leukocytes as well as serum; their parents also had inconclusive tests.

The costs were guaranteed by the Kennedy Foundation but people who attended were given an opportunity to contribute and many did so. The annual cost was considered to be less than the cost of maintaining two or possibly only one child with the disease, and on a national scale to be about one-eighth of maintaining such patients until they died.[2]

Dr Kaback has moved to California and his initial project has continued at a slower rate. The law of diminishing returns operates. A service is provided for those who want it and a few mass screening sessions are arranged. My last information was that there had been some 12 000 tests but there is an implication in the report of the Committee for the Study of Inborn Errors[8] that the figure may have reached 17 000, not perfect but a really considerable success in an at-risk population of 50 000–70 000. In July 1975, Kaback thought that the world total of tests might be 100 000.

Table 7.4 Number of Tay–Sachs screening programmes started[8]

1971	10
1972	17
1973	7

Kaback's original idea and his enthusiasm stimulated others, and he may be regarded as having promoted 34 Tay–Sachs programmes (Table 7.4), 30 in the USA, 2 in Canada, 1 in Britain and 1 (not yet in action) in South Africa. This is probably not the entire sum.

SCREENING IN CANADA AND ELSEWHERE

At the end of 1971, J. A. Lowden started one of the more successful Tay–Sachs screenings, in Toronto. Before the end of the first year 8000 tests had been done.[9] Methods leading on to complete automation were developed and the campaign was carried to other parts of Ontario and as far west as Calgary and Edmonton, yet by June 1975, the total tested has not reached 10 000. The programme in Toronto is 'in a semiquiescent stage.'[10]

Soon after Lowden's effort had been launched, Scriver integrated Tay–Sachs screening with the more general screening arranged by Le Reseau Provincial de Médecine Génétique (The Quebec Provincial Network of Genetic Medicine)[11]. Excluding those who were screened because there was known to be a Tay–Sachs connection in the family, from January 1972 to August 1975, 6791 were tested, and 1 in 26 were found to be carriers. The numbers coming up for tests have not declined annually, probably because recently high school boys and girls have been brought into the scheme.[12]

After a visit to Dr Kaback in December 1971, a screening programme was started in London, but despite brochures, the press, a radio talk and visits to synagogues, to universities, to social centres and even to a party organized at a private house, response was meagre. To give an example, we thought that 3000 had been adequately informed about the situation but only 19 turned up for testing. Altogether 341 individuals (excluding members of known 'Tay–Sachs families') were tested; 181 were male, 160 female; 16 were carriers but none of them were married to one another. About half of the total were unmarried and 20 were under 18 years old. About half were tested by analysis of leucocytes as well as serum. There were eventually no dubious or borderline cases.

There are probably several reasons for this apathy or rejection. One is that British people are not as health-conscious or as health-educated as Americans—even cervical screening for cancer does not go with a swing here; another is that only the Reform and Liberal congregations wanted testing and they constitute only about one-sixth of the Jewish population.[13] Orthodox congregations were not interested. The Chief Rabbi stated that 'No general ruling can be given on the termination of pregnancies in cases where the generation of a diseased child is suspected or established. All such cases would have to be submitted to individual Rabbinic decision.'[14] He was concerned lest the occurrence of the disease in Jews would lead to antisemitism, and he was not alone in this.

In South Africa, Dr Ronald van der Horst has been trying to start a screening programme and has been encouraged and discouraged so that in June 1975 'no screening programme has got off the ground'[15].

Prenatal diagnosis by amniocentesis is carried out in Isreal[6] but I am not at the moment aware of the situation regarding community screening.

GENE FREQUENCY OF TAY–SACHS DISEASE

The occurrence of the Tay–Sachs gene was calculated by Myrianthopoulos[16] to be 1 in 40 in Jews and 1 in 308 in non-Jews, although the figures more often used[1] are 1 in 30 and 1 in 300. Actual measurement of hexosaminidase A has provided different figures. In Baltimore and Washington[2] the overall incidence of the gene for hexosaminidase A deficiency in Jews was 1 in 23.7 and we have found an almost identical incidence in the small numbers tested in London. There were, however, large differences in incidence in Kaback's different samples. His first session showed an incidence of 1 in 30.8 in 1228 subjects; on another occasion it was 1 in 16.5 in 479 subjects. Such differences may have been due to a tendency for members of families to settle in neighbourhood to one another. Lowden[10] found a carrier frequency as high as 1 in 14 in Toronto, but the areas from which the subjects or their parents came were south-west Poland and eastern Germany, instead of north-eastern Poland and the adjacent parts of Russia which appeared to be the source of Tay–Sachs disease occurring in the USA.[17] But in other Canadian cities Lowden found the incidence to be much less than in Toronto, varying from 1 in 26 to 1 in 46. He comments on the tendency in metropolitan Toronto to, as he puts it, 'immigrate in extended families.'

RESPONSE TO SCREENING PROJECTS

The number of people coming forward for screening has varied greatly. One relevant factor has been the personality of investigators;

another their aims, for example are they anxious to include unmarried students, or children, or to limit testing to married people of fecund age. On the other hand, the groups being approached also vary, for they may be closely linked Ashkenazi communities or families living in an integrated society regardless of religious grouping.

Kaback and colleagues [18] and Beck and colleagues[19] have investigated samples in Baltimore and in Montreal. Compliance in Montreal was almost 10% .The Baltimore figure is incalculable as the size of the relevant population is unknown but over a similar period acceptance was probably nearer 20%. In both groups there was a markedly raised incidence of people with higher education. Women outnumbered men in North America (but not in London); women were more likely to have heard of the programme, and as Kaback suggests, may have been more preoccupied with having children and less afraid of blood tests. Previous knowledge of Tay–Sachs disease promoted the demand for testing; the physician was felt to be the preferred informant but was in practice much less influential than pamphlets, newspapers, publicity within the community or word of mouth from a friend. Childs[4] found physicians and their nurses often ignorant about Tay–Sachs disease; of 635 persons who had come for testing, more than 99% had completed high school; 94% had a college degree; 23% had postgraduate degrees; 50% earned more than $50 000 a year. Information provided before screening was not long remembered but carriers recalled more than their non-carrier husbands or wives.

Not surprisingly, most volunteers intended to have children and did not disapprove of abortion. Kaback and colleagues[18] found no correlation with sectarianism, degree of religiosity or overconcern about health.

The pay-off

Interesting and imaginative although the search for Tay–Sachs carriers has been, it is difficult to know how much practical good it has done. 'In Kaback's experience, of 17 000 people screened, 17 couples were found to be at risk. Of these, eight have had pregnancies and one affected fetus has so far been discovered and aborted.[8] The yield is meagre. In London the screening project was a failure but 19 mothers who had previously had babies with Tay–Sachs disease were examined by amniocentesis; four fetuses were found to be affected and were aborted.[20] In

Britain family investigation seems a better bargain than screening, but it does mean letting the first horse escape before shutting the stable door.

REFERENCES

1. O'BRIEN, J. S., OKADA, S., HO, M. W., FILLERUP, D. L., VEATH, M. L. and ADAMS, K. (1971). Ganglioside storage diseases. In J. Bernsohn and H. J. Grossman (eds.), *Lipid Storage Diseases*, p. 225. (New York and London: Academic Press)
2. KABACK, M. M., ZEIGLER, K. J., REYNOLDS, L. W. and SONNEBORN, M. (1974) In A. G. Steinberg and A. G. Bearn (eds,), *Progress in Medical Genetics*, Vol. 10, p. 103. (New York: Grune and Stratton).
3. EVANS, P. R., ELLIS, R. B. and MASSON, P. K. (1973). Testing for Tay–Sachs heterozygotes. *Lancet*, ii, 1143
4. CHILDS, B. (1975). Personal communication
5. LEONARD, C., CHASE, G. and CHILDS, B. (1974). Who shall live? *Johns Hopkins Magazine*, May 23, 16
6. NAVON, R. and PADEH, B. (1971). Prenatal diagnosis of Tay-Sachs genotypes. *Br. Med. J.*, 4, 17
7. SHEBA, C., (1970). Gene frequencies in Jews. *Lancet*, i, 1230
8. Committee for the Study of Inborn Errors of Metabolism (1975). *Genetic Screening Programs. Principles and Research*, pp. 388 ff. (Washington, DC: National Academy of Science)
9. LOWDEN, J. A., SKOMOROWSKI, M. A., HENDERSON, F. J. and KABACK, M. (1973). Automated assay of hexosaminidases in serum. *Clin. Chem.*, 19, 1345
10. LOWDEN, J. A. (1975). Personal communication
11. CLOW, C. L., FRAZER, F. C., LABERGE, C. and SCRIVER, C. R. (1973). In A. G. Steinberg, and A. G. Bearn, (eds.), *Progress in Medical Genetics*, vol. 9, p. 159. (New York: Grune and Stratton)
12. CLOW, C. L. and SCRIVER, C. R. (1975). Personal communication
13. PRAIS, S. J. and SCHMOOL, M. (1968). The size and structure of the Anglo-Jewish population, 1960-65. *Jew. J. Sociol.* 10, 5
14. EVANS, P. R. and ELLIS, R. B. (1974). Screening for Tay-Sachs disease. *Lancet*, i, 575
15. VAN DER HORST, R. L. Personal communications
16. MYRIANTHOPOULOS, N. C. (1962). Some epedemiolic and genetic aspects of Tay-Sachs disease. In: S. M. Aronson and B. W. Volk (eds.) *Cerebral Sphingolipidoses*. p. 359. (New York: Academic Press)
17. MEALS, R. A. (1971). Paradoxical frequencies of recessive disorders in Ashkenazi Jews. *J. Chronic Dis.*, 23, 547
18. KABACK, M. M., BECKER, M. H., RUTH, M. (1974). Compliance factors in a voluntary screening health program. In D. Bergsma, (ed.), *Ethical, Social and Legal Dimensions of Screening for Genetic Disease, Nat. Fed. Birth Defects*, 10, 145
19. BECK, E., BLAICMAN, S., SCRIVER, C. R. and CLOW, C. L. (1974). Advocacy and compliance in genetic screening. *N. Engl. J. Med.*, 291, 1166
20. STEPHENS, R. Personal communications

8

Genetic counselling clinics

Valerie A. Cowie

The medical profession has slowly, over decades, come to recognize the necessity to make available informed genetic counselling. Strong demands are now coming from another source, from the general public. These demands, from the potential consumer, have been stimulated by education mainly through the mass media. There is a fast-growing awareness that levels of risk can be given for a number of deleterious conditions, and that some of these conditions can be detected before birth. In the United Kingdom the facilities for expert genetic counselling fall far short of the demand. It is to be hoped that this will be rectified by the inclusion of medical genetics as an integral part of undergraduate and postgraduate medical training, and by the extensive development of genetic counselling clinics in conjunction with the laboratory back-up services that can be provided by hospitals and universities. Up to now, genetic counselling services in this country have been developed mainly through the efforts of individuals with a special interest in medical genetics. Consequently, these services have grown up in a regrettably haphazard way, and do not give adequate national coverage. Many are threatened by extinction when their present incumbents retire or move away, through lack of successors sufficiently interested or equipped to take their place. This problem will be discussed in the light of experience of the organization of genetic counselling in other countries. Before this, however, it will be helpful to consider some general principles.

The obligations of the genetic counsellor

The role of the genetic counsellor has always been open to question. Today, however, when matters of civil liberties and human rights loom very large, he is more prone than ever to self-conscious appraisal of his work. Furthermore, prenatal detection of genetic conditions has brought him a host of new ethical problems.

Taking first the advice to families into which affected children have already been born, there is a broad spectrum of opinion amongst medical geneticists as to the nature and limits of their obligations. Fraser Roberts[1] states simply that it is no part of the task to tell people whether they should have children or not. He considers the duty of the genetic counselling clinic is to provide estimates of risk in terms of odds, after which it is up to the couple to make up their own minds in the light of this information. His approach is essentially pragmatic, and he even gives a yardstick of good and bad risks by which to measure the estimated risk. He judges bad risks to be those which are worse than 1 in 10, good risks are those better than 1 in 20. Carter[2] considers estimates of recurrence fall into three broad groups: those in which the recurrence risk is little more than the random risk for the outcome of any pregnancy; those in which there is a high risk of recurrence, for example at least 1 in 10, and those in which there is only a moderate risk of recurrence, of about less than 1 in 10. Implicit in his discussion of his collaborative work with Fraser Roberts is the straightforwardness with which the genetic risk was presented to the parents, who were then left to make their own decision. Carter states their findings showed that 'genetic predictions are on the whole reliable, and that parents do on the whole take sensible decisions on the basis of the advice given them'.

These are good guidelines as far as they go, but now that genetic counselling is becoming a more complicated procedure, especially through the development of microbiological and biochemical techniques and with the advent of prenatal diagnosis of genetic disorders, new thought is being given to wider ethical issues. In an international conference on 'ethical issues in genetic counselling and the use of genetic knowledge'[3] the opening address by Sonneborn was focused upon value judgements and the criteria were examined for deciding what is right or good. This bears on the vexed question of eugenic practices. Certain abuses in the name of eugenics undoubtedly created a wary attitude to the practical application of medical genetics. Even today this influence is felt to some extent. Professor Scharfetter in Zurich, speaking mainly from the standpoint of psychiatric genetics, states: 'Genetic counselling is not a generally accepted professional action here—maybe partly because of the terrible "eugenic" acts by the Nazi Germans, which are by far not forgotten today and which arise in people's minds at any time'.[4] Penrose considered that the best antidote to pernicious ideas based upon emotional bias lay in spreading knowledge about established facts.[5] Great advances have been made in medical genetics since Penrose made that pronouncement, and genetic advice now has a more solid scientific basis. The orientation now is certainly not towards altering the gene pool in the population, but it is towards helping the patient and his family.

This is expressed well by Motulsky[6] who points out that most genetic counsellors consider their work to be little different from any other medical practice; they put the interests of the patient and his family before the interests of society and the state, and pursue medical, not eugenic, objectives. Although untoward effects on society may be pointed out, most counsellors do not attempt to give advice based on considerations of the gene pool. Therefore, Motulsky goes on to say, 'genetic counselling has traditionally been non-directive.' Moreover it is usually maintained that every family situation is different, and that the meaning of a given risk varies from family to family, so that in some cases even high recurrence risks may justify a future pregnancy. Motulsky comments that some critics have suggested that families expect more definite advice than is often provided, saying that because a genetic counsellor understands the total impact of the disease and the real meaning of risks better than does the family, he should advise what he thinks would be the best course of action.

This view runs counter to the more generally accepted notion of the obligations of those giving genetic advice. This is summed up by Hall (quoted by Callahan)[3] who notes that the traditional role of the counsellor has been that of the 'neutral educator', essentially doing no more than presenting patients with the odds and the facts. This concept, however, as Callahan indicates, faces increasingly heavy weather, particularly because of the rapidly increasing range of options.

Edwards[7] emphasizes the ease with which the neutral educator may take up the stance of an instructor. In a leading article in the *British Medical Journal*[8] it had been said that parents make sensible use of information on the chances of a particular genetic (or part-genetic) disorder in the family recurring in future children. Edwards points out that this means they respond to information in the way the donor of this information thinks they should; in practice *information* easily becomes degraded into *advice*.

Although the concensus of opinion appears to be in favour of the neutral educator in genetic counselling, as in all medical practice the circumstances of individual cases override generalities. Woolf[9] is of the opinion that it is extremely difficult to avoid swaying the decision of a family with whom one feels empathy while making sure they understand the courses open to them, particularly since genetic counselling is usually sought at moments of great stress. The genetic counsellor must understand himself at least as well as he understands the problems of the families with which he deals. Woolf felt at one time that for this reason the best genetic counsellor would be someone with psychiatric training, but on the whole psychiatrists are not interested in genetics.

My own experience has been in psychiatric genetics, where the enquirer is usually self-selected and has sought or even pressed for expert genetic advice; enquirers seem to be relatively rarely referred spontaneously by their medical advisors. Many such enquirers have already consulted the literature about the condition in question and have a good idea of the genetic risk involved; they come seeking mainly support or guidance, having reached their own decisions. This pre-empts to a large extent the approach of the neutral educator. In many cases the advice rests not so much on genetic risk as on the mental state of the enquirer, who may still be suffering from the effects of a psychiatric disorder, and his or her capacity as a future parent is the central problem. The adviser in such cases must be more than a neutral educator in the strictest sense. Exclusive adherence to the role of neutral educator would preclude the flexibility of approach that is essential in psychiatric genetics, and undoubtedly also in all other branches of medical genetics. Deviation from the role of neutral educator does not by any means imply that the counsellor becomes a dictatorial donor of his own brand of advice. On the contrary, it gives latitude for all the salient aspects of the individual case to be taken into consideration, in the true tradition of good medical practice.

Psychological considerations

Psychological considerations are of great importance in genetic counselling. Not only do they influence the way in which the information is imparted, but also the type and extent of the information that should be given may rest heavily on the psychological needs of the enquirers. For example, in a limited survey quoted by Fraser[10] about half the potential carriers of the Huntington's chorea gene thought they would like to know their carrier state, and half would not. Fraser stresses that much more information is needed on the psychological effects of finding out that one carries a deleterious gene. Motulsky[6] also gives Huntington's chorea as an example, and questions whether or not most persons would want to know many years before symptoms develop that they will die prematurely of an incurable genetic disease. Two years ago a young man came to me for genetic advice because his father had Huntington's chorea. I answered his questions concerning his own chances of developing the disease and the likelihood of its being transmitted to any children he might have. He already knew the answers, having read books on the subject. Recently he returned to the clinic with a severe anxiety state, showing a tremor which he was convinced was a sign he had developed Huntington's chorea. He is now having intensive psychiatric treatment for his anxiety state. I agree with Motulsky that a serious question is posed as to what advice should be given in such cases. On the other hand many enquirers, such as my own enquirer, come already equipped with full information. A judicious psychotherapeutic approach, tailored to the needs of the particular case, seems possibly the only answer.

Little has been written about the psychodynamics of genetic counselling. Shock, denial, guilt and anger may be obstacles to the acceptance, or even to the comprehension, of genetic advice.[10] Genetic information given at the time of diagnosis or shortly after may not be retained because of emotional shock.[11] Careful distinction should be made here between the disclosure of the diagnosis of a deleterious condition when this can be made in the neonatal period or early infancy, and genetic advice. It has been well established in a number of studies, mainly in connection with mongolism, that most parents appreciate information about the diagnosis of their baby's condition as early as possible.[12-14] In connection with genetic advice in phenylketonuria, McBean[15] was interested to see how little parents had understood at the time what was thought to have been an adequate and full explanation. As regards timing, Emery[16] underlines the point that it is wrong to give genetic counselling when the diagnosis of a serious genetic disorder is first made, as parents are often upset and confused. The first step is to remove the parents' feelings of guilt and self-recrimination which often accompany the realization that a child has a genetic disorder, before proceeding to explain the nature of the disease, its prognosis, the possibility of treatment and in simple terms what is meant by *genetic* and the risks of recurrence. In Emery's experience through follow-up studies, genetic counselling in many cases is best given, or at least reinforced, in the home environment. Here the family doctor plays an important role in reinforcing advice given by the geneticist and probably enabling the parents to understand it better.

An important psychological effect of genetical counselling is the possible influence it may have on the social as well as the sexual life of the enquirers.[16] This may be profound. Fraser Roberts[1] remarks on the sense of loneliness in the parents of children with genetic disorders, who feel different from their relatives and friends who have numbers of perfectly normal children. Therefore as well as being able to impart correct information the genetic counsellor should be equipped to recognize and to take into account the possible difficulties that may lie ahead in individual cases. For this reason a psychiatric training is useful for the counsellor, but general clinical acuity in assessing the possibility of emotional hazards is essential.

Genetic counselling problems associated with prenatal diagnosis

Most of the experience that has been gained regarding genetic counselling problems with prenatal diagnosis has been in connection with chromosomal disorders. This is because of the greater scope for determining chromosome abnormalities in the fetus with a high degree of certainty than for determining inborn errors of metabolism. However, the same general principles apply, whatever the nature of the condition that can be diagnosed *in utero*.

Total population screening programmes for prenatal diagnosis are not feasible for obvious reasons: mainly because the technical facilities available would fall far short of the needs, but also because prenatal diagnosis is not acceptable to many prospective parents. Also, it is doubtful whether such screening programmes would have a significant impact on the epidemiology of deleterious conditions that can be detected before birth, although optimism has been expressed. Carter[17] feels it is perhaps not unreasonable to anticipate screening of all mothers over 35 who wish for it within the next 10 years, with a gradual extension to younger age groups, ultimately leading to the prevention of the large majority of births of Down's Syndrome. Griffith[18] believes that in theory at least this condition could be completely eliminated if every pregnant woman had an amniocentesis, but goes on to point out the obstacles, and draws attention to the recommendations of a group of advisers to the Department of Health and Social Security who saw no need for a general screening programme aimed at testing all pregnant women above a specified age, but recommended rather the provision of a service to keep pace with increasing demand.

As regards inborn errors of metabolism, general screening programmes are at present even less feasible owing to the technical difficulties of prenatal diagnosis and the variety of conditions in question, each calling for specialized assay. Therefore, perforce, attempts to diagnose conditions in this category in the fetus are limited and are called for only when a technique is available for diagnosis of a particular disease, and only when there is reason to suppose a mother is at risk for producing an affected child. Polani and Benson[19], however, hold out some hope for population or subpopulation screening which may become possible if in the future simpler, indirect and chemical diagnostic procedures, perhaps safer and less expensive than amniocentesis, were developed. A development in this direction is the attempt to estimate maternal serum alpha-fetoprotein levels, for the prenatal detection of neural tube defects, although the reliability of this method is still open to question.[20] Despite the fact that it is unlikely for prenatal diagnosis to be used for large-scale screening in the foreseeable future, there is nevertheless a growing public demand for it in individual cases, and this is closely linked with genetic counselling.

The value of investigating the level of alpha-fetoprotein in the amniotic fluid of pregnant women who have already produced a child with a neural tube defect has been demonstrated and is now well established. For example, out of a series of 41 such women tested in this way four had their pregnancies interrupted on these grounds, and in each case the fetus had a severe neural tube defect.[20] These workers point out that the predictive efficiency of alpha-fetoprotein in neural tube defects in pregnancy would be greatly enhanced if a critically elevated serum level could be detected; many more women could be tested, and amniocentesis, with its attendant slight risks, would not be necessary. If a satisfactory test could be established using serum, routine screening in all pregnancies could be envisaged, and in theory at least there would be the hope that the number of children born with neural tube defects would be drastically cut, although there would always be some parents who refuse termination of pregnancy.

Many parents have a strong aversion to the procedure of amniocentesis itself, the possible implication of abortion, or to both. In genetic counselling it is wise to ascertain judiciously whether or not the prospective parents have such an aversion before proposing the possibility of amniocentesis. It should be explained that the procedure is not without some risk. The degree of risk is difficult to assess with exactitude. Polani[21] thinks it is small, and would place it at between 1 in 300 and 1 in 100 amniocenteses in early pregnancy, at around 16 weeks. Polani indicates that the risk is abortion, and the difficulty in knowing what happens is that there is an appreciable risk of abortion in *any* pregnancy from the age of 16 to 28 weeks. Thus, the assessment of the increased risk from amniocentesis is difficult; large numbers are needed for an assessment to be made.

The techniques and hazards of amniocentesis have been well reviewed by many writers.[22-25] Trauma to the umbilical cord, premature labour, haemorrhage and infections are possible complications, but harm to the fetus is more a theoretical than practical hazard,[26] and Scrimgeour[27] reports that no evidence of direct trauma to the fetus has been recorded.

The risk, then, in the procedure of amniocentesis is small. Even so, in genetic counselling it is clear that the pregnant mothers who request prenatal diagnosis invariably state that a high risk of miscarriage would be preferable to a low risk of fetal abnormality, a view which is not always appreciated by the obstetrician.[28]

The comfort and reassurance brought by amniocentesis to anxious pregnant women at risk is often overshadowed by the unjustifiably gloomy view that the results are likely to reveal an abnormality in the fetus, and that the procedure is therefore an almost inevitable forerunner of abortion. Experience shows, however, that in the majority of cases no abnormality is detectable in the fetal cells, in series of amniocenteses carried out on mothers at risk for bearing a mongol child.[29,30] With inborn errors of metabolism, most of which are transmitted by an autosomal recessive gene, the proportion of affected fetuses is likely to be much higher, but even so, in theory about three-quarters of the mothers within this category of risk are likely to be found to have unaffected fetuses, and the relief that can be given by this news should not be undervalued.

It is not infrequent that the doctor rather than the patient has qualms about the recommendation of amniocentesis. In genetic counselling it has been my experience that the obstetrician may be the most hesitant.

The medical geneticist and those, such as paediatricians, who are more closely involved with families with severely affected children with genetic defects and who are aware of the often disastrous long-term consequences are more likely to appreciate the value of prenatal diagnosis by this method.

Ferguson-Smith[28] considers the economics of prenatal diagnosis. Leaving aside humane considerations, the cost of providing a comprehensive diagnostic service for pregnancies most at risk is small compared with that involved in the care and management of those at present born with incurable disabilities detectable in early pregnancy; such a service is most economically provided in conjunction with facilities for genetic counselling. The need for a multidisciplinary approach in prenatal diagnosis and genetic counselling is further underlined by Scrimgeour:[31] the primary objective should be that each couple plan to have children in relation to their career and financial prospects and that the children should be as normal as the genetic and physical environment permit. To achieve this objective, the patient at risk should be identified, and medical, surgical and technological expertise should be available.

Facilities for genetic counselling

Emery[16] notes the development of genetic counselling over the past 15 years or so, saying that until the early 1960s little was done and few people appreciated its value or even its need, but now almost every medical school and teaching hospital supports a genetic counselling unit. This, however, is barely reflected in the list of genetic advisory centres in the United Kingdom entitled *Human Genetics* and published by the Department of Health and Social Security.[32] This lists only 35 clinics (Figure 8.1), some of which are specialist clinics dealing only with such conditions as psychiatric, ophthalmological and dermatological disorders.

Although the need and the demand for genetic counselling are obviously linked, they are fundamentally separate issues, and whilst the need is presumably constant, the demand is growing. The proportion of people in the population who might profit from genetic advice is by no means negligible, and it has been estimated that in all countries probably not less than 4% of liveborn individuals suffer from some genetic or partly genetic condition and might benefit from genetic counselling.[33]

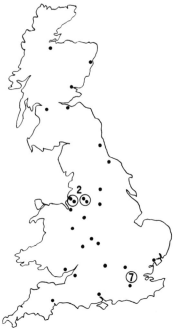

FIGURE 8.1   The distribution of genetic counselling clinics in the United Kingdom
(one clinic in Belfast not shown on map)

As regards public demand for genetic counselling, this is growing
rapidly. Instruction through the mass media has done much to increase
awareness of the genetic aspects of disease and to raise the level of
sophistication in knowledge of special techniques available for investigation. The demand for genetic counselling is hard to quantify and is
governed by a number of variables including the awareness of an
hereditary element in the causation of a condition and the degree of
dread. Spina bifida is an example of a condition in which the general
public has received considerable information recently through the
mass media. There is a growing awareness of its hereditary implications
and the techniques for prenatal diagnosis. In a current study,[34] out of
39 pairs of parents of affected children, 12 pairs recollected having been
given genetic advice without requesting it, and 13 pairs said they had
asked for genetic advice because it had not been forthcoming. The
majority of parents interviewed had now learned through recent television programmes about the prenatal diagnosis of spina bifida. Sly[35]
stresses that increasing public awareness will soon force us to deal not

only with needs for genetic counselling at present unmet, but also to devise ways to handle many new needs created by scientific advances in medical genetics.

Genetic counselling in countries other than Britain

The resources for genetic counselling vary greatly not only from country to country but often from region to region within the same country. Therefore it would be unrealistic to attempt an overall evaluation. It is clear, however, that there are wide international differences in the facilities available.

Denmark is outstanding in the excellence of its genetic counselling services. The demand for genetic advice was intensified at the end of the 1930s, as Danish legislation made abortion and sterilization possible in cases of increased risk to the offspring. Genetic counselling services were organized in Denmark in 1938 when the University Institute of Human Genetics was founded in Copenhagen, attached to the Faculty of Medicine. This Institute was one of the first of its kind in the world. It had three closely linked activities: research, counselling and the teaching of medical students and doctors. Great stress was laid on the necessity for genetic advice to be based on the results of careful research. Advantage was taken of the fact that Denmark was especially suitable for genetic research as the population was stable and homogeneous, the medical services were highly developed and effective public registration systems facilitated family studies. The role of genetic counselling in preventive medicine was also strongly emphasized, with the implication that genetic knowledge is indispensable to any doctor. In Denmark, full cognisance is taken of the increasing need for collaboration between centres of medical genetics and the sharing of expertise and facilities to maintain a counselling service of the highest level of excellence.[36]

The necessity for a close link between the practice of medical genetics, research and teaching is also well recognized in Israel. There, an active genetic counselling service is based on at least four centres. In one of these (Tel Aviv) counselling is carried out by a team consisting of physicians in paediatrics, obstetrics and gynaecology, internal medicine and medical genetics, two geneticists with Doctorates of Philosophy, and one social worker. The need for postgraduate teaching is recognized, to increase the awareness of doctors generally of the role of genetics in medicine, and university-based courses are planned.[37]

In Poland, genetic counselling was first organized in 1963 at the Psychoneurological Institute in Warsaw. Later, at least four other genetic counselling centres were developed, mainly attached to university departments. Services are now rapidly expanding since, in December 1974, the Commission of Human Genetics of the Section of Medical Sciences of the Polish Academy of Sciences recommended a programme of development of genetic units with counselling facilities in the 10 medical schools in Poland.[38]

These are three countries in which the necessity for comprehensive services in medical genetics has been fully envisaged and genetic counselling, teaching and research are closely integrated. Surprisingly, in some other countries notable for their excellence in genetic research, far less provision appears to have been made for genetic counselling on an organized service basis. Switzerland is an example that has already been quoted. Professor Åkesson[39] writes as regards genetic counselling: 'It is almost correct to say that in Sweden services are non-existent'. Genetic counselling is carried out on an *ad hoc* basis at the five Swedish universities by a couple of people at each who did it out of interest. The need for more services for genetic counselling are great; medical geneticists are very rare in Sweden. One exception is the service in Gothenburg for prenatal diagnosis; there, over 600 amniocenteses have been carried out in the past few years.

It is difficult to get an overall picture of genetic counselling services in the USA. About 200 centres are listed in a directory of genetic services published by the National Foundation,[49] including many in the USA. It would seem that there, in comparison with other countries, more genetic counselling is done by non-medical counsellors than by physicians, and the recommendation has been put forward in the USA for fostering the training of non-physicians as genetic associates, but not as independent genetic counsellors.[41] This suggestion carries with it the advantage of increasing the number of personnel in a service where trained workers are universally in short supply.

From the examination of genetic counselling in different countries emerges prominently the necessity of close integration of genetic advisory services with teaching (undergraduate and postgraduate) and with research. This requires planning and foresight, and much can be learned from Denmark as an example of excellence in what can be achieved. This kind of integration has special implication for the genetic management of inborn errors of metabolism, and Raine[42] has shown exceptional vision in setting out the need for a national policy for the management of inherited metabolic disease.

Genetic counselling and inborn errors of metabolism

It has been said that unmet needs in genetic counselling stem more from lack of perceived benefit than from the lack of counselling facilities or personnel.[35] The point has been stressed many times that the effectiveness of genetic counselling is a function of the extent to which the enquirer comprehends it.[11] Emotional barriers to comprehension have already been touched upon, but Leonard and his colleagues[11] place more importance on the lack of grasp of *probability* which can be attributed to a number of factors, including intelligence, education and special experience.

In addition, with inborn errors of metabolism a special obstacle may be the difficulty of grasping that anything is wrong with, for example a phenylketonuric baby, who looks perfectly normal; or that a phenylketonuric mother who was treated herself in her earlier years but who now considers herself normal is, in fact, suffering from a genetic disease and may damage her infant *in utero* unless she herself resumes treatment. An excellent account of the severe clinical effects on the infant associated with maternal phenylketonuria is given by Fisch and Anderson.[43] They give an account of their own clinical observations and tabulate the collated findings of others. They point out that children born of mothers with 'classical' phenylketonuria show intrauterine growth retardation, postnatal growth retardation, microcephaly, mental retardation and severe and varied congenital malformations; early spontaneous abortion also appears more frequent than in non-phenylketonuric pregnancies. There may be a number of mothers, or potential mothers, who are untreated phenylketonurics. One such mother was discovered in a survey based on our own hospital to investigate genetic prognosis in mental handicap.[44] This mother, discovered to be phenylketonuric, had given birth to seven mentally handicapped children all with microcephaly, retardation in growth, abnormal facies, skeletal and ear abnormalities. Two had Fallot's tetralogy; one of these had infantile spasms. Four had EEG abnormalities. The mother herself was backward, with an IQ possibly in the range 65 – 80. Possibly on account of this she was reluctant to give relevant information about her family and was unwilling to cooperate in investigations.[45] This is an example of the special kind of difficulty than may be encountered in genetic counselling in inborn errors of metabolism. It was only by dint of close teamwork between clinicians, biochemists, electrophysiologists, neuropathologists and social workers that the family just quoted was discovered, investigated and given counselling. With inborn errors of metabolism, possibly more than with any other single category of disease, genetic counselling requires the groundwork of close collaboration and recourse to the appropriate sources of special expertise.

It is likely that our present view of conditions that may be regarded as inborn errors of metabolism is restricted by the limitations of our technical abilities. The constancy with which mental subnormality is concomitant with inborn errors of metabolism suggests a causal link, and it is possible that a much wider range of conditions with mental impairment than that at present recognized will be found to be enzymopathies. In turn this will demand more and better facilities to meet increasing needs for genetic counselling. Again, we could learn much from the Danish model, in which research, teaching and genetic counselling exist as a triad.

REFERENCES

1. ROBERTS, J. A. FRASER (1963). *Genetic Counselling and Genetic Clinics*. Reproduced for private circulation for the 44th South African Medical Congress, Johannesburg, 1963, by courtesy of Mer-National Laboratories (Pty) Limited
2. CARTER, C. O. (1971). Genetic counselling. In J. M. Berg (ed.), *Genetic Counselling in Relation to Mental Retardation*. (Oxford: Pergamon Press for the Institute for Research into Mental Retardation)
3. CALLAHAN, D. (1972). Ethics, law and genetic counselling. *Science*, **176**, 197
4. SCHARFETTER, C. (1975). Personal communication
5. PENROSE, L. S. (1946). Phenylketonuria: a problem in eugenics. *Lancet*, **i**, 949
6. MOTULSKY, A. G. (1974). Brave new world? *Science*, **185**, 653
7. EDWARDS, J. H. (1972). Genetic counselling. *Br. Med. J.*, **2**, 229
8. ANONYMOUS. (1972). Genetic counselling. *Br. Med. J.*, **1**, 458
9. WOOLF, L. I. (1975). Personal communication
10. FRASER. F. C. (1974). Genetic counseling. *Am. J. Hum. Genet.*, **26**, 636
11. LEONARD, C. O., CHASE, G. A. and CHILDS, B. (1972). Genetic counseling: a consumer's view. *N. Engl. J. Med.*, **287**, 433
12. DRILLIEN, C. M. and WILKINSON, E. M. (1964). Mongolism: when should parents be told? *Br. Med. J.*, 2, 1306
13. COWIE, V. (1966). Genetic counselling. *Proc. R. Soc. Med.*, **59**, 149
14. STONE, D. H. (1973). The birth of a child with Down's syndrome: a medico-social study of thirty one children and their families. *Scot. Med. J.*, **18**, 182
15. McBEAN, M. S. (1971). The problems of parents of children with phenylketonuria. In H. Bickel, F. P. Hudson and L. I. Woolf (eds.), *Phenylketonuria and Some Other Inborn Errors of Amino Acid Metabolism*. (Stuttgart: Georg Thieme Verlag)
16. EMERY, A. E. H. (1975). Genetic counselling. *Br. Med. J.*, **3**, 219
17. CARTER, C. O. (1974). Public health aspects of prenatal diagnosis. *Proc. R. Soc. Med.*, **67**, 1257
18. GRIFFITH, G. WYNNE (1973). The 'prevention' of Down's syndrome (mongolism). *Health Trends*, **5**, 59

19. POLANI P. E. and BENSON, P. F. (1973). Prenatal diagnosis. *Guy's Hosp. Rep.*, **122**, 65

20. SELLER, S. J., SINGER, J. D., COLTART, T. M. and CAMPBELL, S. (1974). Maternal serum alpha-fetoprotein levels and prenatal diagnosis of neural-tube defects. *Lancet*, **i**, 428

21. POLANI, P. E. (1975). Personal communication

22. BURNETT, R. G. and ANDERSON, W. R. (1958). The hazards of amniocentesis. *J. Iowa Med. Soc.*, **58**, 130

23. FREDA, V. J. (1965). The Rh problem in obstetrics and a new concept of its management using amniocentesis and spectrophotometric scanning of amniotic fluid. *Am. J. Obstet. Gynecol.*, **92**, 341

24. QUEENAN, J. T. (1966). Amniocentesis and transamniotic fetal transfusion for Rh disease. *Clin. Obstet. Gynecol.*, **9**, 491

25. NADLER, H. L. (1969). Prenatal detection of genetic defects. *J. Pediatr.*, **74**, 132

26. GORDON, H. (1969). Amniocentesis. *Br. J. Hosp. Med.*, **2**, 2000

27. SCRIMGEOUR, J. B. (1971). The diagnostic use of amniocentesis: technique and complications. *Proc. R. Soc. Med.*, **64**, 1135

28. FERGUSON-SMITH, M. A. (1974). Prenatal diagnosis of chromosome anomalies. *Proc. R. Soc. Med.*, **67**, 1256

29. FERGUSON-SMITH, M. E., FERGUSON-SMITH, M. A., NEVIN, N. C. and STONE, M. (1971). Chromosome analysis before birth and its value in genetic counselling. *Br. Med. J.*, **4**, 69

30. PHILIP, J., BANG, J., HAHNEMANN, N., MIKKELSEN, M., NIEBUHR, E., REBBE, H. and WEBER, J. (1974). Chromosome analysis of fetuses in risk pregnancies. *Acta Obstet. Gynecol. Scand.*, **53**, 9

31. SCRIMGEOUR, J. B. (1974). Antenatal interference. *Br. Med. J.*, **3**, 237

32. Standing Medical Advisory Committee. (1972). *Human Genetics*. Department of Health and Social Security

33. World Health Organization. (1969). *Genetic Counselling*. Third Report of the WHO Expert Committee on Human Genetics. (*Geneva: WHO Tech. Rep. Ser.* No. 416)

34. ECKSTEIN, H., COWIE, V. and COLLISS, V. (1975). Unpublished observations

35. SLY, W. S. (1973). What is genetic counseling? In: *Contemporary Genetic Counseling. Birth Defects Original Article Series.* **9**, 5. (New York: National Foundation —March of Dimes)

36. HAUGE, M. (1975). Personal communication

37. GOODMAN, R. M. (1975). Personal communication

38. WALD, I. (1975). Personal communication

39. ÅKESSON, H. O. (1975). Personal communication

40. International Directory. Third edition (1971). Birth Defects Genetic Services. (New York: The National Foundation—March of Dimes)

41. EPSTEIN, C. J. (1973). Who should do genetic counselling and under what circumstances? In: *Contemporary Genetic Counselling. Birth Defects Original Article Series*, **9**, (4) 39. (New York: The National Foundation—March of Dimes)

42. RAINE, D. N. (1974). The need for a national policy for the management of inherited metabolic disease. In: *Molecular Variants in Disease*. Symposium organized by the Royal College of Pathologists, February 1974. Published for the Royal College of Pathologists by the *Journal of Clinical Pathology*, London

43. FISCH, R. O. and ANDERSON, J. A. (1971). Maternal phenylketonuria. In H. Bickel, F. P. Hudson and L. I. Woolf (eds.), *Phenylketonuria and Some Other Inborn Errors of Amino Acid Metabolism*. (Stuttgart: Georg Thieme Verlag)

44. ANGELI, E. and KIRMAN, B. H. (1971). Genetic counselling of the family of the mentally retarded child. In D. A. A. Primrose. (ed.), *Proceedings of the Second Congress of the International Association for the Scientific Study of Mental Deficiency*, p. 692. (Warsaw: Polish Medical Publishers)

45. ANGELI, E., DENMAN, A. R., HARRIS, R. F., KIRMAN, B. H. and STERN, J. (1974). Maternal phenylketonuria: a family with seven mentally retarded siblings. *Dev. Med. Child Neurol.*, **16**, 800

9

The coming of the second genetic code: eugenic abortion in the United Kingdom

Gary A. Ratner

The probable response pattern of the American legal system to developing capabilities for medico-social management of human genetics has been previewed by a number of commentators.[1,2]

The United States Congress may soon establish a commission with a broad interdisciplinary base to study the social, legal and ethical problems arising from the New Biology and to make recommendations for possible legislative action regulating the use or otherwise controlling the impact of human genetic technologies;[3] when these recommendations arrive they may amount to a 'Second Genetic Code'. Similar efforts are being undertaken by both private study groups[4] and, in the international arena, by conferences under the auspices of the World Health Organization.[5]

Despite this high level of activity elsewhere, little attention has been paid to legal aspects of the practice of medical genetics in the United Kingdom. Although commentators in the English law journals have dutifully analysed the 'wrongful life' case discussed below[6] and other possibly relevant legal data,[7] their approach has been, with rare exceptions, directed along the lines indicated by traditional, technical legal categories. The Abortion Act of 1967, for example, has been seen primarily as a criminal statute,[8] the role played by the Act in setting up a process of decision-making for abortion usually perceived only in terms of criminal liability for the practitioner. Attempts to formulate an interdisciplinary perspective on the emerging biological future have produced but a single volume on the one topic particularly appropriate in a country which claims a 'test-tube' baby[9] and a number of cloned frogs.[10,11]

That anticipation of an emerging 'Second Genetic Code' should be at such a low level in the United Kingdom is somewhat surprising since Parliament has already enacted one of its more significant chapters. The decision of the United States Supreme Court in *Rowe v. Wade*,[12] which in effect made abortion available 'on demand' in that country, rendered any separate consideration of eugenic abortion unnecessary. In Britain, however, the law allows abortion only when limited conditions specified by the Abortion Act are met. Given this background of restricted abortion, the eugenic abortion section of the Act is quite clearly an important chapter in the new Genetic Code. In fact, few statutes in any jurisdiction are comparable. The barbaric statutes of many of the United States, requiring sterilization of 'mental defectives' and the like, are remnants of an era long before Watson and Crick and, fortunately, have been rarely used. The genetic screening statutes of most of the United States are concerned primarily with the management of genetic disease after birth. Voluntary screening for heterozygote status usually involves the State only in finance and administration. Restricted abortion with a eugenic exception as exists in the United Kingdom goes much further by involving the State in 'unnatural selection'—those fetuses whose probable genotypes do not qualify for eugenic abortion must be born.

When the whole of the context of the Abortion Act is surveyed, something a great deal more important than the convictability of practitioners is seen. A particular process of decision-making for eugenic abortion, allocating authority amongst State, medical profession and parents is there. So, too, is one possible framework for decision-making in the even more complicated situations likely to result from increasing capabilities for human genetic engineering. Since the question of the practitioner's role in decision-making is likely to be of central importance to any system for the delivery of genetic technology, I will attempt to analyse the legal framework surrounding that role in the case of eugenic abortion.

A NOTE ON ABORTION IN GENERAL

Section 1(a) of the Abortion Act of 1967 provides for the lawful termination of pregnancy by a registered practitioner

'. . . if two practitioners are of the opinion, formed in good faith . . . that the continuance of the pregnancy would involve risk to the life of the pregnant woman, or of injury to the physical or mental health of the pregnant woman or any existing child of her family, greater than if the pregnancy were terminated . . .'

Although the broadest view of the Genetic Code would consider the eugenic implications of 'ordinary' abortion and abortion on demand, detailed examination of abortion performed under section 1(a) of the Act is beyond the scope of the present discussion. While the policy considerations relating to conventional abortions, whether for risk or on demand, are closely related to those in eugenic abortion, the two cases are sufficiently distinguishable to permit restricting discussion of ordinary abortion to selected comparative aspects. Before turning to analysis of the structure of decision-making in eugenic abortion, however, one point should be explored. The availability of abortion on demand, as I have suggested, tends to render discussion of eugenic abortion from a legal standpoint somewhat fruitless. Although there is a continuing debate as to whether abortion is *in fact* available on demand in England, it seems sensible to proceed for several reasons. Conviction under the law of abortion is a possibility even for registered practitioners; at least one such conviction has been obtained when the good faith requirement was breached.[13] Next, there can be little doubt that the great bulk of practitioners do attempt to adhere to the statute and, thus, despite the possibility of a 'demand' abortion, the statute continues to shape the practices of a great portion of medical and client communities. Finally, the Act may be studied as a model decision structure. Notwithstanding its arguably limited practical relevance, the model may reveal strengths and weaknesses worth consideration.

Eugenic abortion under the Act: allocation of authority between State and practitioner

Section 1(b) of the Abortion Act of 1967 provides for the lawful termination of pregnancy by a registered medical practitioner:

'. . . if two registered medical practitioners are of the opinion, formed in good faith . . . that there is a substantial risk that if the child were born it would suffer from such physical or mental abnormalities as to be seriously handicapped.'

Since section 5(2) of the Act explicitly declares all terminations not authorized by section 1 unlawful, criminal liability of the participants in a given abortion hinges, not on fulfilment of the risk condition, but on the good faith beliefs of the practitioners involved. That participants in some interaction should make the *initial* interpretation of an Act and, thereby, of the legality of their own conduct is not unusual; the success of legal systems depends largely upon self-enforcement of just this type. What is somewhat surprising is the fact that the practitioner's good faith determination, however badly made, is the *final* determination of his own criminal liability. The practitioner would seem to be making the sort of determination usually reserved for the judiciary. This partial delegation of the interpretive function results, however, in considerably different decision structures for ordinary health risk and eugenic abortions.

The statutory standard for the degree of risk justifying abortion in non-eugenic cases is precisely stated—the risk to the pregnant woman (or existing child) of continuing the pregnancy must exceed the risk of termination. One subject of the standard, risk to the life of the pregnant woman, presents few interpretive difficulties. The remaining subject of the standard, risk of injury to the physical or mental health of the pregnant woman or an existing child, may cause some interpretive problems, but these are comparatively easily resolved. While the meaning of risk to health, especially mental health, may be less than perfectly clear, the apparent reference of the term is familiar enough to allow the presumption that the legal policy coincides with the conventional role of the practitioner. If public and medical policy are in this identical, the medical aspects of any determination and the individualized social decision required by the Act will be fully merged. While section 2 of the Act allows for 'the pregnant woman's actual or reasonably foreseeable environment' to be taken into account in determining the risk to health, the wording of that section makes it clear that 'social' elements are to be considered only as they affect the woman's health. A pregnancy cannot be terminated merely because a woman's job, or even her marriage, might be affected unless health considerations are also present.[14] Although the Act apparently allows considerations of a medico-social nature, the practitioner's opportunity to actually formulate public policy is tethered by his own professional understanding of the concept of health. To the extent that individual cases may lie in a grey area at the boundary between health and social considerations, it is not unreasonable to permit medical men acting in good faith to categorize them.

The policy of Parliament regarding non-eugenic abortion might be put thus: any risk, however slight, to maternal health (or the health of an existing child), as such risk is understood by health experts acting in good faith, will settle the conflict between fetal and maternal claims conclusively. Should an extraordinary case present interpretive difficulties, the ensuing deliberations are, it appears, channelled and confined to but a single issue—whether there is a risk to health. Since the applicable public policy is relatively well-defined by the applicable statutory test and more or less coterminous with medical policy, direct controls in consideration of the moral gravity of abortion can be restricted to the requirements of good faith and a second opinion. Second-guessing of actions actually taken is only slightly different from second-guessing any medical determination and, while proper in ordinary private law procedures such as suits for medical negligence, is not a suitable basis for criminalizing persons who have acted in good faith.

When the identical 'good faith' requirement is combined with the much vaguer language used in the standard for eugenic abortion, a wholly different situation is presented. The purpose of a statutory standard is to separate two zones of factual situations in which different policies are to prevail; any problems of interpretation must be resolved by reference to the policy objectives of the Act. When the standard is precisely stated, that is one risk greater than another, and where it makes explicit reference to particular determinative events, that is health factors, the task of interpretation is relatively easy. When the standard is very broadly stated, meanings cannot be assigned to the words without detailed understanding of the policy implications of the choice to be made.

When the Abortion Act is considered as a Genetic Code, the policy territory on either side of the verbal boundary created by section 1(b) is seen to be quite complex. Where termination is prevented, there lies more than the conventional issues of the sanctity of life and the protection of the fetus from abortion at the hands of its parents, issues which themselves must be considered legitimate since abortion is, in theory, not available 'on demand'. Added to the usual anti-abortion arguments is a whole range of questions arising from the possibility of limited indirect control of the national gene pool. It can be argued, for example, that there may be a legitimate State interest in ensuring the continuance of particular genes, of a sufficient diversity of genotypes, or of given ratios of particular genotypes, XXs/XYs, for example. Although sex selection is not allowed under section 1(b), which provides that the prospective abortus must be at risk of abnormality resulting in handicap, the example is instructive. When the potential interests of persons due to be born into, say, a 60% sexual majority are weighed, they may fall well short of justifying State dictation of the sex of new-borns; when the same interests are added to already recognized claims for the right to life, a powerful case against sex-selective abortion can be made out. That some such argument could also be made for abnormalities is suggested by the sometimes beneficial effects of the sickle cell gene in heterozygous form. To go just one step further, it may be argued that the preservation of genetic diversity may justify limiting eugenic abortions for the same reason that population control objectives are often thought to justify allowing ordinary abortion—the survival of the species.

The policy ground located on the opposite side of the boundary is even more complex. First, there is the counterpart to the claims for right to life, the claim on behalf of the child *in utero* for freedom from state-required birth. The claim represents an unusual twist to traditional relationships among parent, child and state, as typified by those cases in which the state will override the parents' religiously based opposition to life-saving therapy. The more familiar view is that the life of the child can be protected from danger at the hands of the parents by some form of state intervention. For eugenic abortion, this relationship is turned inside out; it is the parents who claim the right to protect the fetus from harm arising from the State's requirement that he be born. Next come the claims of the parents on their own behalf. Excluding bona fide claims of risk to the health of the mother or an existing child which can be accommodated by section 1(a), there are still important interests of the parents at stake. Handicap can be a tremendous economic and social burden; the need for special treatment or diets, for example, may lead to heavy costs, fewer opportunities to take holidays or eat in restaurants, restrictions on hours worked and even geographical relocation.[15] Finally there may be interests of the state weighing for allowing abortion as well, including items as cynical as the protection of the national treasury from the burden of aid to the handicapped, as practical as the maintenance of a healthy work-force, and as idealistic as the protection of future generations from a Mullerian dysgenic horror.

Though a nearly comparable range of issues can be drawn from the implications of the ordinary abortion law, especially if population size objectives are considered, the Parliamentary resolution of that issue rather clearly channels individual decision along the lines of conventional medicine. On the other hand, beyond stating that the child *in utero* must be at risk of abnormality, the standard for eugenic abortion gives little guidance to the decision-maker. The words 'serious' and 'substantial' both imply a weighing up of interests. Yet nowhere does the Act clearly indicate from whose perspective these interests are to be evaluated or which may be legitimately considered. May a risk be considered 'substantial' by virtue of the strength of a parental desire for only the most perfect of specimens? Should the determination of 'serious'-ness consider the cost to the State of the particular treatment available? or the value of the gene in the heterozygous form to future generations? What is clear is that, while the issues at stake involve a large medical and technical component, they also have major social, political, economic and ethical dimensions. Determining the facts concerning health risks to an individual is a legitimate medical task. Determining whether some health risk is greater than another, though highly subjective in many cases, is a medical task in a conventional sense. Determining whether a given risk is 'substantial' or a handicap 'serious', for the purpose of drawing lines between the sort of complex policy alternatives present in eugenic abortion cases, is not a medical function; it is a policy task of the sort usually left to agencies of public authority.

The problem created by the good faith clause and the vagueness of section 1(b), the over-broad policy role placed in the medical community, cannot be cleared up by simply making the assumption that only the interests of the child *in utero* are to be considered in applying the standard. Most counsellors believe strongly that decisions arising in the course of genetic counselling should be taken with a view to the overall welfare of the family;[16] that a practitioner will be able to segregate considerations of the welfare of the unborn child from the welfare of the parents should it become necessary to apply the statute is doubtful. Known medical practice in respect of certain genetic conditions is a relatively clear indication that the policy pursued is family oriented; abortion of fetuses with Down's syndrome, for example, is common; yet it seems that a great number of children born with that condition are in fact happy and content in spite of their handicap.

Even were it feasible to consider only the interests of the fetus in determining the substantiality of the risk and the seriousness of the handicap, the determination called for stands quite apart from mere 'medicine'. In no purely medical sense, after all, can the fetus be considered healthier dead; from the abortee's point of view there can be no solely medical indication for the treatment of abortion. Even were we to admit that this particular barrier might be overcome for very sharp cases such as Tay–Sachs disease, a vast ground remains in which the seriousness of the handicap, e.g., Down's syndrome, can only be properly evaluated on behalf of the child *in utero* in social, psychological, economic and environmental terms. Curiously, section 2 of the Act, which allows consideration of environmental factors in ordinary abortion, does not apply to eugenic abortion. Even if the eugenic abortion standard had been cast in terms which could be interpreted as asserting only that the child would be better off dead, which it was not, the policy questions can no more be left to be answered by medical men alone than can the question of euthanasia.

The very broad policy-making role of the medical practitioner in respect of eugenic abortion is the result of the relatively narrow objectives of the Abortion Act of 1967, which was enacted primarily for the protection of doctors performing abortions.[8] Nothing in the Parliamentary debate suggests that genetic code considerations played an important part. It is not surprising, therefore, that no distinction is drawn in respect of the all-important good faith clause between the two grounds for abortion. Since doctors were performing eugenic abortions prior to the Act by treating such terminations as falling within the then-existing common law exemption for risk to the health of the mother, the abortion for handicap section served to secure their position against being forced to this sometimes shaky assumption. Once abortion is conditionally legalized, of course, it is difficult to criminalize good faith efforts to comply with the conditions. As a matter of criminal law, the good faith clause, even in conjunction with the vague standard for eugenic abortion, is defensible. But national policy opposes abortion on demand; if any particular species of abortion is to form an exception, the conditions triggering that exception are matters of public policy. For eugenic abortions, these conditions touch issues far beyond the fairness of prosecuting individual practitioners. While the criminal justice issues present adequate reason for retaining the good faith device for criminal law purposes, they cannot justify substituting the consensus of medical men for publicly-made public policy. Parliament seems to have inadvertently delegated critical policy-making powers by treating the first chapter of the Second Genetic Code as just another item of criminal law.

The wrongful life case: allocation of authority among practitioner, parent and State

Whether one is concerned that ordinary abortion will be too easy or too difficult to obtain will, of course, depend on one's own preference and beliefs. For many, perhaps most, of the participants in traditional abortion politics, any compromise standard will inevitably be either too high or too low. Yet, if the reason for restricting abortion lies in protection of fetal interests, eugenic abortion calls for a position somewhere between forced birth and forced termination. Such a position may in fact be acceptable to a very broad segment of the community, excluding only those who believe that life is always better than death or non-existence, that life is absolutely sacred, or that abortion should be available on demand. When the full range of eugenic issues is considered, including, for example, any State eugenic objectives, the setting of the standard for eugenic abortion calls for more than a compromise between the poles of the traditional abortion debate in the form of a loosely-worded doctor protection statute. Some precision in stating and developing standards is to be recommended.

The protection afforded the practitioner under the good faith clause effectively blocks efforts to use the criminal law to insure that the standard is not set too low. On the other hand, if the standard is set so high that desirable abortions do not go forward, no question of criminal liability can arise. A recent American case, however, suggests that the private law of physical injuries may be available to develop limits to the practitioners' discretion. The plaintiffs in the case of *Gleitman v. Cosgrove*[17] were an infant, Jeffrey, and his parents. The infant's complaint arose from his birth defects; the mother and father complained respectively for the effects on her emotional state caused by her son's condition and for the costs of caring for Jeffrey. The defendants were specialists in obstetrics and gynaecology. Mrs Gleitman consulted the defendants and was found to be 2 months pregnant. She informed Dr Cosgrove that she had had rubella 1 month previously. On receipt of this information Dr Cosgrove told her that the rubella would have no effect on the child. The child was subsequently born with substantial defects in sight, hearing and speech.

For present purposes we may also assume the following; that the defects were causally connected with the infection; that the risk that the child would be born with the defects was roughly 1 in 4; that the parents would have sought and obtained an abortion had they known the degree of risk; and that Dr Cosgrove withheld the information because of his belief that it was improper to destroy three healthy babies because the fourth might suffer these handicaps. The court dismissed the action on the basis that 'the conduct complained of does not give rise to damages recognizable in law'.

In his discussion of this case, Capron[18] has stated that:

'The relationship between a genetic counsellor and his patients is a delicate, complex and important one. Treating, as it does, subjects of great moment—the prevention of crippling diseases, and even life and death themselves—it commands growing public interest and scrutiny, especially as the counsellor's predictive skills increase. It involves not only parents but also geneticists, physicians, clergymen and others in more lengthy and careful contemplation of the conception and birth of a child than occurs in any other type of "planned parenthood". Its highly charged subject matter and deeply involved participants open it to the internal and external pressures which encumber all significant decisions.'

Shaw,[19] having emphasized that the counsellor must accept the counsellee as the ultimate decision-maker, has expressed the faith that the law will provide any needed checks upon misbehaviour. The capacity of the law to supervise subtle interpersonal relationships, however, has been seen as subject to severe limitations.[20] Pound[21] suggested a number of such limitations on effective legal action; among them are the difficulties involved in ascertainment of fact, the subtlety of modes of infringing important interests, and the necessity of appealing to individuals to set the law in motion.

Consider a case in which a crusading and rather directive genetic counsellor improperly persuades counsellee-parents, both heterozygous for an autosomal recessive inborn error which can only be treated at great expense, to adopt a child rather than proceed with their own pregnancy. The counsellor might be a Mullerian pessimist worried about long-term dysgenic consequences, or he might see himself as conservator of the state treasury. More simply, he might be an anti-abortionist convinced that the parents, if they proceed with conception and subsequently learn through prenatal diagnosis that they have lost the Mendelian lottery, will have the pregnancy terminated by another practitioner. Assuming for the moment that the counsellor has indeed misbehaved in these circumstances, corrective action may run foul of the limits suggested above. Firstly, there is the problem of setting legal machinery in motion. Since the parents have already been persuaded, it will not occur to them to scrutinize the events that transpired. The never-born child is, of course, unavailable to act as plaintiff. The only likely initiators of legal action would have to come from a class of paternalistic counter-crusaders. This additional load of good intentions is unlikely to be of service. Next, there may be considerable difficulty in reconstructing the relevant events—private conferences likely to have been held in an emotionally-charged atmosphere. Yet even these difficulties seem relatively manageable when compared with the more fundamental problem of evaluating the propriety of the counsellor's persuasive behaviour. Assuming that the counsellor is asked for his own view, and is allowed to answer, judgmental separation of legitimate advice from improper advocacy might require knowledge of such subtle considerations as the effects of gesture and tone of voice, or perhaps even a consideration of the entire psychodynamic relationship among the participants.[22]

One might, therefore, be legitimately sceptical of the law's capacity to provide checks on the misbehaviour of genetic counsellors. But not all factual situations arising from genetic counselling present as many of the contraindications to legal treatment as that hypothesized. When, for example, the counsellor actually withholds crucial information from the counsellees, the mode of infringement of their interest is anything but subtle; the importance of the interests at stake may render coarse legal action better than no action at all.

Whether the alleged behaviour of Dr Cosgrove is characterized as wilful imposition of his own moral views or as merely a negligent failure to make available the full range of treatment is not too important to our considerations. In either case, if the other legal barriers to Jeffrey Gleitman's complaint of 'wrongful life' can be avoided, the court would be unable to escape applying the statutory standard for eugenic abortion to this and subsequent cases. The threat of liability for negligent or wilful failure to authorize eugenic abortion would, in theory, serve as a check on the setting of too high a standard. In addition the court would have the opportunity to interpret, clarify and develop the standard for eugenic abortion. Each decision of the court for or against the legality of a particular eugenic abortion could cut down the range of discretion available to the medical profession. Since even criminal liability would be a possibility for a doctor who knowingly ignored judicial opinion that a given sort of eugenic abortion is not within the terms of the standard, the wrongful life action might also help to assure that the standard is not set too low. The wrongful life action may, therefore, play an important role in re-allocating authority between the State and the practitioner, in addition to its more apparent function of controlling the distribution of decision-making power between parents and practitioner.

Under English law, a plaintiff in an action like *Gleitman* would have to build his case on the ground that the relationship between himself and the defendant was such that the defendant owed him a duty of care and that as a result of conduct breaching that duty of care the plaintiff suffered foreseeable harm. That the plaintiff's situation was foreseeable and that it was a result of the doctor's conduct poses no difficulty. Of course, Dr Cosgrove did not cause Jeffrey's birth defects in the same sense as the original infection did; most events in the physical world have a multiplicity of causes. In Jeffrey's case his mother's selection of an obstetrician is one cause among others. The law, however, will ignore causal events which are beyond its power to control, instead focussing on causal conduct likely to be responsive to rule-making and sanctioning.

Turning to the question of harm, what the New Jersey court did find decisive in the *Gleitman* case was its own inability to 'weigh the value of life with impairment against the non-existence of life itself'; the court found it impossible 'to measure the difference between plaintiff's life with defects against the utter void of non-existence'. Critics of the decision invariably attack these statements with vigour, pointing out that the courts daily make necessarily subjective assessments of such intangibles as pain and suffering, mental anxiety and even the value of life cut short. Yet there is a difference between the assessment of Jeffrey's damages and these more typical examples of judicial assessment of intangibles. In the more conventional cases, the court begins with a notion of something being lost. The thing or things lost are all things that, although they may be intangible, have been known to the conscious mind and can therefore be given some subjective value. Each such case has the form: the difference between the value of something intangible, but within human experience, and the value of something else intangible. But non-existence by definition cannot be experienced. The comparison of non-existence and life impaired, therefore, has the form: the difference between the value of something intangible, but not experienced, and the value of something else intangible. Indeed, since non-existence is unknowable, we cannot be certain whether, after a subjective value has been assigned to life with impairments, the latter quantity has a positive or negative value. The determination suggested compounds intangibility with unknowability. On the other hand, the comparison to be made is necessarily similar to that already made by every parent and practitioner involved in eugenic abortions, which now total approximately 3000 annually in the United Kingdom.[23] Moreover, British courts in particular have shown a willingness to undertake a wide variety of subjective calculations and would probably experience little difficulty in making a *Gleitman*-like computation. In one recent case,[24] an English justice was called upon to consider the difference in damages due to one plaintiff who had been reduced to the state of a 'human vegetable' and those due to another in substantially the same condition with the sole difference that the latter had a slight possibility of conscious knowledge of his state; the difference was judicially computed with little apparent difficulty—£2500. The determination in that case seems intuitively, if not analytically, comparable to the calculation of Jeffrey's damages.

The court and its supporters have raised another problem, the so-called 'logico-legal' difficulty. Citing Professor Tedeschi,[25] the court adopts the view that 'by his very cause of action, the plaintiff cuts from under himself the ground upon which he needs to rely in order to prove his damage'. Lord Kilbrandon,[26] one of the few British jurists to comment on the case, has said that those who say, 'it would be preferable not to exist!', have been 'forced into the use of an indefinite pronoun which conceals a semantic vacuum', since the 'subject, being *ex hypothesi* non-existant in one alternative, cannot predicate his preference for another alternative'.

On close inspection, the logico-legal difficulty appears to be a hyper-analytical vacuum. It cannot be, as Professor Tedeschi seems to suggest, that in a suit for denial of a preferred result the plaintiff is barred if the result denied was of a sort which would have rendered a suit impossible. Suppose an alien who sought to leave the jurisdiction was unlawfully detained by the authorities; the legal action to win his freedom can surely not be dismissed on the basis that, had he been allowed to leave originally, he would have been unable to 'predicate his preference' in court. This, indeed, is nonsense. Nor can the logico-legal difficulty be satisfactorily explained on the basis that, were the plaintiff to have been accorded his wish, he would have been unable to predicate his satisfaction. Under English law, very substantial damages may be awarded to persons reduced to 'vegetable' status, and even, in strict logico-legal theory, to the dead. If those who can't 'enjoy' money are not denied damages, it makes little sense to say that a plaintiff who could enjoy such damages can not receive them because he might not have 'enjoyed' the non-existence for which they substitute. Logic might admit such a result; commonsense would not.

If the logico-legal difficulty is indeed a hyper-analytical vacuum, it should be pointed out that it too conceals something. Policy-oriented lawyers have long realized that when logical derivations and linguistic sleight of hand dominate a legal argument what is usually being concealed is the policy preference of the speaker. In this case what is being concealed is no more nor less than the belief that life, even life with severe handicap, is always preferable to death or non-existence. Yet this policy judgement is hardly consistent with the legality of eugenic abortion; even Lord Kilbrandon admits that for this reason the result of the *Gleitman* case might well be different in the United Kingdom.

The remaining doctrinal issues, whether the defendant owed the plaintiff a duty of care and whether that duty was breached by the defendant, are closely connected. Under English law, the traditional starting point for determination of the question of duty is the test laid down by Lord Atkin in *Donoghue v. Stephenson*[27]:

'... You must take reasonable care to avoid acts or omissions which you can reasonably foresee would be likely to injure your neighbour. Who, then, in law is my neighbour? The answer seems to be—persons who are so closely and directly affected by my act that I ought reasonably to have them in contemplation as being affected when I am directing my mind to the acts or omissions which are called into question.'

One obvious example of the sort of relationship required is that between practitioner and patient. That the relationship between the obstetrician and the child *in utero* also fits the test of *Donoghue v. Stephenson* cannot seriously be doubted.*

---

* While there is little English authority on the question of liability for prenatal injuries, scholarly opinion has left little doubt that such an action can be recognized.[6,28] Furthermore, the Law Commission[29] has recommended that Parliament enact clarifying legislation favourable to this position. Whether the matter is finally settled by judicial or Parliamentary initiative, it seems highly unlikely that recovery by a plaintiff like Jeffrey Gleitman will be denied solely on the theory that his injuries, being sustained *in utero*, cannot give rise to a cause of action.

The usual standard for evaluating the conduct of a practitioner with regard to his patient is whether the course taken by the practitioner is one which no practitioner of ordinary skill would have taken had he been taking ordinary care.[30] This standard would be applied to a practitioner whose lack of expertise led him to fail to diagnose a genetic disease, or whose careless computation led him to seriously underestimate the probability of affliction. In cases like *Gleitman*, however, the defendant does not stand accused of the failure to exercise the required degree of medical skill; rather the complaint is founded on the failure to inform the parents. The duty of the practitioner to obtain the informed consent of his patient was firmly established in *Slater v. Baker and Stapleton, C.B.*[31] Obviously, the fetus itself cannot be informed of its condition and the alternatives of treatment. In this, however, he is no different from a new-born and would seem to fall under the ordinary requirement of parental consent. While there are two exceptions to the requirement of informed consent, neither is applicable here. The exception for emergency is of no apparent relevance. The other exception, known to American lawyers as therapeutic privilege, has been adequately discussed in only a single English case.[32] The rule of that case seems to allow the physician to proceed with less than fully informed consent only when the mental condition of the patient renders him unable to make an informed decision. When the decision will necessarily be made by someone other than the patient, incapacity and, correspondingly, therapeutic privilege are irrelevant.

The purpose behind the informed consent rule is to assure that it is the patient or, in the case of a minor, his parent who makes the choice between available courses of action. Can Dr Cosgrove claim that the child *in utero* is to be treated differently, that the decision is his to make?

In a fascinating line of American cases[33] the courts have been called upon by practitioners to override parental objections, usually based on religious grounds, to particular forms of treatment. Where the decision involves the alternatives of life and almost certain death, the decision to save the life will be taken by the court almost solely on the medical evidence. In these extreme cases, however, it is clear that it is the State which takes the decision, not the practitioner. Where, as in the United Kingdom, the State itself will not protect the life of a child *in utero* at serious risk of substantial handicap, the claim that the doctor may do so on his own initiative is unlikely to succeed.

Although a practitioner who conscientiously objects to abortion will not be compelled to participate,[34] he will not be permitted to fore-close the possibility of legally available 'treatment'.[14] The possibility of such foreclosure has usually been thought of in the context of the practitioner imposing his own moral views. Where, however, there is restricted abortion with statutory exceptions, it is possible for the same result to be reached through a failure to take care in applying the statutory standard to the facts of the case. While detailed consideration of the precise standard of care which will be required of a doctor in interpreting this rather vague statute would raise technical issues beyond the scope of this paper, there can be little doubt that in the sort of circumstances envisaged by the *Gleitman* case, a court can and would conclude that a practitioner should have a relatively high degree of competence in dealing with the legal aspects of medical practice, and it seems unlikely that Dr Cosgrove could be successfully defended on that point.

There is, however, one avenue of defence left to Dr Cosgrove. He can argue that he has deprived neither Jeffrey of his abortion, nor his parents of their choice, merely by asserting that the proposed abortion did not in fact fall within the statutory exemption. Once all the other doctrinal and policy barriers have been dealt with and overcome, the court can get down to the important policy task of interpreting the statute and deciding when the option of eugenic abortion should be made available.

Assuming that the court decides that the abortion would have been legal, it is relatively easy to dispose of the parental claims in the *Gleitman* case. If Jeffrey's damages are, as I have argued, cognizable in law, so too are those of his parents. It is possible that the court will, when it comes to evaluate a complainant's injuries, decide that birth in the particular case was the preferred alternative. An interesting question is whether the court could then award damages to the parents. The answer, it is submitted, is yes. Even though Jeffrey would not have been better off dead, his parents are clearly worse off. If the court finds that the abortion would have been illegal at the time it took place because, for example, there was virtually no risk of serious handicap, both cases must fail. If the court finds that the abortion would have been legal, it must necessarily evaluate the damages suffered as a result. But a determination that Jeffrey was in fact better off alive, does not defeat the claim that the earlier existing risk justified the abortion. To deny the parents damages arising from deprivation of the opportunity for legal abortion would amount to a retrospective denial of the legality of the abortion itself. Yet nothing can be clearer than that it is the Act and nothing else that determines the legality of the abortion. Moreover, to the extent that the Act decriminalizes abortion under appropriate standards, it is consistent with the general policy of family freedom in procreation; any judicial limitation on this type of suit by the parents would tend to restore an element of intervention already cast aside by Parliament and would be very difficult to justify.

Our discussion of the *Gleitman* case and its importance may be summarized briefly. A complaint for wrongful life would probably survive the application of English legal doctrine. If that is true, the court in such a case would be virtually unable to avoid interpreting the eugenic abortion statute. In terms of the decision structure for eugenic abortion, such a suit might serve several purposes. Firstly, by allowing the court to determine whether given risk conditions fall within or beyond the terms of the Act, the wrongful life suit provides a vehicle for limiting the practitioner's discretion which is unavailable under the criminal law. When applying the standard the court will be able to consider the full range of important eugenic, social and economic issues, issues which go far beyond the normal portfolio of medical practitioners. The issues would be scrutinized by a public agency with highly developed techniques of policy analysis. Decisions in individual cases could be related to each other and to the whole flow of decisions involving like issues arising in other contexts. The results would likely be more coherent and consistent than any alternative emerging from the disorganized consensus of practitioners. Finally, the wrongful life action would tend to assure that, in cases in which eugenic abortion is socially acceptable, parents and not practitioners have the final word.

SOME DISADVANTAGES OF THE WRONGFUL LIFE ACTION

Despite its theoretical potential, there are a number of reasons why an action for wrongful life is likely to be of limited value as an instrument for developing public policy on eugenic abortion. Firstly, the peculiar emotional atmosphere of a personal injury action would itself tend to distort the resolution of important public policy issues. The court would have to shape its judgement almost literally in the face of the victim (but in the absence of Dr Cosgrove's three healthy babies). Secondly, the major focus of the case will usually be on the practitioner's conduct. Unless the practitioner actually questions the legality of the proposed abortion, the trial will be concerned with whether the practitioner should have realized that the proposed abortion would have been legal, the question of the actual legality of the abortion taking up a secondary position. Thirdly even if the court reaches the point of interpreting the statute, wrongful life cases will probably be few and far between. Only a handful have been reported in the USA, a jurisdiction roughly four times the size of Great Britain and a good deal more prone to invoke the tort law for any sort of misfortune. With only two or three cases with which to work the courts would probably be unable to develop the kind of specificity needed to guide future decision-makers. Finally, the presentation of data to the court by committed adversaries will be client oriented; important issues, especially those of a complex and far-reaching nature, e.g., social eugenic considerations, may be overlooked if not of particular relevance to either side.

All of these objections and others of similar nature are well known to analysts of the legal process and reflect the limited capacity of courts, confined to a case by case approach, to formulate broad principles of public policy.[35] As Waltz and Thigpen[36] have pointed out:

> 'A piecemeal evolution of the law from *ad hoc* decisions in individual cases would be undesirable as a means of setting public policy because of the unforeseeable and wide-ranging side-effects that might be produced; therefore the entire area should be comprehensively reviewed and a general policy should be formulated. Since the law is largely a reflection of the values of the society which it regulates, and since the area in question is so closely tied to the religious and moral feelings of society, the major responsibility for the formulation of policy in this area should be assumed by the people's elected representatives.'

Parliament, however, has already acted, but without that necessary comprehensive review. Against the background of the Abortion Act of 1967, a wrongful life action may even have a distorting effect on the development of eugenic abortion, since practitioners may lower the barriers to these abortions in an effort to avoid civil liability.[37] Since the good faith clause makes criminal prosecution nearly impossible, except perhaps for a practitioner who actually ignores an as yet non-existent judicial interpretation of the standard, and because of the fact that the aborted are incapable of vindicating their position, the legal forces will be pushing in one direction only, towards easy eugenic abortion. Such are the consequences of using the wrong legal tool for an important job.

Although the wrongful life action will probably fail as a tool for developing criteria for eugenic abortion, the value of even a single such law suit towards assuring that parents and not practitioners make the final decision for eugenic abortion is likely to be fairly high. While too large a role should not be assigned to the threat of legal action *per se*, a finding of liability in a case like *Gleitman* would clearly impress upon the medical community the limits of their authority. Since *Slater v. Baker and Stapleton, C.B.*,[31] probably the first informed consent case on record, that issue has been raised only rarely in the English courts. Once a court clarifies public policy with regard to the relative authority of the practitioner and parent in eugenic abortion cases, self-enforcement by the medical community and the demands of medical consumers should be adequate to assure execution.

Conclusion

The legal framework surrounding the practitioner's role in eugenic abortion marks an inauspicious beginning to the development of the genetic code. Neither the wrongful life lawsuit nor the criminal law of abortion can provide an adequate vehicle for working out details of public policy on eugenic abortion. Indeed, the threat of a wrongful life law suit may be a distorting influence. What remains is only the vaguest of parliamentary guidelines, resulting in an over-broad discretion in the hands of individual practitioners of probably widely varying views, and, on the brighter side, some hope that the wrongful life action will help support the position of parents.

Yet, it is certain that over the next few years technical advance and consumer interest will lead to increased demand for genetic control over offspring through the technique of selective abortion. In view of the importance and scope of the public and private interests at stake, it would be unwise to leave the effective control of policy in this area to even a united medical community confined only by the requirements of second opinion and good faith. Moreover, the decision-making role of the practitioner is only one feature of eugenic abortion requiring attention. Whether a wrongful life action lies against a parent who declines to abort a child known to be at risk, and whether consent to abortion should be required from both parents, are just two examples of questions I have not discussed, but which also raise important and disturbing issues which have no satisfactory answer in existing law. The time for comprehensive review of the first chapter of the Second Genetic Code is at hand.

REFERENCES

1. *eg* GREEN, H. (1973). Genetic technology: law and policy for the Brave New World. *Indiana Law J.*, **48**, 559
2. *eg* PARKER, W. C. (1970). Some ethical and legal aspects of genetic counseling. *Birth Defects, Orig. Art. Ser.*, **6**, 52
3. TUNNEY, J. and LEVINE, M. (1972). Genetic engineering. *Saturday Review*, **55**, Issue 32, 23
4. *eg* BERGSMA, D. (1974). *Ethical, Social and Legal Dimensions of Screening for Human Genetic Disease.* (Miami: Symposia Specialists)
5. Btesh, S. (ed.). (1974). *Protection of Human Rights in the Light of Scientific and Technological Progress in Biology and Medicine.* 8th CIOMS (Council for International Organizations of Medical Science) Round Table Conference. (Geneva: CIOMS Publications)
6. *eg* LOVELL, P. and GRIFFITH-JONES, R. (1974). 'The Sins of the Fathers'—tort liability for prenatal injuries. *Law Q. Rev.*, **90**, 531
7. O'NEILL, P. and WATSON, I. (1975). The father and the unborn child. *Mod. Law Rev.*, **38**, 174
8. HOGGETT, A. (1968). The Abortion Act 1967. *Criminal Law Rev.*, **247**
9. BEVIS, H. (1974). Press conference. *Washington Post*, 17th July, p. 1
10. GURDON, J. (1962). Multiple genetically identical frogs. *Heredity*, **53**, 5
11. CIBA FOUNDATION. (1973). *Law and Ethics of A.I.D. and Embryo Transfer.* Symposium No. 17. (Amsterdam: Elsevier)
12. *Rowe v. Wade*, (1973). 410 U.S. 113
13. *Regina v. Smith (John)*, (1973). 2 W.L.R. 1510
14. Abortion Law Reform Association (1968). *A Guide to the Abortion Act 1967.* pp. 14–15. (London: Alra)
15. WAMBERG, E. (1976). This volume, p. 63
16. COWIE, V. (1976). This volume, p. 103
17. *Gleitman v. Cosgrove*, (1967). 49 N.J. 22, 227 A. 2d 689
18. CAPRON, A. (1973). Informed decision-making in genetic counseling: a dissent to the 'Wrongful Life' debate. *Indiana Law J.*, **48**, 581
19. SHAW, M. W. (1974). Genetic counseling. *Science*, **184**, 751
20. GOLDSTEIN, J., FREUD, A. and SOLNIT, A. (1973). *Beyond the Best Interests of the Child*, pp. 49–52. (New York: Free Press)
21. POUND, R. (1916). The limits of effective legal action. *Int. J. Ethics*, **27**, 161
22. KATZ, J. (1972). *Experimentation with Human Beings*, pp. 635–51. (New York: Russell Sage Foundation)
23. COWIE, V. (1975). Personal communication
24. *West (H.) v. Shepherd*, (1967). A.C. 326
25. TEDESCHI, G. (1966). On tort liability for 'Wrongful Life'. *Israel Law Rev.*, **1**, 513
26. LORD KILBRANDON (1972). The comparative law of genetic counseling. In Hilton *et al.* (eds.), *Ethical Issues in Human Genetics.* (New York: Plenum)
27. *Donoghue v. Stephenson*, (1932). A.C. 562
28. *eg* VEITCH, E. (1973). Delicta in Uterum. *Northern Ireland Legal Q.*, **24**, 40
29. Law Commission. (1974). *Report on Injuries to Unborn Children.* Cmnd. 5709. (London: HMSO)
30. PERCY, R. (1971). *Charlesworth on Negligence*, 5th ed., p. 84. (London: Sweet & Maxwell)
31. *Slater v. Baker and Stapleton*, C.B., (1767). 95 Eng. Rep.
32. *Bolam v. Friern Hospital Committee*, (1957). 2 All E.R. 118
33. *Clarke, In re*, (1962). 90 O.L.A. 21, among others
34. *Abortion Act 1967.* Section 4

35. HART, H. and SACKS, A. (1958). *The Legal Process.* Tentative Ed. (Cambridge, USA: informal publication)

36. WALTZ, J. and THIGPEN, C. (1973). Genetic screening and counseling: the legal and ethical issues. *Northwestern University Law Rev.*, **68**, 696

37. WRIGHT, P. (1975). The dangers of using existing law to protect the rights of the unborn child. *The Times*, 12th December

ASPECTS OF MANAGEMENT REQUIRING CENTRAL POLICY

10

The basis for prescriptive screening

T. W. Meade

Prescriptive screening is the provision of a service for detecting pre-symptomatic or established disease with the intention of making a direct contribution to the health of individuals.[1] This provision implies that prior research has indicated screening will confer some benefit on those with the condition in question; it places a special responsibility on the health professions that is perhaps not so evident in day-to-day clinical practice. For when a patient with symptoms consults a doctor it is usually the patient who has taken the initiative; if, in the present state of knowledge, the accuracy of diagnosis for his illness is limited, or if there is no treatment for the illness, or if the treatment is uncomfortable or painful, it can hardly be said that the doctor is to blame. However, if the doctor takes the initiative, and in effect invites the patient (who may feel perfectly well) to undergo an examination or a test, the position is very different. The individual concerned now has every right to expect several things; firstly, that if he has the condition in question, this will be detected; secondly, that he can be effectively treated, if necessary; and thirdly, that if he does not have the condition, he will not be diagnosed as having it. Others also have the right to expect that resources are not being wasted in the provision of the relevant screening and treatment services. In brief, the doctor who advocates prescriptive screening must be sure of his ground to a degree that cannot always be expected of the clinician. These general principles are now fairly widely accepted, though their practical application to any individual condition has led to widely differing interpretations of the value of screening in that particular case; the current controversy about detecting hypertension[2-4] is a good example of this.

The following 10 headings[5] are often used as a framework within which to test proposals for the introduction of a prescriptive screening service. The application of some of these headings may be considered in the context of disorders which can now be detected perinatally, including conditions like mongolism and neural-tube defects, as well as inborn errors of metabolism.

1. *The condition sought should be an important problem.* Obviously, some considerable attention must be paid to the incidence, prevalence and consequences of the condition concerned. While very rare but disabling or lethal disorders are of the greatest importance to those who have them, and to their families, it is usually difficult to justify a screening service for their detection, bearing in mind the competing claims of other options. Even phenylketonuria, probably the most frequent inborn error of metabolism, occurs only once in about 10 000 births. The comparative rarity of inborn errors is an argument which tends to militate against screening for them even though their consequences are severe. On the other hand, the cumulative burden of all the inborn errors is a point which protagonists of perinatal screening rightly emphasize. On the whole, the larger the number of disorders that can be sought on the basis of a procedure such as amniocentesis and the examination of liquor, for example, the stronger the case becomes for screening for conditions that can be detected in this way. Another way of enhancing the 'importance' of a disorder is by some initial selection of those mothers who are especially likely to have affected children. Advanced maternal age is the definition of 'high risk' for mongolism. It may be that estimations of maternal serum alpha-fetoprotein levels will prove to be a better means of pre-selecting those who ought to have liquor samples examined for the detection of fetal neural-tube defects than the present criterion, which is a previously affected child.

2. *There should be an accepted treatment for patients with recognized disease.* The fact that a condition can be described as 'important' does not, however, automatically, and on its own, justify a screening service; one of the reasons for this is that there may not be any effective, accepted and acceptable treatment. Ischaemic heart disease is clearly extremely 'important', but those who believe that it can be successfully prevented on any scale (through manipulation of the factors by which its onset can to some extent be predicted, e.g. hypercholesterolaemia), are at least equalled, if not outnumbered, by those who do not. There are two components to the scepticism of the latter group; one is that the measures concerned are in any case ineffective in preventing the onset of the disease—the other is doubt that the measures will be carried out (even if they are effective) because they are unacceptably difficult to adhere to. The same applies to the perinatal screening situation; the treatment

must be acceptable as well as effective. Not all would necessarily accept that the treatment for phenylketonuria, for example, meets these criteria, although screening for phenylketonuria is now routine. For an increasing number of conditions, however, selective abortion—both effective and generally acceptable, almost by definition—is becoming the alternative to treatment by diets or surgical procedures of doubtful value.

3. *Facilities for diagnosis and treatment should be available.* It is self-evident that a routine service cannot be introduced unless diagnostic facilities, at least, are available. Routine facilities for treatment may not be quite so critical, especially for rare conditions, but there should be some means, even if they are rather *ad hoc*, or depend on a few specialized centres, of providing treatment where necessary.

4. *The natural history of the condition to be sought should be adequately understood.* This is also really self-evident. If a disease always regressed quickly, painlessly and completely, or if it always proved fatal, whatever was done, there would be probably little point in screening for it, even though other criteria for screening were met. In practice, of course, the real situation usually lies between the two extremes.

It is necessary to understand the natural history of the pre-symptomatic stages of disease, as well as of established illness with clinical manifestations. What, for example, is the relationship between high blood pressure and cerebrovascular disease, and at what point on the blood pressure scale is intervention necessary in order to prevent complications? At what stage should a high fasting blood sugar be regarded as indicating diabetes and what are the nature and risks of complications in diabetes? Is enough known about the frequency with which cervical carcinoma *in situ* proceeds to invasive cancer?

5. *There should be a recognizable latent or early symptomatic stage.* The detection of latent or early disease implies the possibility of preventing late, florid manifestations. However, it would still be reasonable to consider a screening service for a disease which could only be detected when fairly advanced, if other criteria, especially the availability of effective treatment, are met.

6. *There should be a suitable test or examination.* This is crucial and complex. A test must be repeatable, that is, give the same or similar results in the same person on different occasions (assuming, of course, that the variable concerned has not truly altered in the interim; individual biological variation is one of the features of the test that must be

properly understood). The test must be *sensitive*, and detect a very high proportion of those who do indeed have the disease under consideration. It must also be *specific* in accurately identifying those who do not have the disease; this is especially important if those with a positive test are to be put through further investigations that are unpleasant or painful. There could today rarely, if ever, be a good case for introducing a screening service where these aspects of the relevant test had not been fully worked out beforehand.

7. *The test or examination should be acceptable.* A proportion of rectal cancers could probably be detected earlier than would otherwise be the case, and with a greater chance of successful treatment, if proctoscopy and sigmoidoscopy were made a regular practice in those over the age of, say, 40. Whether this proposition would find general acceptance is obviously doubtful. Again, the point is really obvious; we need to be sure that the test will not be unpleasant or painful, to the extent that it will seriously put people off. Considerations of this sort could be a factor in the poor take-up rate of cervical cytology among women in social classes IV and V.

8. *There should be an agreed policy on whom to treat.* In screening for hypertension or diabetes, for example, we are dealing with continuously distributed variables, which are associated with a continuous rise in the chances of the development of complications, such as a stroke. There is, in the case of these and many other variables, no clear and obvious cut-off point, one side of which we can regard as indicating health, and the other, disease. In these circumstances, the decision as to what level is regarded as an indication for treatment is largely arbitrary; it depends to a considerable extent on a balance between the risk of overloading treatment services, if the cut-off point is set at too low a level, and the likelihood of not treating many who might benefit from intervention if it is set at too high a level.

9. *Case-finding should be a continuous process.* In many cases, it is not enough simply to persuade people to have one check, and leave it at that. If screening for hypertension becomes established, suggestions have already been made, based on epidemiological data, as to the frequency with which individuals in different groups should have their blood pressure measured.[6] Similarly, a single cervical cytology test at the age of 35 is not adequate, and a programme of repeat examinations is needed. (This criterion is less crucial in perinatal screening, where we are concerned almost entirely with congenital diseases which can be

adequately confirmed or excluded on the basis of a single examination.)

10. *The cost of early diagnosis and treatment should be economically balanced in relation to total expenditure on medical care.* Screening services are not cheap. Today, as never previously, and whether we like it or not, attention does have to be paid to the relationship between the costs and benefits of various health services. A new health centre here means that someone goes without a pathology laboratory there. Many of the costs and benefits in the perinatal screening field are imponderable; no one can measure the personal or family anguish that follows the birth of a child with a serious congenital disorder. Techniques are, however, now being quite rapidly developed by which to estimate the overall balance between the costs and benefits to the health and social services involved. These techniques are still rather rough and ready, but provided their results are not over-interpreted, they are useful. It is quite clear, for example, that immunization against *rubella* and other maternal infections associated with congenital deformities is cost-beneficial, the benefits outweighing the costs by 20 to 1 or more, that is, by an order of magnitude; in the case of amniocentesis and liquor examination in the detection of mongolism or neural-tube defects, however, the balance is very much more equal. It is a hard but inevitable fact that cost-benefit considerations will increasingly be taken into account in decisions about the provision of services.

These ten criteria may seem to many to be no more than stating the obvious, especially now that some lessons have been learned from early experiences. The issues were not, however, so obvious 15 or 20 years ago, when the whole subject seemed much more straightforward than it has turned out to be. In many ways, the whole subject has actually become more, rather than less, complex, as experiences over breast cancer screening have shown.[7] Current pressures for screening services in an increasing number of fields too often take little or no account of the scientific, organizational and financial conditions that ought to be met, and are supported more by enthusiasm than a reasoned case. It is in fact surprising how few procedures satisfy all, or even most, of the 10 criteria; prenatal care is a form of screening often cited as most nearly doing so. The possibility of routinely detecting neonatal hypothyroidism is a recent development which may turn out to have many of the prerequisites for prescriptive screening.[8,9]

Decisions about perinatal screening depend on answers to a number of inter-related questions, some of which cannot at present be answered;

they are considerably influenced by special pressure groups and political interests, as well as by purely scientific considerations. The field is developing rapidly, and it seems likely that the next 5 or 10 years will see a rapid growth in perinatal screening, even in spite of economic constraints on health services as a whole.

REFERENCES

1. McKeown, T. (1968). Validation of Screening Procedures. In: Lord Cohen of Birkenhead, Williams, E. T. and McLachlan, G. (eds.), *Screening in Medical Care*, (Oxford University Press) p. 1.
2. Sackett, D. L. (1974). Screening for disease: cardiovascular diseases. *Lancet*, **ii**, 1189
3. Coope, J. (1974). Screening for hypertension. *Lancet*, **ii**, 1380
4. Hart, J. T. (1974). Screening for hypertension. *Lancet*, **ii**, 1380
5. Wilson, J. M. G. (1968). *Presymptomatic Detection and Early Diagnosis*. (London: Pitman Medical Publishing Company Limited)
6. Miall, W. E. and Chinn, S. (1974). Screening for hypertension; some epidemiological observations. *Br. Med. J.*, **3**, 595
7. McKeown, T. (1976). An approach to screening policies. *J. R. Coll. Phys.*, **10**, 145
8. Lancet. (1975). Mass screening for cretinism. *Lancet*, **ii**, 356
9. Buist, N. R. M., Murphey, W. F., Grandon, G. R., Foley, T. P. and Penn, R. L. (1975). Neonatal screening for hypothyroidism. *Lancet*, **ii**, 872

11

Resources for nutritional treatment: basic principles and a national 'Food Bank'

Carol L. Clow and C. R. Scriver

Genetic screening has broadened the spectrum of disease open to early medical intervention and it has also led to an increase in the cumulative number of patients who require treatment at any given time. In the following discussion, we will consider, first, some essential resources for treatment of the patient; we will then consider some desirable resources to support the treating agent who may be a physician, a nutritionist, a team at a genetics centre, or otherwise. Although the two types of resource are interdependent, they are not the same and they deserve independent development and consideration. We will confine our comments to the inborn errors of amino acid metabolism, but the principles are applicable to other forms of hereditary metabolic disease.

Resources for the patient

KNOWLEDGE OF MODES OF TREATMENT

Treatment of a patient with an hereditary metabolic disease, to offset the effects of the mutant gene, involves euthenic, environmental engineering, that is, neutralization of the phenotypic effects of the mutant allele without altering the genome which continues to express itself and to be transmitted to future generations. The basic modes of treatment involve either some mechanism, singly or in combination, of substrate restriction, product replacement, or amplification of residual apoenzyme activity by coenzyme supplementation; or of enzyme replacement.[1] *A knowledge of the pathogenetic mechanism and how to offset it is, therefore, a primary resource for the patient.* The likelihood that such a resource will be more available in genetic centres than in an individual medical practice is discussed elsewhere in this volume.[2]

When disease results primarily because of substrate accumulation, constraint on its accumulation, beginning in the newborn period, may prevent disease. This result may be achieved by blocking the endogenous synthesis of the substrate, if biosynthesis is the major source of substrate, an example of this approach is the use of allopurinol to block uric acid synthesis in the Lesch–Nyhan syndrome. Or we may be able to remove a substrate which is 'toxic', by chemical means as in cystinuria or Wilson's disease with the drug D-penicillamine; and in cystinosis with dithiothreitol. Finally, we may use special dietary methods to prevent accumulation of the substrate, particularly when it is derived from an essential nutrient found only in the diet. *Knowledge about nutritional requirements is an important resource for the latter mode of therapy.*

KNOWLEDGE OF NUTRIENT REQUIREMENTS

Mutants are consumers with special needs.[3] Many have need of special diets and their unusual and specific nutrient requirements must be met.* Let us imagine a patient with inborn error X whose customary intake of a critical offending substrate is in excess of the mutant tolerance (column A, Figure 11.1) so that it accumulates in the patient. The hypothetical Recommended Dietary Allowance (RDA) for this particular nutrient is also indicated in Figure 11.1. The RDA is defined as that quantity of nutrient which meets the requirement for all persons in a normal population.[4] Let us suppose a semi-synthetic diet is available for treatment of disease X, and that it contains a very low and, therefore, unnatural amount of the nutrient under consideration; this desirable therapeutic relationship is indicated by the hatched area in column A. The difference between the amount of the nutrient provided by the therapeutic diet and the patient's actual requirement must then be met either by providing a supplement in purified form or in natural foods which contain it. Another hypothetical nutrient whose metabolism is not affected by the same inborn error of metabolism is symbolised in column B of Figure 11.1. Should this nutrient be abundant in the semi-synthetic diet and in the natural foods comprising the total therapeutic diet, its intake is likely to be higher than its hypothetical Recommended Dietary Allowance. The point of Figure 11.1 is to emphasize the need for day-to-day titration of nutrients in the treatment of the patient, to

---

* A detailed statement concerning treatment of patients with inborn errors of amino acid metabolism, by means of special diets is forthcoming from the American Academy of Pediatrics Committee on Nutrition and will be published in *Pediatrics* in 1976

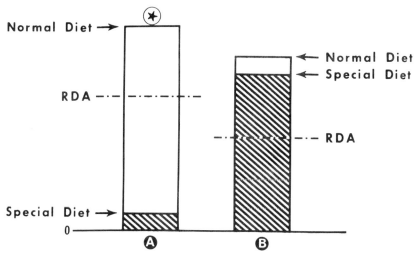

FIGURE 11.1   Diagram of principles applying to treatment of inborn error of metabolism involving a substance which accumulates in body fluids and is 'toxic'. Special
diet provides restricted intake (hatched area) of critical substance (column A) and
adequate intake of other nutrients (represented by column B). RDA is the recommended dietary allowance of nutrients A and B (see text for further discussion)

avoid depletion or excess of nutrients. Accordingly, *mechanisms for
titration and constant supervision are another essential resource for the
patient.*[5]

The actual requirement for each nutrient, in the final analysis, will be
a function of the patient's chemical individuality. General statements
about age-specific requirements[4] (Table 11.2) are a starting point for
therapy; but in themselves they are not sufficient for the treatment of
patients with inborn errors of metabolism. While the general principles
of dietary treatment are simple [1,6] their application is not and treatment
must be individualized. In addition to the multifactorial events which
determine biochemical individuality in normal persons,[7] and control
nutrient requirements for all persons, the inborn errors are themselves
heterogeneous[8] and requirements for offending nutrients may vary
according to the genetic variant inherited by the patient.

The need to acquire knowledge about the specific nutrient requirements for individual probands cannot be over-emphasized at this stage
of our experience with treatment of patients with inborn errors of
metabolism; to illustrate this theme we have compiled representative
data on the dietary tolerance for L-phenylalanine, L-leucine and L-
methionine among probands with the classical forms of phenylketonuria,

Table 11.2   Approximate daily requirements for various nutrients in infancy and childhood (NAS/NRC[14], amino acid data[16], CDS 1975[18] and UK 1969[19]

Nutrient	Source	Age (months)			Age (years)					
		0–2	2–5	6–12	1–2	2–3	3–4	4–6	6–8	8–10
Calories[a]	NAS/NRC (kcal)	120/kg	110/kg	100/kg	1100/kg	1250/kg	1400/kg	1600/kg	2000/kg	2200/kg
	CDS '75 (kcal)	117/kg	117/kg	108/kg	1400/kg	1400/kg	1800/kg	1800/kg	M–2200/kg F–2000/kg	M–2500/kg F–2300/kg
	UK '69 (kcal)	800	800	800	1200	1400	1600	1800	2100	M–2500 F–2300
Volume (H₂O) (ml/day)		120/kg	110/kg	100/kg	1100	1250	1400	1600	2000	2200
Carbohydrate[b] (g/day)		Calories × 0.50 →								
Protein[c]	NAS/NRC (g)	1.8–2.2/kg	1.8–2.0/kg	1.8/kg	25	25	30	30	35	M–40 F–41
	CDS '75 (g)	1.67/kg	1.67/kg	1.67/kg	1.67/kg	1.67/kg	1.41/kg	1.41/kg	1.23/kg	→
	UK '69 (g)	20	20	20	30	35	40	45	53	M–63 F–58
Fat (g)		Calories × 0.35 →								
Sodium	NAS/NRC (mg/kg)	69	69	69	69	69	69	69	69	69
	CDS '75 (mg/kg)	30	30	30	30	30	30	30	30	30
	UK '69 (mg/kg)	48	48	48	48	48	48	48	48	48
Potassium	NAS/NRC (mg/kg)	117	117	117	117	117	117	117	117	117
	CDS '75 (mg/kg)	60	60	60	60	60	60	60	60	60
	UK '69 (mg/kg)	80	80	80	80	80	80	80	80	80
Calcium	NAS/NRC (mg)	400	500	600	700	800	800	800	800	800
	CD '75 (mg)	500	500	500	500	500	500	600	700	M–900 F–1000
	UK '69 (mg)	600	600	600	500	500	500	500	500	700
Phosphorus	NAS/NRC (mg)	200	400	600	700	800	800	800	900	1000
	CDS '75 (mg)	250	250	400	500	500	500	500	700	M–900 F–1000

Nutrient	Source									
Magnesium	NAS/NRC (mg)	40	60	70	100	150	200	200	250	M−250 / F−175
	CDS '75 (mg)	50	50	50	75	75	100	150	150	200
Iron	NAS/CDS (mg)	6	10	15	15	15	10	10	10	10
	CDS '75 (mg)	7	7	7	8	8	9	9	10	10
	UK '69 (mg)	6	6	6	7	7	8	8	10	13
Iodine	NAS/NRC (µg)	25	40	45	55	60	70	80	M−100 / F−110	M−110 / F−120
	CDS '75 (µg)	35	35	50	70	70	90	90	100	130
Phenylalanine	(mg)	47–90	[20–50]*/kg	→			[250–500]*	[400–800]+	(> 800)[d]	
Histidine	(mg)	16–34/kg	[?]	→			[300–600]*	[1000–1500]−		
Leucine	(mg)	76–150	[30–70]*/kg	→						
Isoleucine	(mg)	79–110	[15–35]*/kg	→			[200–400]*	[1000]+		
Valine	(mg)	65–105	[20–50]*/kg	→						
Methionine[e]	(mg)	20–45	[15–30]*/kg	→			[400–600]*	[600–900]+		
Cyst(e)ine[f]	(mg)	15–50/kg	[?]	→			[200–300]+	[400–800]+		
Lysine	(mg)	90–120/kg	[?]	→			[400–800]+	[1200–1600]+		
Threonine	(mg)	45–87/kg	[?]	→				[800–1000]+		
Tryptophan	(mg)	13–22/kg	[?]	→				[60–120]−		
Vitamin B₁ (thiamine)	NAS/NRC (µg)	200	400	500	600	600	700	800	1000	1100
	CDS '75 (µg)	300	300	500	700	700	700	900	1100	M−1200 / F−1100
	UK '69 (µg)	300	300	300	500	600	600	700	800	M−1000 / F−900
Vitamin B₂ (riboflavin)	NAS/NRC (µg)	400	500	600	600	700	800	900	1100	1200
	CDS '75 (µg)	400	400	600	800	800	800	1100	1300	M−1500 / F−1400
	UK '69 (µg)	400	400	400	600	700	800	800	1000	1200
Vitamin B₆ (pyridoxine)	NAS/NRC (µg)	200	300	400	500	600	700	900	1000	1200
	CDS '75 (µg)	300	300	400	800	800	800	1300	1600	M−1800 / F−1500

		Age (months)			Age (years)					
		0–2	2–5	6–12	1–2	2–3	3–4	4–6	6–8	8–10
Vitamin B₁₂	NAS/NRC (μg)	1.0	1.5	2.0	2.0	2.5	3.0	4.0	4.0	5.0
	CDS '75 (μg)	0.3	0.3	0.3	0.9	0.9	0.9	1.5	1.5	3.0
Folic acid	NAS/NRC (μg)	50	50	100	100	200	200	200	200	300
	CDS '75 (free folate) (μg)	40	40	60	100	100	100	100	100	100
Niacin	NAS/NRC (mg)	5	7	8	8	8	9	11	{M–13, F–14}	{M–15, F–17}
	CDS '75 (NE)	5	5	6	9	9	9	12	13	15
	UK '69 (mg equiv.)	5	5	5	7	8	9	10	11	{M–14, F–13}
Vitamin C (ascorbic acid)	NAS/NRC (mg)	35	35	35	40	40	40	40	40	40
	CDS '75 (mg)	20	20	20	20	20	20	20	30	30
	UK '69 (mg)	15	15	15	20	20	20	20	20	25
Vitamin A	NAS/NRC (IU)	1500	1500	1500	2000	2000	2500	2500	3500	3500
	CDS '75 RE[h]	400	400	400	400	400	500	500	700	800
	UK '69 RE[h]	450	450	450	300	300	300	300	400	575
Vitamin D	NAS/NRC (IU)	400	400	400	400	400	400	400	400	400
	CDS '75 (μg)[i]	10	10	10	10	10	10	5	2.5	2.5
	UK '69 (μg)[i]	10	10	10	10	10	10	2.5	2.5	2.5
Vitamin E	NAS/NRC (IU)	5	5	5	10	10	10	10	15	15
	CDS '75 (d-α-tocopherol) (mg)	3	3	3	4	4	4	5	6	7

(a) The caloric requirement is increased when a protein is provided as a mixture of the corresponding free L-amino acids
(b) Minimum fraction is 15% of total calories; optimum value given
(c) Minimum fraction is 14% of total calories; optimum value given
(d) More phenylalanine is required in the absence of tyrosine
(e) More methionine is required in the absence of cyst(e)ine
(f) More cyst(e)ine is required in the presence of a blocked transsulphuration outflow pathway for methionine metabolism
(g) Niacin Equivalent = 1 mg niacin or 60 mg tryptophan
(h) Retinol Equivalent corresponds to a biological activity in humans equal to 1 μg retinol (3.33 IU) or 6 μg β-carotene (10 IU)
(i) μg Cholecalciferol = 40 IU Vit.D activity

* Data obtained from study of actual probands with blocked catabolic pathways for phenylalanine, branched-chain amino acid or homocystine oxidation respectively
† Data derived from studies in normal patients with 'open' catabolic pathways (compiled from Irwin & Hegsted[17])

maple syrup urine disease and homocystinuria (Table 11.1). The wide range of amino acid tolerances in such patients (expressed as mg/kg/day) is indicated in the left-hand column of data. Corresponding data are also given for normal infants in the first year of life. The data reveal that age-dependent amino acid requirements vary several-fold among probands with phenylketonuria, maple syrup urine disease and homocystinuria. If we then consider total daily amino acid intakes tolerated by probands at any time during the first 5 years of life (right-hand column, Table 11.1), we find two-fold variation between the upper and lower tolerance limits in these three inborn errors of metabolism. We notice also that as the patient grows tolerances tend to fall behind the requirements of normal subjects.

These observations indicate that nutrient requirements related to weight are influenced by the rate of growth in young patients with inborn errors of metabolism; they are also individualized phenomena

Table 11.1 Amino acid tolerances and requirements in probands with inborn errors of metabolism*

		Intake	
Trait	*Amino acid*	mg kg^{-1}day^{-1}*	mg day^{-1}§
Phenylketonuria	phenylalanine	20–125	250–500
Normal infant†	phenylalanine	47–94	
Normal child†	phenylalanine		>400
Maple syrup urine disease	leucine	30–145	300–600
Normal infant	leucine	76–226	
Normal child	leucine		>1000
Homocystinuria	methionine (met. + cystine)	10–40	~200–300
Normal infant	methionine (met. + cystine)	15–50	
Normal child	methionine (met. + cystine)		>400

* Data compiled from literature cited[9] for specific diseases
† Normal infant and child data[9,16,17]
‡ Data cover period of infancy (predominantly) but extend to 5 years of age
§ Newborn–5 years age range

and they are related to the total genotype of the patient. Consequently, any significant discrepancy between a recommended intake derived from theoretical considerations and the precise tolerances demanded by the actual patient, may have dire consequences in the long term if the patient experiences uncorrected overtreatment or undertreatment. The further impact of heterogeneity, at the genetic locus affected by the mutation causing the inborn error, upon substrate tolerances and treatment has been well documented, particularly in the hyperphenylalanin-aemias and in the branched-chain hyperaminoacidaemias.[9]

RECOMMENDATION

Since physicians usually have had only a modest exposure to nutrition theory and practice and almost no exposure to the subtle art of feeding probands with inborn errors of metabolism, a regionalized diagnosis and treatment service is an effective resource to translate general knowledge about nutritional requirements into specific terms for probands with inborn errors of metabolism. Knowledge about nutritional requirements and how to apply it to specific patients, and knowledge about genetic heterogeneity and phenotypic manifestations in the individual proband, can also be considered as basic resources for the treatment of patients with inborn errors of metabolism.

Two types of information are required for treatment. One is the composition analysis of treatment products in use (examples of amino acid products are given in Table 11.3). This information will allow the treating agent to know what the patient receives in his treatment product (equivalent to the hatched areas in Figure 11.1). The other is an estimate of the nutrient requirements that must be met during treatment of the patient (Table 11.2). Specific monitoring of metabolic levels and day-to-day titration of nutrient intake is necessary to determine the patient's individual requirement and progress.

These principles have been developed from practical experience at treatment centres in Europe and North America. In our experience it has been relatively easy to avoid significant nutrient deficiency or undesirable accumulation of offending metabolites and to meet nutritional requirements for growth during several hundred patient-treatment years; we should emphasize that treatment is performed in the home and not in a hospital or by means of repeated clinic visits.[5]

Resources for the treating agent

We have now to consider how the physician or treating agent may obtain special diets and how he can be assisted in the use of these products.

The prevalence of patients with hereditary metabolic disease is likely to be low in any one physician's practice and there are usually multiple sources of therapeutic diet products which can benefit his patient. The typical relationship between the physician, his treatment resource, and

RESOURCE

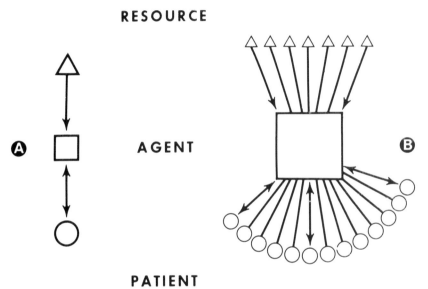

AGENT

PATIENT

FIGURE 11.2 Diagram of typical relationships for physician in practice (A) and for genetics centre between supplies of treatment products (resources) and the patient (see text for further discussion)

his patient with an inborn error of amino acid metabolism is depicted in Figure 11.2; there is usually a dearth of interaction between the components of the relationship. The distributors of special dietary products may not be able to reach the physician who needs these resources; the physician may not know about the existing spectrum of resources; the physician's whole practical experience may be limited to one patient.

Alternate mechanisms to bridge the 'resource gap' are shown on the right of Figures 11.2 and 11.3. The resource or structure which serves

Table 11.3 Approximate nutritive composition* of special dietary products (per 100 g powder)

	Lofenalac (M-J)	Albumaid-XP (MSMR)	Aminogran (GM)	3229-A (MJ)	3200-AB (MJ)	MSUD-Aid (MSMR)	Metinaid (MSMR)	3200-K (MJ)	Histidine-Low (MSMR)	80056 (MJ)
Calories	454	370	400	406	460	393	384	464	360	486
Protein (equivalent) (g)	15	40	100	20.3	15	98.2	40	14	40	0
Fat (g)	18	1	0	6.8	18	0	0	19	0	22.5
CHO (g)	60	47	0	66	60	0	56.1	60	50	73.5
L-Amino Acids (g)										
Essential:										
Isoleucine	0.75	1.1	8.5	1.08	0.86	0	0.8	0.67	1.2	
Leucine	1.41	3.5	9.9	1.70	1.76	0	1.8	1.16	2.0	
Lysine	1.57	3.4	(7.3)§	1.85	1.91	10.4	3.7	0.87	3.0	
Methionine	0.45	0.5	2.9	0.62	0.56	2.2	0	0.16	0.8	
Phenylalanine	0.08	0	0	0	0.08	4.3	2.4	0.76	1.2	
Threonine	0.77	2.8	5.7	0.93	0.86	4.3	1.8	0.52	1.6	
Tryptophan	0.19	0.4	1.5	0.28	0.20	1.6	0.4	0.16	0.6	
Valine	1.20	2.5	7.0	1.24	1.38	0	1.9	0.71	1.6	
Histidine	0.39	0.9	3.8	0.46	0.40	3.2	1.6	0.34	N.L.†	
Non-Essential:										
Arginine	0.34	1.7	(4.3)‡	0.68	0.39	6.5	2.4	0.96	2.4	
Alanine	0.64	2.3	2.4	N.L.	0.76	8.8	3.2	0.60	3.2	
Aspartate	1.34	4.4	6.1	5.15	1.60	15.3	5.3	1.72	5.6	
Cystine	0.025	1.7	1.5	0.34	0.042	5.4	2.0	0.107	2.0	
Glutamate	3.78	5.1	(12.9)§	1.85	4.31	17.5	6.0	2.76	6.4	
Glycine	0.35	1.7	6.1	3.30	0.40	8.8	2.4	0.59	3.2	
Proline	1.13	2.1	4.3	N.L.	1.13	2.8	0.9	0.68	1.0	
Serine	1.02	2.8	8.4	N.L.	1.09	2.8	1.0	0.72	1.0	
Tyrosine	0.81	3.1	6.4	0.93	<0.04	4.3	2.4	0.49	2.4	
Glutamine	N.L.	N.L.	N.L.	4.75	N.L.	N.L.	N.L.	N.L.	N.L.	

Vitamins										
Vitamin A (IU)	1160	0	0	2030	1160	0	0	1450	0	1440
Vitamin D (IU)	284	0	0	406	284	0	0	290	0	360
Vitamin E (IU)	7.1	0	0	10	7.1	0	0	7.2	0	9
Vitamin C (mg)	37	0	0	53	37	0	0	38	0	45
Thiamin (μg)	428	2000	0	609	428	5000	2000	440	2000	450
Riboflavin (μg)	714	2000	0	1015	714	5000	2000	720	2000	540
Vitamin B_6 (μg)	290	1000	0	508	290	2500	1000	360	1000	360
Vitamin B_{12} (μg)	1.4	20	0	2.5	1.4	50	20	1.8	20	1.8
Niacin (μg)	5714	10 000	0	8122	5714	25 000	10 000	5820	10 000	7200
Folic Acid (μg)	72	200	0	51	72	500	200	36	0	90
Pantothenic Acid (μg)	2142	4000	0	3046	2142	10 000	4000	2200	4 000	2700
Choline (mg)	61	0	0	86	61	0	0	62	0	76
Biotin (μg)	36	49	0	30	36	130	50	22	50	45
Vitamin K (μg)	72	0	0	102	72	0	0	71	0	90
Inositol (mg)	72	0	0	102	72	250	100	73	100	90
Minerals										
Calcium (mg)	435	1000	8200	634	435	none	700	650	700	540
Phosphorus (mg)	326	637	3837	508	326	254	1500	450	1500	300
Magnesium (mg)	51	148	970	76	51	200	80	54	80	63
Iron (mg)	8.6	20	50	12	8.6	10	4	8.7	4	11
Iodine (μg)	32	77	700	66	32	150	60	47	60	41
Copper (μg)	429	2000	6300	609	429	1250	500	430	500	540
Manganese (mg)	0.7	1.2	5.7	2	0.7	1250	500	1.4	0.5	0.9
Zinc (mg)	2.9	2.2	10.5	4.1	2.9	2.5	0.9	2.9	0.9	3.6
Sodium (mmol)	9	43	172	10	9	N.L.	33	10	34	3
Potassium (mmol)	12	23	213	18	12	N.L.	19	15	19	9
Chloride (mmol)	9	114	N.L.	14	9	N.L.	N.L.	N.L.	N.L.	4

* Composition may vary between batches of individual product
† N.L. = Not listed
‡ Offered as glutamate salt
§ Includes glutamate from lysine and arginine salts
¶ Provided in separate package insert

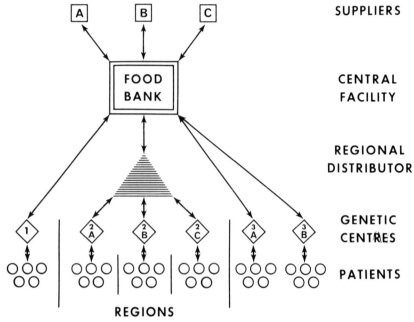

FIGURE 11.3   Diagram of 'Food Bank' process in Canada serving three types of regions: (1) with one (genetics) treatment centre per region; (2) with three regional centres and one supra-regional depot; and (3) with independent centres served directly by Food Bank. Bidirectional arrows indicate flow of information, orders and deliveries of treatment products from supplies to patients (see text for further discussion)

the physician is the genetics centre (Figure 11.2). The resource or structure which serves the genetics centre is a 'Food Bank' (Figure 11.3). The process implemented by the Food Bank is the supply of a variety of treatment diets. The objectives of the Food Bank structure are to control, facilitate and evaluate the usage of treatment products.

THE GENETIC CENTRE AS RESOURCE

A genetics treatment centre[2] can achieve broad access to a range of treatment products through the Food Bank. Furthermore, the spectrum of inborn errors of metabolism which is likely to be encountered by the genetics centre, will be larger than that encountered by the physician in practice. Accordingly, a treatment centre can capitalize on a larger experience in a shorter time, and it can regionalize its influence to facilitate communication between the treatment source and the patients.

The 'Food Bank' concept

Until recently in Canada, for example, there was no uniform national system to provide access to special dietary products for the treatment of inborn errors of amino acid metabolism in a population of 23 million people. Only a few semi-synthetic dietary products were easily available and usually only in certain regions of the country. Moreover, these dietary products could be prescribed by physicians without a requirement for follow-up procedures to avert hazards in their use. With medical emergencies, such as maple syrup urine disease or hereditary tyrosinaemia, it was often difficult to obtain the treatment products rapidly at a time of crisis. Labelling is also a problem; if the label is not approved by the Food and Drug Directorate of Canada, the product cannot be imported. In some countries, these products are liable for classification as drugs and therefore are not even available as foods.

These obvious deficits in treatment resources have been met in Canada by the establishment of an *ad hoc* committee of nutritionists, geneticists, physicians, members of government and representatives of the public. The committee has developed a structure called the National Food Distribution Center for the Management of Hereditary Metabolic Disease[10,11] to bridge the gap between the supply of special diet products and the patients who need them. The 'Food Bank' also provides a mechanism whereby government and physician can invest some confidence in the supervision of the difficult modes of treatment to our patients with inborn errors of metabolism.

A centralized facility for the Food Bank was established in January 1974. The main distribution centre is located in Montreal. It receives products from over 15 suppliers, and distributes them to the regional depots around the nation. This network of Food Bank depots reduces delivery points to a manageable number and accordingly reduces the costs of operation.

The semi-synthetic dietary products and other food items distributed by the Food Bank have been classified as foods by the Federal Food and Drug Directorate in Ottawa. This simple expedient of removing nutrient treatment products from the drug list, because their use could be supervised at recognized treatment centres, and would be distributed only through the auspices of the Food Bank, was one of the single most effective measures taken. A similar action by the Food and Drug Administration in the USA is pending and should pave the way towards a broader range of semi-synthetic diet products being available to patients in that country as well. If there are restrictive food laws in other countries, perhaps the Canadian Food Bank may prove to be an effective model for them also.

A national network of treatment centres came about through the influence of the Food Bank. The network now comprises 16 centres from coast to coast in Canada (the four centres in Quebec province are serviced by one regional depot); the centres serve regions in some parts of the USA along the Canadian border. Treatment centres are allocated by the committee to medical genetic programmes where there are persons with expertise in diagnosis, counselling and treatment of hereditary metabolic disease.

With regard to produce approval, each food item is reviewed by a member of the committee in the nutrition division of the Federal government and a decision is made as to whether the item can be stocked by the Food Bank. Suppliers are identified and approved by the committee. The sources of our information are by word of mouth from physicians, from articles in the literature,[12] from the suppliers themselves, and from contacts with the amino acid subcommittee of the Committee on Nutrition of the American Academy of Pediatrics. The original *ad hoc* committee has assumed a supervisory role on a national and regional basis and it provides guidance and support to the on-going operation of the Food Bank.

The advantages of the Food Bank have been made evident from the experience gained since it began operation:

1. It has facilitated centralization of treatment services for patients who are widely scattered across Canada, and within regions around the treatment centres.

2. It encourages regionalization of treatment mechanisms at a time when expertise in treatment is still limited. Centralization of expertise resources and regionalization of influences in line with the current recommendations of the World Health Organization concerning diagnosis, counselling, rehabilitation and treatment of patients with genetic disease.[13]

3. It provides a method for regulating the use of modified food products, which if used improperly, could be hazardous; they are distributed only to the approved regional treatment centres.

4. It facilitates distribution of information about new products.

Absence of such information has been a serious constraint to the quality of treatment in the past.

5. It provides an unusual opportunity to identify the epidemiology of hereditary metabolic disease in regions across our country, and to co-ordinate follow-up on patients.

6. It is an efficient mechanism for the provision of emergency service to patients who are likely to appear only at an unpredictable and low frequency in any region in the country.

The Food Bank maintains a catalogue of treatment products which is under continuous revision and updating; about 25 products are currently listed in the catalogue. Resource information about their composition is provided (see Table 11.3).

The Food Bank budget is approximately $15 000 per year to maintain inventory, to receive and fill orders, and to distribute the information. Funding of the Food Bank is by a donation from the Steinberg Co., which acts as manager of the operation, and a grant from the Federal Minister of Health. Shipment costs are paid by the clients; in this case, the treatment centres.

Comment

We have chosen to highlight two limbs of the problem of resources for the treatment of patients with inborn errors of metabolism. One limb concerns the individual patient; the other, the treating agent. Genetic disease with its low frequency for any given trait, and with its high degree of heterogeneity within any particular phenotype, places un-usual demands upon the practising physician who is directly responsible for the care of the patient. We suggest that a treatment centre, which is likely to be a component of any major regional genetics centre, is an important resource for the patient. By means of the knowledge and experience accumulated at such centres, and by the use of allied health personnel, as well as physicians, to maintain day-to-day contact with the patients and to provide frequent biochemical monitoring, it is possible to sustain informed day-to-day care of probands with rare forms of hereditary metabolic disease.

On the other hand, the treatment centre itself needs its own re-sources. They comprise semi-synthetic diet products, which without adequate supervision, are potentially dangerous in their use. The availability of these products is limited; and relatively few suppliers manufacture them. The manufacturing process is difficult and there is little incentive to enhance their organoleptic properties,[3] when the market is as small as it is. Some advances in the food technology of protein hydrolysates has been reported,[14,15] and national food banks servicing patients with genetic and allied disease could benefit from such improved products. On the other hand, without adequate treatment resources there is little merit in pursuing genetic screening activities and other related genetic services in communities. We have described a mechanism which we believe bridges the 'treatment gap'. We suggest that with appropriate and imaginative variation, the Food Bank concept can be applied to countries other than our own, so that patients elsewhere will benefit from the advantages which we ourselves have experienced.

Summary

Resources for nutritional treatment of inborn errors of metabolism are of two types: those for the patient, and those for the treating agent. The former include knowledge about pathogenetic mechanisms and the optimal mode of treatment to offset the mutant allele; knowledge about the patient's genotype and his nutritional individuality; and mechanisms for titration of nutritional requirements and the response to therapy. The latter include genetic centres with expertise to assist the treatment agent and the authority to regionalize their treatment programmes so as to increase its efficiency; and a 'Food Bank' network which facilitates access to a wide range of treatment products whose composition is known and whose use can be controlled and evaluated systematically.

Mme Huguette Ishmael, Dr Keith Murray, Dr James Haworth and Dr Margaret Cheney in particular helped to develop the National 'Food Bank' in Canada; the parents of patients stimulated us to develop the idea; and Mr Arnold Steinberg and his colleagues made it a reality. The Quebec Network of Genetic Medicine supported the research and development behind the project. We are grateful to Dr J. Hopkin who helped us in the early stages.

REFERENCES

1. SCRIVER, C. R. (1969). Treatment of inherited disease: Realized and potential. *Med. Clin. N. Am.*, **53**, 941

2. SCRIVER, C. R. and CLOW, C. L. (1976). Genetic screening and allied services: Structure, process and objective. This volume Chapter 2
3. SCRIVER, C. R. (1971). Mutants: Consumers with special needs. *Nutr. Rev.*, **29**, 155
4. National Acad. Sci. (1974). Nat. Res, Council: Food and Nutrition Bd. *Recommended Dietary Allowances*. 8th revised ed. (Washington, D.C.: Nat. Acad. Sci.)
5. CLOW, C., READE, T. and SCRIVER, C. R. (1971). Management of hereditary metabolic disease. The role of Allied Health Personnel. *N. Engl. J. Med.*, **284**, 1292
6. LOWE, C. U. *et al.* Committee on Nutrition, American Academy of Pediatrics. (1967). Nutritional management in hereditary metabolic disease. *Pediatrics*, **40**, 289
7. WILLIAMS, R. J. (1963). *Biochemical Individuality. The Basis for the Gene Trophic Concept*. Science ed. (New York: J. Wiley & Son)
8. CHILDS, B. and DER KALOUSTIAN, M. (1968). Genetic heterogeneity. *N. Engl. J. Med.*, **279**, 1205 and 1267
9. SCRIVER, C. R. and ROSENBERG, L. E. (1973). *Amino Acid Metabolism and its Disorders*. (Philadelphia: W. B. Saunders Ltd.)
10. MURRAY, T. K., CLOW, C. and SCRIVER, C. R. (1974). National Food Distribution center for patients with hereditary metabolic disease. *Rx Bulletin* (HPB NH & W. Gov't. of Canada), **5**, 79
11. CLOW, C. L., ISHMAEL, H., SCRIVER, C. R., MURRAY, K., CAMPEAU, H., LONG, D. and STEINBERG, H. A. (1975). The National Food Distribution Center for Management of Patients with Hereditary metabolic disease *Nutrition Today*.
12. RAINE, D. N. (1972). Management of inherited disease. *Br. Med. J.*, **2**, 329
13. World Health Organization (1972). *Genetic Disorders: Prevention Treatment, and Rehabilitation*. Techn. Rep. Ser. No. 497, (Geneva: WHO)
14. CLEGG, K. M. and McMILLAN, A. D. (1974). Dietary enzymic hydrolysates of protein with reduced bitterness. *J. Fed. Technol.*, **9**, 21
15. CLEGG, K. M., SMITH, G. and WALKER, A. L. (1974). Production of an enzymic hydrolysate on casein on a kilogram scale. *J. Fed. Technol.*, **9**, 425
16. HOLT, Jr. L. E., GYORGY, P., PRATT, E. L., SNYDERMAN, S. E. and WALLACE, W. M. (1960). *Protein and Amino Acid Requirements in Early Life*. (New York: University Press)
17. IRWIN, M. I. and HEGSTED, D. M. (1971). A conspectus of research on amino acid requirement of man. *J. Nutr.*, **101**, 539
18. Bureau of Nutritional Sciences. (1975). *Dietary Standard for Canada* (Ottawa: Department of National Health and Welfare)
19. Department of Health and Social Security. (1969). *Recommended Intake of Nutrients for the United Kingdom* Rep. Publ. Hlth. No. 120 (London: HMSO)

12

Detection of heterozygotes

A. Westwood

An individual homozygous for a pathogenic recessive gene will have gross clinical or biochemical abnormalities which can usually be easily recognized. However, the heterozygote, carrying one abnormal (mutant) gene and one normal (wild-type) gene, will be, at least superficially, phenotypically normal because the normal gene ordinarily masks the presence of the abnormal gene. Some qualification with respect to the normality of heterozygotes is necessary because slight clinical manifestations, collectively recognizable but in the individual difficult to distinguish from the normal variation are known in some diseases and are suspected in others. These are more common in the sex-linked inherited metabolic diseases such as glucose-6-phosphate dehydrogenase deficiency, where the female carrier may have increased susceptibility to drug-induced anaemia[1] or Fabry's disease, where the carrier may have corneal opacity.[2] This may be explicable in terms of sex-chromosome inactivation (discussed later), but there are examples for autosomally inherited diseases. Electroencephalographic abnormalities in phenylketonuria heterozygotes have occasionally been noted[3,4] and Gaucher cells have been found in the bone marrow of healthy relatives of patients with Gaucher's disease.[5]

In addition to clinical abnormalities in heterozygotes there are large numbers of reports of biochemical abnormalities.[6] These are also slight, but are more easily quantitated and consequently more simply demonstrated. Most success has been achieved in those diseases in which the primary gene product can be determined, since the loss of one normal gene in heterozygotes may lead to synthesis of approximately half the normal quantity. In the inherited metabolic diseases the gene product is an enzyme which, if it can be assayed in a suitable tissue, may be a good test of genotype (Figure 12.1). This was first demonstrated in the parents (obligate heterozygotes) of children with galactosaemia, who were found to have galactose-1-phosphate uridyl transferase activities

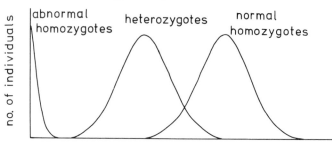

FIGURE 12.1   Distribution of enzyme activity in the three genotypes for an inherited metabolic disease

intermediate between those of their galactosaemic children (mutant homozygotes) and normal individuals (normal homozygotes).[7]

Similar partial enzyme deficiencies in the heterozygous carriers have now been established in a number of inherited metabolic diseases and provisional evidence (one or two family studies) has now been obtained in several others. Usually, direct enzyme assays on tissues from the parents of known cases are compared with those from normal individuals with no family history of the disease. When a suitable tissue cannot be easily obtained indirect assays, such as measurement of the enzyme substrate or product in blood or urine, perhaps after a loading dose of the substrate, may sometimes be used. However, it is not always necessary to be aware of the primary enzyme defect in order to demonstrate biochemical deviations from the norm in heterozygotes, and in the brief review which follows three other methods, in addition to these two types of enzyme assay, are recognized. One, the demonstration of a secondary biochemical abnormality not necessarily directly related to the primary enzyme defect, has been used in both autosomal and sex-linked diseases, but the other two, demonstration of cellular mosaicism and use of genetic linkage analyses, have so far only been used in sex-linked diseases.

Tests of heterozygosity

DIRECT ENZYME ASSAY

Clearly, heterozygotes can only be studied by these methods when the enzyme deficiency associated with a disease has been unequivocally established. In addition, since heterozygous carriers of inherited metabolic disease are clinically normal, with the slight qualifications already mentioned, only tissues obtainable with the minimal risk to the subject can be used for these assays. Peripheral blood erythrocytes, leukocytes or plasma are most convenient and have been widely used, but when this has not been possible, because the enzyme is not measurable even in normal blood or because the deficiency is masked by the presence of interfering isoenzymes, inhibitors or activators, other body fluids or tissues (urine, tears, saliva, cultured cells and some tissue biopsies) have been used. Those diseases known to the author in which at least a single family study has indicated that heterozygotes have lower than normal enzyme activities in one or more of these fluids or tissues are listed in Table 12.1.

Table 12.1 Inherited metabolic diseases in which a partial enzyme deficiency in the heterozygote has been demonstrated by direct enzyme assay in at least one family study

Disease	Enzyme	Tissue used*
Acatalasaemia	catalase	eryth.[119]
		clt. fib.[120]
Adenylate kinase deficiency	adenylate kinase	eryth.[121]
Argininaemia	arginase	eryth.[122]
Argininosuccinic aciduria	argininosuccinase	eryth.[123]
Ataxia, intermittent	pyruvate decarboxylase	clt. fib.[124]
		leuk.[124]
Carnosinaemia	carnosinase	plasma[125]
Combined immuno-deficiency disease	adenosine deaminase	eryth.[126]
Crigler–Najjar syndrome	glucuronyl transferase	liver[38]
Diphosphoglycerate mutase deficiency	2,3-diphosphoglycerate mutase	eryth.[127]
Fabry's disease	α-galactosidase	leuk.[128]
		plasma[129]
		urine[130]
	ceramide trihexosidase	int. mucosa[43]
Fucosidosis	α-fucosidase	leuk.[131]
Galactokinase deficiency	galactokinase	eryth.[132]
Galactosaemia	galactose-1-phosphate uridyl transferase	clt. fib.[133] eryth.[7]

Disease	Enzyme	Tissue used*
Galactose epimerase deficiency	uridine diphospho-galactose-4-epimerase	eryth.[134]
γ-Glutamyl-cysteine synthetase deficiency	γ-glutamyl-cysteine synthetase	eryth.[135]
Gaucher's disease	β-glucosidase	clt. fib.[136] leuk.[137]
	glucocerebrosidase	clt. fib.[17] leuk.[17]
Glucose-6-phosphate dehydrogenase deficiency	glucose-6-phosphate dehydrogenase	eryth.[138] clt. fib.[139] leuk.[140]
Glutathione peroxidase deficiency	glutathione peroxidase	eryth.[141]
Glutathione synthetase deficiency	glutathione synthetase	eryth.[142]
Glycogen storage disease type 1	glucose-6-phosphatase	int. mucosa[41] platelets[35]
Glycogen storage disease type 2	α-glucosidase	clt. lymph.[31] clt. fib.[143] leuk.[143]
	acid maltase	leuk.[144]
Glycogen storage disease type 3	amylo-1,6-glucosidase	leuk.[20]
Glycogen storage disease type 4	brancher enzyme	clt. fib.[145]
Glycogen storage disease type 7	phosphofructokinase	eryth.[146]
Glycogen storage disease type 8	phosphorylase kinase	leuk.[147]
GM1 gangliosidosis	β-galactosidase	leuk.[148]
GM2 gangliosidosis type 1	β-N-acetylhexosaminidase	leuk.[149] plasma[150] saliva[37] tears[37]

Disease	Enzyme	Tissue used*
GM2 gangliosidosis type 2	β-*N*-acetylhexosaminidase	plasma[151]
Hereditary disaccharide intolerance	disaccharidase	int. mucosa[42]
Hexokinase deficiency	hexokinase	eryth.[152]
Hexose phosphate isomerase deficiency	hexose phosphate isomerase	eryth.[153] leuk.[153]
Histidinaemia	histidase	epidermis[36]
Homocystinuria	cystathionine synthase	clt. lymph.[34] clt. fib.[196] liver[39]
Hyperammonaemia type 1	ornithine carbamyl transferase	int. mucosa[40] liver[154]
Hyperlipoproteinaemia type 1	lipoprotein lipase	plasma[155]
Hypophosphatasia	alkaline phosphatase	plasma[156]
Krabbe's disease	galactocerebrosidase	clt. fib.[157] leuk.[157] plasma[157]
Lactosylceramidosis	lactosylceramidase	clt. fib.[158]
Lysosomal acid phosphatase deficiency	acid phosphatase	clt. lymph.[32]
Maple syrup urine disease	α-ketoacid decarboxylase	leuk.[22]
Metachromatic leukodystrophy	arylsulphatase	clt. fib.[159] leuk.[160]
Methaemoglobin reductase (NADP-linked) deficiency	NADP-linked methaemoglobin reductase	eryth.[161]
Methaemoglobinaemia	NAD-linked methaemoglobin reductase	eryth.[162]
Mucopolysaccharidosis type 3B	α-*N*-acetylhexosaminidase	plasma[163]
Mucopolysaccharidosis type 7	β-glucuronidase	clt. fib.[164]
Myeloperoxidase deficiency	myeloperoxidase	leuk.[165]

Disease	Enzyme	Tissue used*
Niemann–Pick disease	sphingomyelinase	leuk.[17]
Orotic aciduria type 1	orotidine-5'-pyrophosphorylase and orotidine-5'-phosphate decarboxylase	eryth.[166]
Orotic aciduria type 2	orotidine-5'-phosphate decarboxylase	eryth.[167]
Pentosuria	xylitol dehydrogenase	eryth.[168]
Phosphoglycerate kinase deficiency	phosphoglycerate kinase	eryth.[169] leuk.[169]
Propionic acidaemia	propionyl-CoA-carboxylase	clt.fib.[170]
Pyrimidine-5'-nucleotidase deficiency	pyrimidine-5'-nucleotidase	eryth.[171]
Pyruvate kinase deficiency	pyruvate kinase	eryth.[8]
Refsum's disease	phytanic acid oxidase	clt.fib.[172]
Suxamethonium sensitivity	cholinesterase	plasma[173]
Triose phosphate isomerase deficiency	triose phosphate isomerase	eryth.[174] leuk.[174]
Wolman's disease	acid esterase	leuk.[175]

* Abbreviations for tissues used: clt. fib. = cultured fibroblasts; clt. lymph. = cultured lymphocytes; eryth. = erythrocytes; int. mucosa = intestinal biopsy; leuk. = leukocytes. Plasma includes serum.

Two of the major difficulties of the use of such enzyme assays to reflect genotype, genetic heterogeneity and tissue specificity, are well illustrated by the congenital non-spherocytic haemolytic anaemia due to pyruvate kinase deficiency. Clinical heterogeneity for this condition has been known for some time since even in the initial reports of the condition it was noted that some patients might have a mild fully-compensated anaemia while others had a severe haemolytic disease presenting in the first weeks of life.[8] Biochemical heterogeneity has been established more recently, however, following investigations of patients, sometimes called type 2 (or type B), with normal erythrocyte pyruvate kinase activity when this is measured using the conventional optimal kinetic conditions. Although the majority of patients, called type 1 (or type A), have 5–30% of the normal activity, and heterozygotes have activities intermediate between this and that of normal homozygotes,[8] the defect in the type 2 patients is not in maximal activity but includes decreased affinity for the substrate phospho-enol pyruvate[9] or for the allosteric effector fructose-1,6-diphosphate,[10] altered pH optimum[11] or electrophoretic mobility[12] and instability either at 37 °C [13] or at higher temperatures.[14]

Another difficulty in the diagnosis of pyruvate kinase deficiency and in the study of heterozygotes, arises because the L (liver) isoenzyme defect in erythrocytes is not accompanied by a defect of the M (muscle) isoenzyme in leukocytes.[8] The erythrocyte defect may therefore be masked by the very high leukocyte activity unless adequate precautions to remove leukocytes are taken.[15] Erythrocyte enzyme activities may vary slightly according to cell age,[16] but leukocyte preparations, often used in the study of lysosomal enzyme deficiencies,[17] contain a number of cell types and enzyme activities may be very variable indeed. This will increase the overlap between all three genotypes, and while it may be possible to minimize the variability,[18,19] significant overlap may still remain. This may be why in glycogen storage disease type 3 some[20] report partial deficiency of amylo-1,6-glucosidase in leukocytes while others[21] do not, and in maple syrup urine disease there are reports both that the measurement of leukocyte α-ketoacid decarboxylase does[22] and does not[23] detect the defect in heterozygotes.

Some studies of heterozygotes have been made using blood plasma or urinary enzyme assays, but these may be complicated by variability in dilution or the presence of inhibitors or other interfering substances. Thus, arylsulphatase should be determined in plasma after separation from interfering phosphate ions by ion-exchange chromatography,[24] but this method has not yet been applied to the study of metachromatic leukodystrophy. The enzyme can be measured in plasma and urine without this ion-exchange step[25,26] but these methods, while useful for the diagnosis of abnormal homozygotes, are not considered to be suitable for heterozygote detection.[25,27,28]

Cultured cells are being increasingly used in the study of inherited metabolic diseases, including heterozygote detection by enzyme assay. Small pieces of skin can now be obtained as simply as a venepuncture, and fibroblasts cultured from such biopsies have revealed partial enzyme deficiencies in the carriers of a number of inherited metabolic diseases (Table 12.1). However, several weeks of culture are normally necessary in order to obtain sufficient cells for biochemical analysis, and the limit of cell growth may be reached before these have accumulated. To date this has limited the usefulness of this technique, but if the culture time can be shortened and microtechniques for enzyme assay in small numbers of cells[29] can be perfected it would have great potential use in heterozygote studies, particularly in those diseases in which the enzyme deficiency cannot be detected in blood or urine.

Blood cells can be cultured much more quickly than fibroblasts because mitosis can be stimulated by phytohaemagglutinin,[30] but unlike fibroblasts the cell lines are not easily maintained. It is therefore difficult to collect sufficient cells for analysis, and very sensitive enzyme assays are required. Nonetheless, Hirschhorn and his colleagues[31] and Nadler and Egan[32] were able to demonstrate partial deficiencies of α-glucosidase and acid phosphatase respectively in lymphocytes cultured from carriers of Pompe's disease and lysosomal acid phosphatase deficiency, in the latter case when the trait in carriers was not demonstrable using uncultured leukocytes. In addition, cystathionine synthase, an enzyme not present in leukocytes, can be measured in cultured lymphocytes[33] allowing the demonstration of intermediate activities in the heterozygous carriers of homocystinuria.[34]

Other tissues have occasionally been used for heterozygote studies. Platelet glucose-6-phosphatase activity is lower than normal in carriers of glycogen storage disease type I[35] and in histidinaemia carriers tend to have lower than normal histidase activity in clippings of epidermal tissue.[36] There is a recent report of β-N-acetyl-hexosaminidase assays in the tears and saliva of carriers of Tay–Sach's disease[37] and one or two groups have even used biopsies of liver in the Crigler–Najjar syndrome,[38] homocystinuria[39] and hyperammonaemia type I[40]; or intestinal mucosa in glycogen storage disease type I,[41] hereditary disaccharide intolerance,[42] Fabry's disease[43] and hyperammonaemia type I.[40]

INDIRECT ENZYME ASSAY

When a suitable tissue for assay of enzyme activity is not available but the enzyme deficiency in the disease has been well characterized, it is sometimes possible to demonstrate heterozygosity by indirect estimation of the *in vivo* enzyme activity. These tests usually take the form of measurements of the enzyme substrate or product in the blood or urine either in standardized conditions such as fasting or after a loading dose of the substrate to stress the enzyme activity.

The first loading test to be used in this way was described by Hsia and his colleagues[44] who gave an oral dose of phenylalanine to the parents (obligate heterozygotes) of children with phenylketonuria. The higher and more prolonged plasma phenylalanine concentrations observed in these parents overlapped to some extent with those of their homozygous phenylketonuric children. Many small modifications of this test have been made in attempts to reduce the overlap between heterozygotes and normal homozygotes, including improved methods of amino acid analysis,[45] larger doses of phenylalanine,[46] intravenous loading[47] and discriminant function analysis.[48] These have met with varying degrees of success, but the overlap cannot be eliminated in this way and the search for qualitative differences between the response of carriers and normals to phenylalanine loads has continued. Recent reports[49,50] suggest that increased urinary o-hydroxy-phenylacetic acid, measured by gas chromatography, after the load, particularly after pretreatment with prednisolone, is characteristic of heterozygotes and distinguishes them from normal homozygotes.

Brown and colleagues[51] have criticized the format of the commonly-used phenylalanine loading test on two counts. Firstly, if a dose based on body weight is used then there is a positive correlation with the degree of obesity, so that more obese subjects are more likely to be considered to be heterozygotes, and secondly, since plasma tyrosine concentration is depressed by pregnancy and oral contraceptives[52,53] and fluctuates during the menstrual cycle, plasma tyrosine should not be included with phenylalanine concentration in assessing the response to the load.

Although by far the most experience has been obtained in phenylketonuria, heterozygotes for some other diseases, when subjected to the same type of loading test, have exhibited diminished tolerance to a substrate load, usually after oral administration of the substrate followed by plasma or urinary substrate (or product, or a related metabolite) determinations (Table 12.2). However, loading tests are time consuming and expensive for the subject, because they may last several days, and for the laboratory, because they may involve many biochemical analyses. Demonstration of the partial deficiency of hepatic cystathionine synthase in carriers of homocystinuria, for example, requires a test lasting 24 hours with at least three blood and two timed urine collections and

Table 12.2   Indirect demonstration of partial enzyme deficiencies in heterozygotes by means of loading tests

Disease	Load*	Abnormality in heterozygotes
Crigler–Najjar syndrome[176]	salicylate	reduced urinary salicyl-glucuronide
Cystathioninuria[177]	methionine	increased urinary cystathionine
Histidinaemia[178]	histidine	delayed fall in plasma histidine
Homocystinuria[54]	methionine	increased plasma and urinary sulphur amino acids
Hydroxykynureninaemia[179]	tryptophan	increased urinary xanthurenic acid
Hyperammonaemia type I[40]	protein	increased plasma ammonia
Methionine malabsorption syndrome[180]	methionine	increased urinary α-hydroxybutyrate
Pentosuria[181]	glucuronolactone	increased plasma and urinary xylulose
Phenylketonuria[44]	phenylalanine	increased plasma phenylalanine
Sarcosinaemia[182]	sarcosine	increased plasma and urinary sarcosine
Wilson's disease[183]	^{64}Cu-copper acetate	reduced plasma ^{64}Cu-caeruloplasmin

* All are oral except for histidinaemia which is intravenous

involving some 16 amino acid analyses.[54] Consequently some groups have developed simpler methods of indirect enzyme assay using single analyses of samples obtained in standardized, usually fasting, conditions (Table 12.3).

SECONDARY BIOCHEMICAL ABNORMALITIES

In those diseases in which the primary enzyme defect is not yet known it may still be possible to demonstrate small biochemical devia-

Table 12.3 **Indirect demonstration of partial enzyme deficiencies in heterozygotes**

Disease	*Abnormality in heterozygotes*
Argininosuccinic aciduria[184]	increased urinary argininosuccinic acid
Cystathioninuria[185]	increased urinary cystathionine
Cystinosis[186]	increased leukocyte and fibroblast cystine
Glycogen storage disease type 6[187]	increased erythrocyte glycogen
Hyperammonaemia type 1[40]	increased fasting plasma ammonia
Iminoglycinuria[188]	increased urinary glycine
Mucopolysaccharidoses[189,190]	increased or abnormal urinary mucopolysaccharides
Nephrogenic diabetes insipidus[191]	decreased urine concentration
Phenylketonuria[192]	increased fasting plasma phenylalanine/tyrosine ratio
Prolinaemia type 1[193]	increased plasma proline
Renal glycosuria[194]	increased urinary glucose
Valinaemia[195]	increased urinary valine

tions from the norm in heterozygotes. Unlike enzyme assays, however, these are not necessarily directly related to the presence or absence of a gene, and therefore lack specificity. Thus, while female carriers of the sex-linked Duchenne[55] and Becker[56] types of muscular dystrophy may have higher than normal plasma creatine kinase activities, this may also be the result of other physiological conditions such as strenuous exercise,[57] psychological conditions, such as acute psychosis,[58] or pathological conditions, such as myocardial infarction.[59]

In addition to problems of specificity the differences between heterozygotes and normal homozygotes are usually not marked. Some 30% of muscular dystrophy carriers have creatine kinase activities within the upper 95% confidence limit of the normal range[60] and there is a marked negative correlation of plasma creatine kinase with age in Becker-type carriers but not in Duchenne-type carriers or normal women, so that the abnormality in older Becker-type carriers may be even less marked.[56] These difficulties have led some groups to abandon the test,[61] and a new test is based on the observation that carriers of this disease have increased protein synthesis in muscle ribosomes.[62] However, this is technically difficult and time consuming and requires muscle biopsy, and it has recently been discovered that pregnancy may interfere with this test by increasing the synthesis rate in normal women into the heterozygote range[63] and it remains to be seen whether oral contraceptives will have the same effect.

It has been reported that heterozygous carriers of the mucopolysaccharidoses and some other diseases can be recognized because their cultured fibroblasts contain metachromatic granules after staining with Toluidine Blue.[64-66] However, the fibroblasts cultured from as many as 30% of patients in paediatric hospitals may exhibit metachromasia in this way, especially after prolonged culture.[67] In addition, both heterozygotes and homozygotes for the mucopolysaccharidoses have these metachromatic cells, so that distinction between these two genotypes is not possible.[68]

Both the cultured fibroblasts[65] and cultured leukocytes[69] of carriers of cystic fibrosis exhibit metachromasia with Toluidine Blue, and slightly higher than normal sweat electrolyte concentrations have also been reported in carriers of this disease.[70] Metachromasia is not specific and the increase in sweat concentration is not marked, however, and it may be that new tests based upon the presence, in the serum of both heterozygotes and homozygotes, of a ciliary dyskinesis factor[71] will be more useful. Similarly, it has recently been reported that urine of both heterozygotes and homozygotes of Leigh's subacute necrotising encephalopathy contains an inhibitor of thiamin pyrophosphate synthesis.[72] In chronic granulomatous disease, thought to be due to a leukocyte NADPH oxidase deficiency[73] carriers have recently been shown to have increased leukocyte phagocytic activity to some organisms but not to the extent seen in patients.[74]

ENZYME MOSAICISM

This method can only be used to demonstrate heterozygosity for sex-linked diseases. It is based upon the phenomenon of X-chromosome inactivation, first postulated by Lyon[75] to explain the occurrence of dosage compensation, or sexual equality in phenotypic expression of sex-linked genes in spite of their duplication in females. One X-chromosome in each female cell is genetically inactivated early in embryogenesis, and since the process is completely random, the normal female is a mosaic for functional maternal and paternal X-chromosomes.

In the sex-linked inherited metabolic diseases the X-chromosome carries an abnormal gene, causing an enzyme deficiency in all the cells of the male hemizygote. In the female carrier, either the X-chromosome carrying the normal gene or the abnormal gene may be inactivated, so that some cells will have deficient enzyme activity and some will be normal. This was first demonstrated in the female heterozygotes for glucose-6-phosphate dehydrogenase deficiency.[76] Clearly then, there is a fundamental difference between the heterozygous carriers of auto-somal and sex-linked diseases, since the approximately half-normal enzyme activity in the former is roughly equally divided between all the cells, but in the latter roughly half the cells have normal activity and the other half have none.

Attempts were soon made to utilize this phenomenon in heterozygote detection for the sex-linked inherited metabolic diseases. In glucose-6-phosphate dehydrogenase deficiency this has been achieved by means of specific staining techniques for the enzyme in erythrocytes.[76-78] Blood from affected hemizygotes, or homozygotes, has no or few positively-stained cells, and from normal homozygotes has entirely positively-stained cells. Heterozygotes have a mixture of both types of cell.

Specific cytochemical stains have not yet been used to demonstrate the heterozygous state for any other sex-linked inherited metabolic disease, but other techniques have been used. Davidson and colleagues[79] showed that it was possible to derive two populations of fibroblasts from skin biopsies of the female carriers of glucose-6-phosphate dehy-drogenase deficiency. Individual fibroblasts were separated from the cultures and grown in clones, some of which had the enzyme activity while others did not. Fibroblast cloning of this type has also revealed enzyme mosaicism in carriers of the Lesch–Nyhan syndrome,[80] phos-phoglycerate kinase deficiency[81] and Fabry's disease.[82] However, cloning is a technically difficult and time-consuming procedure, and mosaicism in the Lesch–Nyhan syndrome has been more simply demonstrated by incubating fibroblasts with radioactively labelled (^{3}H) hypoxanthine. This is a substrate for the enzyme hypoxanthine-guanine phosphori-bosyl transferase deficient in this disease, and two cell types can be demonstrated autoradiographically because the deficient cells do not incorporate the label into the cell nucleic acid.[83]

Some hair follicles are monoclonal, and these have also been used to demonstrate enzyme mosaicism in carriers of the Lesch–Nyhan syndrome.[84] A number of scalp hairs were plucked and the root cells attached to the base analysed for hypoxanthine-guanine phosphoribosyl transferase activity. None of the follicles of affected hemizygotes, and all of those of normal individuals, had activity, while in female heterozygotes there were three types of follicle, some with normal activity, some with no activity and some derived from more than one cell with intermediate activities.

A recent development is the use of a selective medium which favours growth of either the normal or deficient fibroblasts. Migeon[85] showed that inclusion of the purine analogue, 6-thioguanine, in the culture medium selects against normal cells and in favour of those carrying the gene for the Lesch–Nyhan syndrome because the latter are not able to incorporate the analogue into their nucleic acids, and are therefore protected from its disruptive action. Similarly, a difference in viability between fibroblasts with the Hunter's syndrome gene (mucopolysaccharidosis type II) and normal fibroblasts was observed accidentally when it was noticed that the former retain their viability in long-term tissue culture or deep-freeze storage longer than the latter.[86]

Cellular mosaicism for sex-linked genes can sometimes be demonstrated non-enzymically. Fibroblasts grown from the carriers of Hunter's syndrome are mosaic with respect to metachromatic staining with Toluidine Blue[87] and carriers of chronic granulomatosis have two types of leukocyte with respect to bactericidal activity.[88] Pinkerton[89] has demonstrated the presence of two morphological types of erythrocyte in carriers of the sex-linked hypochromic anaemia, and two types of muscle cell have been found in some carriers of the Duchenne-type of muscular dystrophy.[90]

LINKAGE ANALYSES

This method of demonstrating heterozygosity is based upon the measurement of linkage between genes on human chromosomes. However, few linkages are known with accuracy in man, and genes for the inherited metabolic diseases have been assigned with certainty only to the X-chromosomes.[91] The method is therefore only of use in the sex-linked diseases as yet, and even then only in some specific family situations. Examples of the use of this method for genetic counselling purposes are in the literature[92] however, and a good example is that reported by McCurdy.[93] A negro woman carrying the A+ and B+

genes for glucose-6-phosphate dehydrogenase activity (determined electrophoretically) had a son with classical haemophilia (Factor VIII deficiency). Since he carried the A+ dehydrogenase gene, the genetic composition of the mother was established as A+ h/B+ H (where h is the mutant gene for haemophilia and H is the wild-type gene). Examination of the erythrocytes from her daughter revealed only the B+ type of dehydrogenase, so that she was very unlikely to carry the haemophilia gene (her genotype most probably being B+ H/B+ H, and that of her untested father probably being B+ H/Y). In fact the recombinant frequency between the glucose-6-phosphate dehydrogenase and haemophilia loci has been estimated at 0.038,[94] from which it can be calcu lated that the daughter had an approximately 92% probability of being a non-carrier of haemophilia.

Evaluation and interpretation of tests of heterozygosity

Most methods of heterozygote detection measure a variable which is continuously distributed in heterozygotes and normal homozygotes. There is invariably some overlap between these two distributions (Figure 12.1), leading to an element of uncertainty in the interpretation of these tests in individual cases, especially when they fall in or near the overlap region. It may not be clear whether some individuals are heterozygotes even after repeated tests[95] and it has been pointed out that these tests were initially designed not to genotype individuals but to demonstrate the collective partial enzyme deficiency in heterozygotes.[96] Consequently, relatively few applications of tests of heterozygosity have been reported.

The ability of a test to discriminate between the genotypes can be determined by measurement of the overlap between them. This is important both to assess the fallibility of the test in assigning genotype and to evaluate different methods of enzyme assay, since some will be more discriminating than others. When the enzyme activity has a Gaussian distribution in both heterozygotes and normal homozygotes a good measure of the discriminatory ability is given by the generalized distance between the means of the two distributions.[97] This function,

$\dfrac{m_2 - m_1}{s}$ where m_2 and m_1 are the normal and heterozygote distribution

means and s is an estimate of the within-group standard deviation, will increase in magnitude with the discriminatory ability as the means are separated or the standard deviation reduced, either of which will result in decreased overlap (Figure 12.2). It is a standardized deviate, and the distance from each mean to the mid-point $\dfrac{m_2 - m_1}{2s}$ gives, from tables of the normal probability integral, the single tail area of each distribution overlapping this mid-point.

The standard deviation, s, used to calculate the generalized distance is best determined as the arithmetic mean of the heterozygote and normal homozygote standard deviations, $\dfrac{s_1 + s_2}{2}$. As Penrose[97] points out, this gives a better estimate of the within-group standard deviation than the more conventional methods for pooling variances used in significance tests since, in this application where the variances will usually differ markedly, these would give too much weight to the group with the larger variance. The generalized distance determined in this way has a sampling variance given by:

$$\frac{\left(1 + \dfrac{(m_2 - m_1)^2}{8s^2}\right)\left(\dfrac{s_1^2}{n_1} + \dfrac{s_2^2}{n_2}\right)}{s^2}$$

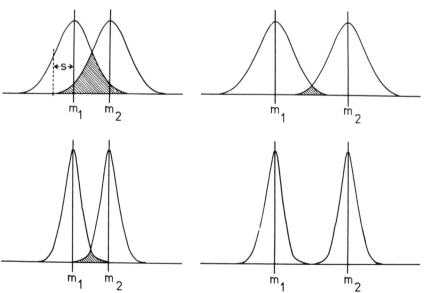

FIGURE 12.2   The effect of variance (s^2) and of the distance between the means ($m_2 - m_1$) on the ability of a discriminant to distinguish between two populations

from which 95% confidence limits for the generalized distance and overlap (%) can be determined.

Overlap between the heterozygote and normal homozygote distributions can also be estimated by a non-parametric method based on percentiles.[98] In this graphical method each test result (enzyme activity) in each distribution is plotted against its estimated percentile, from 100 to 0 for the distribution with the lower median and from 0 to 100 for that with the higher median. The point at which the two distributions intersect is that at which there is the smallest equal percentage overlap between them. This method has been illustrated for the fasting ratio technique to detect heterozygotes for phenylketonuria (Figure 12.3).

A number of methods of assigning genotype from the results of enzyme assays have been proposed. The simplest takes a critical value (C) of the enzyme activity about which classification or allocation can be made. The value most often used is equidistant (in standard deviations) between the means of the two groups in comparison, so that an equal

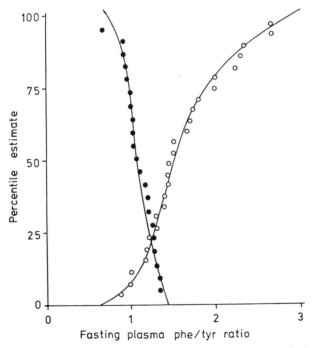

FIGURE 12.3 Percentile method used to measure the ability of the fasting plasma phenylalanine/tyrosine ratio to discriminate between normal homozygotes (●) and phenylketonuria heterozygotes (○)

fraction of each group falls on the wrong side and is consequently mis-classified (Figure 12.4). It is given by $C = \dfrac{(m_1 s_2 + m_2 s_1)}{(s_1 + s_2)}$ where m_1 and m_2 are the means and s_1 and s_2 the standard deviations of the two groups.[97] This value will not give an equal number of misclassifications in each genotype if the distributions in comparison are not the same size, however, and it is not the value at which an individual has an equal chance of heterozygosity or normal homozygosity (Figure 12.4). The latter point is at the intersect of the distributions and will only be at C if they have the same variance and size. For m_1 and m_2, standard deviations s_1 and s_2, and sizes (frequency of each genotype in the population under test) f_1 and f_2, the intersect I, is given by solving the quadratic[99]:

$$I^2 \left(\frac{1}{s_1^2} - \frac{1}{s_2^2} \right) + 2I \left(\frac{m_2}{s_2^2} - \frac{m_1}{s_1^2} \right) + 2In \left(\frac{s_1 \left(1 - \dfrac{f_1}{f_1 + f_2} \right)}{s_2 \left(\dfrac{f_1}{f_1 + f_2} \right)} \right)$$

$$+ \left(\frac{m_1}{s_1} \right)^2 - \left(\frac{m_2}{s_2} \right)^2 = 0$$

I can then be used like the critical value, C, to allocate individuals to one or other genotype.

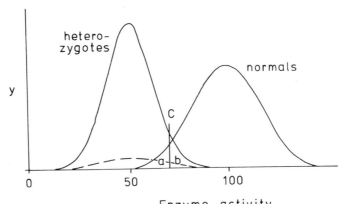

FIGURE 12.4   Interpretation of enzyme assays in assigning genotype. Individuals in the outer tails of the distributions are the most likely to be correctly classified. If the heterozygotes are much less common (interrupted line) than the normal homozygotes they may be difficult to distinguish from normal homozygotes in the lower tail of the normal distribution

These allocation methods have been used to classify individuals even when they fall in the overlap region, whose genotype is consequently in some doubt. In order to avoid this, normal ranges for the distributions, usually the 95% confidence limits, have been defined, so that individuals falling in the overlap region for the two ranges may be left unclassified (Figure 12.5). The size of the unclassified zone will, of course, increase as the discriminatory power of the enzyme assay decreases, and a proportion of individuals will still be wrongly classified (2.5% of each genotype if the 95% limits are used). For this reason more refined limits within which the probability of misclassification is greater than 91% (odds of less than 10 to 1 on either genotype) the following equation is solved for x with y_1/y_2 equal to 10 and 0.1 respectively[100]:

$$2 s_1^2 s_2^2 \log_e \left(\frac{y_1}{y_2} \cdot \frac{f_2}{f_1} \cdot \frac{s_1}{s_2} \right) = s_1^2 (x - m_2)^2 - s_2^2 (x - m_1)^2$$

A deficiency common to all these methods of interpretation is their generality in assigning genotype. Results in a given range are classified with equal certainty, while in fact the possibility of misclassification depends upon the test result (Figure 12.4). This can be avoided by determination of the heterozygote likelihood ratio (HLR), which is the ratio of the probability density functions (y) of the heterozygote and normal distributions (Figure 12.6), calculated for the given test result

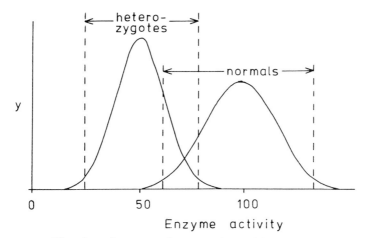

FIGURE 12.5 Allocation of genotype by comparison with ranges derived for the heterozygotes and normal homozygotes. The ranges here are 95% confidence limits, which overlap so individuals with enzyme activities which fall into both ranges are not classified

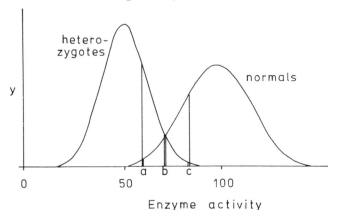

FIGURE 12.6   Determination of the heterozygote likelihood ratio which is the probability density function (i.e. 'height') for the heterozygote distribution at the given
test result divided by that for the normal homozygote distribution at the same result.
Individual a has high odds on heterozygosity, while c has high odds against heterozygosity. Individual b is equally likely to be heterozygous or normal

(enzyme assay). This ratio, which gives the precise odds on heterozygosity, can be found from:

$$\text{HLR} = \frac{s_2 f_1}{s_1 f_2} \cdot \frac{\dfrac{(x - m_2)^2}{2s_2{}^2} \log e}{\dfrac{(x - m_1)^2}{2s_1{}^2} \log e}$$

where e is the natural base

Like the intersect and probability limit methods described above, the
HLR determined in this way allows for differences in the frequency of
each genotype in the population under this test.

The acceptability, to the subjects tested, of the data from these
enzyme assays as probabilities or odds on a given genotype is entirely
unknown, and the opinions of a number of genetic counsellors differ
markedly. Some feel that data in this form is now well understood by
most individuals[101,102] but others consider that the problems of presenting this data are almost insuperable[99,103] or that families expect
more definite advice than this provides.[104] Even if the latter is the case,
it is probably better to present the complete and accurately determined
probability data to the counsellor, so that he at least realizes the certainty with which genotype can be assigned in any particular case.

The role of tests of genotype in preventive medicine

In spite of these difficulties it is now theoretically possible to genotype individuals for some inherited metabolic diseases, to locate couples at risk of bearing affected children, and to eliminate, by prenatal diagnosis and selective abortion or by artificial insemination, the birth of children with the disease.[104-106] The desirability of such a scheme is, of course, open to question and is becoming the subject of considerable discussion,[104,106 108] but it is of interest to examine here the efficiency with which tests of genotype, assuming that they eventually reach a high level of sophistication with no incorrect classifications, could detect abnormal genes in the apparently normal population.

Application of the tests to whole communities, as in some pilot projects to detect carriers of GM2 gangliosidosis[109-111] will allow detection of all heterozygotes but is wasteful because couples at risk could be identified by examining only prospective mothers, who must be heterozygous to conceive a child affected with either an autosomal or sex-linked recessive disease. Fathers need only be tested for autosomal diseases, once the heterozygous mother has been identified. The main difficulty with this type of whole-population screening lies in the large number, and individual rarity, of the diseases, so that testing would be very expensive. In addition, many parents might feel that the inconvenience and anxiety generated bears no relationship to their slight chance of having an affected child, so that voluntary testing would almost certainly result in a poor yield of heterozygotes.[112]

Even for those diseases which have high incidence in small, well-defined communities and for which simple, accurate and inexpensive tests can be developed there are many problems and pitfalls in such screening programmes,[107,113] many of which have been illustrated by the widespread screening for sickle cell anaemia and its carrier status in the USA.[114] These include the delineation of populations at sufficient risk to warrant screening, education to prevent social stigmatization and psychological invalidism in carriers, undue anxiety in perfectly normal parents, and the problem of revealing illegitimacy.

It is now widely felt that tests of genotype should not be applied to the general population until their feasibility, benefits and potential hazards have been carefully investigated in closely monitored pilot programmes.[104,107] Even if they are proved to be financially and socially viable the wisdom of eliminating abnormal genes, some of which may offer a selective advantage to the heterozygote, has quite correctly been questioned.[106] A more practical proposition would appear to be the identification of relatives at risk in families in which a particular disease has already been located.[115] Computerized registers of affected families would facilitate the ascertainment of these relatives, and are already in preparation.[116,117] The maximum proportion of autosomal. recessive disorders that could be prevented in this way would be 15–20%, and of sex-linked disorders would be 20–50% according to their severity[118] but this would be a high yield from tests on very small proportions of the total population.

It is unlikely that prenatal or postnatal treatment of inherited diseases will reach an advanced stage in the foreseeable future[104] and preventive measures of this type currently offer the only alternative. In spite of the difficulties especially in interpretation of quantitative data, formation of genetic registers, education and counselling of families at risk, progress is continuing to be made in this area.[117] The final resolution of the difficulties in genotyping will come with the development of quantitative tests which directly indicate the presence or absence of an abnormal gene, or of tests in which the separation between the genotypes is so great that overlap is negligible. Such negligible overlap is unlikely to be achieved using tests based on enzyme assays, however, because the activities determined only indirectly reflect the presence or absence of an abnormal gene and the enzyme may be subject to genetic and environmental controlling factors and will itself be metabolized.

REFERENCES

1. Trujillo, J., Fairbanks, V., Ohno, S. and Beutler, E. (1961). Chromosomal constitution in glucose-6-phosphate dehydrogenase deficiency. *Lancet*, **ii**, 1454
2. Wise, D., Wallace, H. J. and Jellinck, E. H. (1962). Angiokeratoma corporis diffusum: a clinical study of eight affected families. *Q. J. Med.*, **31**, 177
3. Cowie, V. (1951). Phenylpyruvic oligophrenia. *J. Ment. Sci.*, **97**, 505
4. Fisch, R. O., Sines, L. K., Torres, F. and Anderson, J. A. (1965). Studies on families of phenylketonurics. Observations on intelligence and electroencephalographic changes. *Am. J. Dis. Child.*, **109**, 427
5. Wiedemann, H. R. and Gerken, H. (1964). Gaucher cells in healthy relatives of patients with Gaucher's disease. *Lancet*, **ii**, 866
6. Hsia, D. Y. Y. (1969). The detection of heterozygous carriers. *Med. Clin. North. Am.*, **53**, 857
7. Hsia, D. Y. Y., Huang, I. and Driscoll, S. G. (1958). The heterozygous carrier in galactosaemia. *Nature, (London)*, **182**, 1389
8. Tanaka, K. R., Valentine, W. N. and Miwa, S. (1962). Pyruvate kinase deficiency hereditary non-spherocytic haemolytic anaemia. *Blood*, **19**, 267
9. Paglia, D. E., Valentine, W. N., Baughan, M. A., Miller, D. R., Reed, C. F. and McIntyre, O. R. (1968). An inherited molecular lesion of erythrocyte pyruvate kinase. Identification of a kinetically aberrant isozyme associated with premature haemolysis. *J. Clin. Invest.*, **47**, 1929

10. BUSH, D., HOFFBAUER, R. W., BLUME, K. G. and LOHR, G. W. (1969). Kinetic properties of pyruvate kinase and problems of therapy in different types of pyruvate kinase deficiency. In B. Ramor (ed.), *Red Cell Structure and Metabolism*, p. 193. (London and New York: Academic Press)
11. PAGLIA, D. E., RUCKNAGEL, D. L. and VALENTINE, W. N. (1972). Defective erythrocyte pyruvate kinase with impaired kinetics and reduced optimal activity. *Br. J. Haematol.*, **22**, 651
12. LÖHR, G. W., BLUME, K. G., RÜDIGER, H. W., SOKAL, G. and GULBIS, E. (1968). A new type of pyruvate kinase deficiency of human erythrocytes. *Lancet*, **i**, 753
13. BRANDT, N. J. and HANEL, H. K. (1971). Atypical pyruvate kinase in a patient with haemolytic anaemia. *Scand. J. Haematol.*, **8**, 126
14. STAAL, G., KOSTER, J. and NIJESSEN, J. (1972). New variant of red blood cell pyruvate kinase deficiency. *Biochim. Biophys. Acta*, **258**, 685
15. WESTWOOD, A. (1975). Rapid micro-method for the preparation of leucocyte-free haemolysates for the determination of pyruvate kinase and other erythrocyte enzymes. *Ann. Clin. Biochem.*, **12**, 263
16. POWELL, R. D. and DEGOWIN, R. L. (1965). Relationship between activity of pyruvate kinase and age of the normal human erythrocyte. *Nature (London)*, **205**, 507
17. BRADY, R. O., JOHNSON, W. G. and UHLENDORF, B. W. (1971). Identification of heterozygous carriers of lipid storage diseases. *Am. J. Med.*, **51**, 423
18. HARZER, K. (1973). Inheritance of the enzyme deficiency in three neurolipidoses: variant O of Tay–Sach's disease (Sandhoff's disease), classic Tay–Sach's disease and metachromatic leucodystrophy. Identification of heterozygous carriers. *Hum. Genet.*, **20**, 9
19. YOUNG, E., WILCOX, P., WHITFIELD, A. G. and PATRICK, A. D. (1975). Variability of acid hydrolase activities in cultured skin fibroblasts and amniotic fluid cells. *J. Med. Genet.*, **12**, 224
20. WILLIAMS, C. and FIELD, J. B. (1968). Studies in glycogen storage disease. III Limit dextrinosis: a genetic study. *J. Pediatr.*, **72**, 214
21. HUIJING, F., KLEIN OBBINK, H. J. and VAN CREVELD, S. (1968). The activity of the debranching enzyme system in leucocytes. *Acta Genet.*, **18**, 128
22. DANCIS, J., HUTZLER, J. and LEVITZ, M. (1965). Detection of the heterozygote in maple syrup urine disease. *J. Pediatr.*, **66**, 595
23. MCKNIGHT, M. T. and SPENCE, M. W. (1972). Attempted detection of heterozygotes for maple syrup urine disease. *Clin. Genet.*, **3**, 458
24. RINDERKNECHT, H., GEOKAS, M. C., CARMACK, C. and HAVERBACK, B. J. (1970). The determination of arylsulphatases in biological fluids. *Clin. Chim. Acta*, **29**, 481
25. BERATIS, N. G., ARON, A. M. and HIRSCHHORN, K. (1973). Metachromatic leucodystrophy: detection in serum. *J. Pediatr.*, **83**, 824
26. SINGH, J., TAVELLA, D. and DI FERRANTE, N. (1975). Measurement of arylsulphatases A and B in human serum. *J. Pediatr.*, **86**, 574
27. AUSTIN, J., ARMSTRONG, D., SHEARER, L. and McAFEE, D. (1966). Metachromatic form of diffuse cerebral sclerosis. VI A rapid test for the sulphatase A deficiency in metachromatic leucodystrophy (MLD) urine. *Arch. Neurol.*, **14**, 259
28. THOMAS, G. H. and HOWELL, R. R. (1972). Arylsulphatase A activity in human urine: quantitative studies on patients with lysosomal disorders including metachromatic leucodystrophy (MLD). *Clin. Chim. Acta*, **36**, 99
29. GALJAARD, H., VAN HOOGSTRATEN, J. J., DE JOSSELIN DE JONG, J. E. and MULDER, M. P. (1974). Methodology of the quantitative cytochemical analysis of single or small numbers of cultured cells. *Histochem. J.*, **6**, 409
30. NOWELL, P. C. (1960). Phytohaemagglutinin: an initiator of mitosis in cultures of normal human lymphocytes. *Cancer Res.*, **20**, 462
31. HIRSHHORN, K., NADLER, H. L., WAITHE, W. I., BROWN, B. I. and HIRSHHORN, R. (1969). Pompe's disease: detection of heterozygotes by lymphocyte stimulation. *Science (N.Y.)*, **166**, 1632
32. NADLER, H. L. and EGAN, T. J. (1970). Deficiency of lysosomal acid phosphatase. A new familial metabolic disorder. *N. Engl. J. Med.*, **282**, 302
33. GOLDSTEIN, J. L., CAMPBELL, B. K. and GARTLER, S. M. (1972). Cystathionine synthetase activity in human lymphocytes: induction by phytohaemagglutinin. *J. Clin. Invest.*, **51**, 1034
34. GOLDSTEIN, J. L., CAMPBELL, B. K. and GARTLER, S. M. (1973). Homocystinuria:

heterozygote detection using phytohaemagglutinin-stimulated lymphocytes. *J. Clin. Invest.*, **52**, 218

35. NEGISHI, H., MORISHITA, Y., KODAMA, S. and MATSUO, T. (1974). Platelet glucose-6-phosphatase activity in patients with Von Gierke's disease and their parents. *Clin. Chim. Acta*, **53**, 175

36. LA DU, B. N., HOWELL, R. R., JACOBY, G. A., SEEGMILLER, J. E., SOBER, E. K., ZANNONI, V. G., CANBY, J. P. and ZIEGLER, L. K. (1963). Clinical and biochemical studies on two cases of histidinaemia. *Pediatrics*, **32**, 216

37. SINGER, J. D., COTLIER, E. and KRIMMER, R. (1973). Hexosaminidase A in tears and saliva for rapid indentification of Tay–Sach's disease and its carriers. *Lancet*, **ii**, 1116

38. ARIAS, I. M. (1962). Chronic unconjugated hyperbilirubinaemia without overt signs of haemolysis in adolescents and adults. *J. Clin. Invest.*, **41**, 2233

39. FINKELSTEIN, J. D., MUDD, S. H., IRREVERRE, F. and LASTER, L. (1964). Homocystinuria due to cystathionine synthetase deficiency: the mode of inheritance. *Science (N.Y.)*, **146**, 785

40. LEVIN, B., ABRAHAM, J. M., OBERHOLZER, V. G. and BURGESS, E. A. (1969). Hyperammonaemia: a deficiency of liver ornithine transcarbamylase. Occurrence in mother and child. *Arch. Dis. Child.*, **44**, 152

41. FIELD, J. B., EPSTEIN, S. and EGAN, T. (1965). Studies in glycogen storage diseases. I Intestinal glucose-6-phosphatase activity in patients with Von Gierke's disease and their parents. *J. Clin. Invest.*, **44**, 1240

42. PRADER, A. and AURICCHIO, S. (1965). Defect of intestinal disaccharide absorption. *Ann. Rev. Med.*, **16**, 345

43. BRADY, R. O., GAL, A. E., BRADLEY, R. M., MARTENSSON, E., WARSHAW, A. L. and LASTER, L. (1967). Enzymatic defect in Fabry's disease, ceramide trihexosidase deficiency. *N. Engl. J. Med.*, **276**, 1163

44. HSIA, D. Y. Y., DRISCOLL, K. W., TROLL, W. and KNOX, W. E. (1956). Detection by phenylalanine tolerance tests of heterozygous carriers for phenylketonuria. *Nature (London)*, **178**, 1239

45. RAMPINI, S., ANDERS, P. W., CURTUIS, H. C. and MARTHALER, T. (1969). Detection of heterozygotes for phenylketonuria by column chromatography and discriminatory analysis. *Pediatr. Res.*, **3**, 287

46. JERVIS, G. A. (1960). Detection of heterozygotes for phenylketonuria. *Clin. Chim. Acta*, **5**, 471

47. BREMER, H. J. and NEUMANN, W. (1966). Tolerance of phenylalanine after intravenous administration in phenylketonurics, heterozygous carriers, and normal adults. *Nature (London)*, **209**, 1148

48. WANG, H. L., MORTON, N. E. and WAISMAN, H. A. (1961). Increased reliability for the determination of the carrier state in phenylketonuria. *Am. J. Hum. Genet.*, **13**, 255

49. BLAU, K., SUMMER, G. K., NEWSOME, H. C., EDWARDS, C. H. and MAMER, O. A. (1973). Phenylalanine loading and aromatic acid excretion in normal subjects and heterozygotes for phenylketonuria. *Clin. Chim. Acta*, **45**, 197

50. KOEPP, P. and HOFFMAN, B. (1975). Detection of heterozygotes for phenylketonuria and hyperphenylalaninaemia by gas chromatographic analysis of aromatic acid excretion in urine. *Clin. Chim. Acta*, **58**, 215

51. BROWN, E. S., WAISMAN, H. A., SWANSON, M. A., COLWELL, R. E., BANKS, M. E. and GERRITSEN, T. (1973). Effects of oral contraceptives and obesity on carrier tests for phenylketonuria. *Clin. Chim. Acta*, **44**, 183

52. ROSE, D. P. and CRAMP, D. G. (1970). Reduction of plasma tyrosine by oral contraceptives and oestrogens: a possible consequence of tyrosine aminotransferase induction. *Clin. Chim. Acta*, **29**, 49

53. YAKYMYSHYN, L. Y., REID, D. W. J. and CAMPBELL, D. J. (1972). Problems in the biochemical detection of heterozygotes for phenylketonuria. *Clin. Biochem.*, **5**, 73

54. SARDHARWALLA, I. B., FOWLER, B., ROBINS, A. J. and KOMROWER, G. M. (1974). Detection of heterozygotes for homocystinuria: study of sulphur-containing amino acids in plasma and urine after L-methionine loading. *Arch. Dis. Child.*, **49**, 553

55. OKINAKA, S., SUGITA, H., MOMOI, H., TOYOKURA, Y., KUMAGAI, H., EBASHI, S. and FUJIE, Y. (1959). Serum creatine phosphokinase and aldolase activity in neuromuscular disorders. *Trans. 84th Ann. Meet. Am. Neurol. Ass.*, p. 62

56. SKINNER, R., EMERY, A. E. H., ANDERSON, A. J. B. and FOXALL, C. (1975). The

detection of carriers of benign (Becker-type) X-linked muscular dystrophy. *J. Med. Genet.*, **12**, 131

57. GRIFFITHS, P. D. (1966). Serum levels of ATP: creatine phosphotransferase (creatine kinase). The normal range and effect of muscular activity. *Clin. Chim. Acta*, **13**, 413

58. ENGEL, W. K. and MELTZER, H. (1970). Histochemical abnormalities of skeletal muscle in patients with acute psychoses. *Science (N.Y.)*, **168**, 273

59. HUGHES, B. P. (1962). A method for the estimation of serum creatine kinase and its use in comparing creatine kinase and aldolase activity in normal and pathological sera. *Clin. Chim. Acta*, **7**, 597

60. THOMPSON, M. W., MURPHY, E. G. and McALPINE, P. J. (1967). An assessment of the creatine kinase test in the detection of Duchenne muscular dystrophy. *J. Pediatr.*, **71**, 82

61. MILHORAT, A. (1974). Cited in SIMPSON, J., ZELLWEGER, H., BURMEISTER, L. F., CHRISTIE, R. and NIELSEN, M. KAY. Effect of oral contraceptive pills on the level of creatine phosphokinase with regard to carrier detection in Duchenne muscular dystrophy. *Clin. Chim. Acta*, **52**, 219

62. IONASESCU, V., ZELLWEGER, H., SHIRK, P. and CONWAY, T. W. (1973). Identification of carriers of Duchenne muscular dystrophy by muscle protein synthesis. *Neurology*, **23**, 497

63. IONASESCU, V., WHITE, C., ZELLWEGER, H., LEWIS, R. and CONWAY, R. W. (1974). Muscle ribosomal protein synthesis in normal pregnancy: implication for carrier detection in Duchenne muscular dystrophy. *J. Med. Genet.*, **11**, 114

64. DANES, B. S. and BEARN, A. G. (1967). Cellular metachromasia, a genetic marker for studying the mucopolysaccharidoses. *Lancet*, **i**, 241

65. DANES, B. S. and BEARN, A. G. (1968). A genetic cell marker in cystic fibrosis of the pancreas. *Lancet*, **i**, 1061

66. DANES, B. S. and BEARN, A. G. (1968). Gaucher's disease: A genetic disease detected in skin fibroblasts, *Science (N.Y.)*, **161**, 1347

67. TAYSI, K., KISTENMACHER, M. L., PUNNETT, H. H. and MELLMAN, W. J. (1969). Limitations of metachromasia as a diagnostic aid in paediatrics. *N. Engl. J. Med.*, **281**, 1108

68. MATALON, R. and DORFMAN, A. (1969). Acid mucopolysaccharides in cultured human fibroblasts. *Lancet*, **ii**, 838

69. McMANUS, S. P. and MASTERSON, J. (1974). Cellular metachromasia with toluidine blue O in cultured white cells of cystic fibrosis heterozygotes. *J. Med. Genet.*, **11**, 216

70. DI SANT'AGNESE, P. A. and POWELL, G. F. (1962). The eccrine sweat defect in cystic fibrosis of the pancreas (mucoviscidosis). *Ann. N. Y. Acad. Sci.*, **93**, 555

71. BOWMAN, B. H., LOCKHART, L. H. and COMBS, M. L. (1969). Oyster ciliary inhibition by cystic fibrosis factor. *Science (N.Y.)*, **164**, 325

72. MURPHY, J. V. (1973). Subacute necrotizing encephalomyelopathy (Leigh's disease): detection of the heterozygous carrier state. *Pediatrics*, **51**, 710

73. HOHN, D. C. and LEHRER, R. I. (1974). Identification of the defect in X-linked chronic granulomatous disease. *Clin. Res.*, **22**, 394

74. BIGGAR, W. D. (1975). Phagocytosis in patients and carriers of chronic granulomatous disease. *Lancet*, **i**, 991

75. LYON, M. F. (1961). Gene action in the X-chromosome of the mouse. *Nature (London)*, **190**, 372

76. BEUTLER, E., YEH, M. and FAIRBANKS, V. F. (1962). The normal human female as a mosaic of X-chromosome activity: studies using the gene for G-6-PD deficiency as marker. *Proc. Natl. Acad. Sci. U.S.A.*, **48**, 9

77. GALL, J. C., BREWER, G. J. and DERN, R. J. (1965). Studies of glucose-6-phosphate dehydrogenase activity of individual erythrocytes: the methaemoglobin-elution test for identification of females heterozygous for G-6-PD deficiency. *Am. J. Hum. Genet.*, **17**, 359

78. FAIRBANKS, V. F. and LAMPE, L. T. (1968). A tetrazolium-linked cytochemical method for estimation of glucose-6-phosphate dehydrogenase activity in individual eyrthrocytes: applications in the study of heterozygotes for glucose-6-phosphate dehydrogenase deficiency. *Blood*, **31**, 589

79. DAVIDSON, R. G., NITOWSKY, H. M. and CHILDS, B. (1963). Determination of the two populations of cells in the human female heterozygous for G-6-PD variants. *Proc. Natl. Acad. Sci. U.S.A.*, **50**, 481

80. MIGEON, B. R., DER KALOUSTIAN, V. M., NYHAN, W. L., YOUNG, W. J. and CHILDS, B. (1968). X-linked hypoxanthine-guanine phosphoribosyl transferase deficiency: heterozygote has two clonal populations. *Science* (*N.Y.*), **160**, 425
81. DEYS, B. F., GRZESCHICK, K. H., GRZESCHICK, A., JAFFE, E. R. and SINISCALCO, M. (1972). Human phosphoglycerate kinase and inactivation of the X chromosome. *Science* (*N.Y.*), **175**, 1002
82. ROMEO, G. and MIGEON, B. R. (1970). Genetic inactivation of the alpha-galactosidase locus in carriers of Fabry's disease. *Science* (*N.Y.*), **170**, 180
83. ROSENBLOOM, F. M., KELLEY, W. N., HENDERSON, J. F. and SEEGMILLER, J. E. (1967). Lyon hypothesis and X-linked disease. *Lancet*, **ii**, 305
84. GARTLER, S. M., SCOTT, R. C., GOLDSTEIN, J. L., CAMPBELL, B. and SPARKES, R. M. (1971). Lesch–Nyhan syndrome: rapid detection of heterozygotes by use of hair follicles. *Science* (*N.Y.*), **172**, 572
85. MIGEON, B. R. (1970). X-linked hypoxanthine-guanine phosphoribosyl transferase (HGPRT) deficiency: detection of heterozygotes by selective medium. *Biochem. Genet.*, **4**, 377
86. BOOTH, C. W. and NADLER, H. L. (1974). Demonstration of the heterozygous state in Hunter's syndrome. *Pediatrics*, **53**, 396
87. DANES, B. S. and BEARN, A. G. (1967). Hurler's syndrome: a genetic study of clones in cell culture with particular reference to the Lyon hypothesis. *J. Exp. Med.*, **126**, 509
88. WINDHORST, D. B., HOLMES, B. and GOOD, R. A. (1967). A newly defined X-linked trait in man with demonstration of the Lyon effect in carrier females. *Lancet*, **i**, 737
89. PINKERTON, P. H. (1967). X-linked hypochromic anaemia. *Lancet*, **i**, 1106.
90. PEARSON, C. M., FOWLER, W. M. and WRIGHT, S. W. (1963). X-chromosome mosaicism in females with muscular dystrophy. *Proc. Natl. Acad. Sci. U.S.A.*, **50**, 29
91. MCKUSICK, V. A. (1975). *Mendelian Inheritance in Man*. 4th ed. (Baltimore: Johns Hopkins University Press)
92. ROBERTS, J. A. F. (1973). *An Introduction to Medical Genetics*. 6th ed. (London: Oxford University Press)
93. MCCURDY, P. R. (1971). Use of genetic linkage for the detection of female carriers of haemophilia. *N. Engl. J. Med.*, **285**, 218
94. BOYER, S. H. and GRAHAM, J. B. (1965). Linkage between the X-chromosome loci for glucose-6-phosphate dehydrogenase electrophoretic variation and haemophilia A. *Am. J. Hum. Genet.*, **17**, 320
95. ROSENBERG, L. E. (1970). In M. Harris (ed), *Early Diagnosis of Human Genetic Defects*, p. 121. (Bethesda, Maryland: H.E.W. Publication No. (NIH) 72–75)
96. HSIA, D. Y. Y. (1970). In M. Harris (ed.), *Early Diagnosis of Human Genetic Defects*, p. 121, (Bethesda, Maryland: H.E.W. Publication No. (NIH) 72–75)
97. PENROSE, L. S. (1951). Measurement of pleiotropic effects in phenylketonuria. *Ann. Eugenics*, **16**, 134
98. WESTWOOD, A. and RAINE, D. N. (1975). Heterozygote detection in phenylketonuria. Measurement of discriminatory ability and interpretation of the phenylalanine loading test by determination of the heterozygote likelihood ratio. *J. Med. Genet.*, **12**, 327
99. GOLD, R. J. M., MAAG, U. R., NEAL, J. L. and SCRIVER, C. R. (1973). The use of biochemical data in screening for mutant alleles and in genetic counselling. *Ann. Hum. Genet.*, **37**, 315
100. WALKER, F. A., HSIA, D. Y. Y., SLATIS, H. M. and STEINBERG, A. G. (1962). Galactosaemia: a study of twenty-seven kindreds in North America. *Ann. Hum. Genet.*, **25**, 287
101. CARTER, C. O., EVANS, K. A., ROBERTS, J. A. F. and BUCK, A. R. (1971). Genetic clinic: a follow-up. *Lancet*, **i**, 281
102. CLARKE, C. A. (1972). Genetic counselling. *Br. Med. J.*, **1**, 606
103. LEONARD, C. O., CHASE, G. A. and CHILDS, B. (1972). Genetic counselling: a consumers view. *N. Engl. J. Med.*, **287**, 433
104. MOTULSKY, A. G. (1974). Brave New World? *Science* (*N.Y.*), **185**, 653
105. SPAETH, G. L. (1974). The carrier state. In M. F. Goldberg (ed.), *Genetic and Metabolic Eye Disorders*, p. 3. (Boston: Little, Brown and Company)
106. JONES, A. and BODMER, W. F. (1974). *Our Future Inheritance: Choice or Chance?* (London: Oxford University Press)

107. KABACK, M. M. (1973). Heterozygote screening—a social challenge. *N. Engl. J. Med.*, **289**, 1090
108. ROSNER, F. (1973). Screening for genetic disease. *N. Engl. J. Med.*, **289**, 221
109. KABACK, M. M. and ZEIGLER, R. S. (1972). Heterozygote detection in Tay–Sach's disease: a prototype community screening programme for the prevention of recessive genetic disorders. *Adv. Exp. Med. Biol.*, **19**, 613
110. EVANS, P. (1973). Testing for Tay–Sach's heterozygotes. *Lancet*, **ii**, 391
111. LOWDEN, J. A., SKOMOROWSKI, M. A., HENDERSON, F. and KABACK, M. M. (1973). Automated assay of hexosaminidases in serum. *Clin. Chem.*, **19**, 1345
112. KABACK, M. M. and O'BRIEN, J. S. (1973). Tay–Sacks': a prototype for prevention of genetic disease. *Hosp. Pract.*, **8**, 107
113. EDWARDS, J. H. (1973). Testing for Tay–Sach's heterozygotes. *Lancet*, **ii**, 1143
114. MOTULSKY, A. G. (1973). Screening for sickle cell haemoglobinopathy and thalassaemia. *Isr. J. Med. Sci.*, **9**, 1341
115. SMITH, C., HOLLOWAY, S and EMERY, A. E. H. (1971). Individuals at risk in families with genetic disease. *J. Med. Genet.*, **8**, 453
116. EMERY, A. E. H., ELLIOTT, D., MOORES, M. and SMITH, C. (1974). A genetic register system (RAPID). *J. Med. Genet.*, **11**, 145
117. RAINE, D. N. (1974). The need for a national policy for the management of inherited metabolic disease. *J. Clin. Pathol.*, 27 (Suppl.), **8**, 156
118. SMITH, C. (1970). Ascertaining those at risk in the prevention and treatment of genetic disease. In A. E. H. Emery (ed.), *Modern Trends in Human Genetics—1*, p.350. (London: Butterworths)
119. NISHIMURA, E. T., HAMILTON, H. B., KOBARA, T. Y., TAKAHARA, S., OGURA, Y. and DOI, K. (1959). Carrier state in human acatalasaemia. *Science (N.Y.)*, **130**, 333
120. KROOTH, R. S., HOWELL, R. R. and HAMILTON, H. B. (1962). Properties of acatalasic cells growing *in vitro*. *J. Exp. Med.*, **115**, 313
121. SZEINBERG, A., KAHANA, D., GAVENDO, S., ZAIDMAN, J. and BEN-EZZER, J. (1969). Hereditary deficiency of adenylate kinase in red blood cells. *Acta Haematol.* **42**, 111
122. TERHEGGEN, H. G., SCHWENK, A., LOWENTHAL, A., VAN SANDE, M. and COLOMBO, J. P. (1969). Argininaemia with arginase deficiency. *Lancet*, **ii**, 748
123. TOMLINSON, S. and WESTALL, R. G. (1964). Argininosuccinic aciduria. Argininosuccinase and arginase in human blood cells. *Clin. Sci.*, **26**, 261
124. BLASS, J. P., AVIGAN, J. and UHLENDORF, B. W. (1970). A defect in pyruvate decarboxylase in a child with an intermittent movement disorder. *J. Clin. Invest.*, **49**, 423
125. HEESWIJK, P. J., TRIJBELS, J. M. F., SCHRETLEN, A. M., VAN MUNSTER, P. J. J. and MONNENS, L. A. H. (1969). A patient with a deficiency of serum carnosinase activity. *Acta Paediatr. Scand.*, **58**, 584
126. SCOTT, C. R., CHEN, S. H. and GIBLETT, E. R. (1974). Detection of the carrier state in combined immunodeficiency disease associated with adenosine deaminase deficiency. *J. Clin. Invest.*, **53**, 1194
127. SCHROTER, W. (1965). Kongenitale nichtspharocytare hamolytische anamie bei 2,3-diphosphoglyceratmutose-mangel der erythrocyten im fruhen sauglingsalter. *Klin. Wochenschr.*, **43**, 1147
128. KINT, J. A. (1970). Fabry's disease: alpha-galactosidase deficiency. *Science (N.Y.)*, **167**, 1268
129. DESNICK, R. J., ALLEN, K. Y., DESNICK, S. J., RAMEN, M. K., BERNLOHR, R. W. and KRIVIT, W. (1973). Fabry's disease: enzymatic diagnosis of hemizygotes and heterozygotes. *J. Lab. Clin. Med.*, **81**, 157
130. RIETRA, P. J. G. M., TAGER, J. M. and DE GROOT, W. P. (1972). Detection of Fabry hemizygotes and heterozygotes by measurement of alpha-galactosidase in urine. *Clin. Chim. Acta*, **40**, 229
131. MATSUDA, I., ARASHIMA, S., ANAKURA, M. and OKA, Y. (1973). Alpha-L-fucosidase and alpha-D-mannosidase activity in the white blood cells in the disease and carrier state of fucosidosis. *Clin. Chim. Acta*, **48**, 9
132. GITZELMANN, R. (1967). Hereditary galactokinase deficiency, a newly recognised cause of juvenile cataracts. *Pediatr. Res.*, **1**, 14
133. KROOTH, R. S. and WEINBERG, A. N. (1961). Studies on cell lines developed from the tissues of patients with a galactosaemia. *J. Exp. Med.*, **113**, 1155
134. GITZELMANN, R. and STEINMANN, B. (1973). Uridine diphosphate galactose-4-epimerase deficiency. II Clinical follow-up, biochemical studies and family investigation. *Helv. Paediatr. Acta*, **28**, 497

135. KONRAD, P. M., RICHARDS, F., VALENTINE, W. N. and PAGLIA, D. E. (1972). Gamma-glutamyl-cysteine synthetase deficiency: a cause of hereditary haemolytic anaemia. *N. Engl. J. Med.*, **286**, 557

136. BEUTLER, E., KUHL, W., TRINIDAD, F., TEPLITZ, R. and NADLER, H. (1970). Detection of Gaucher's disease and its carrier state from fibroblasts cultures. *Lancet*, **ii**, 369

137. BEUTLER, E. and KUHL, K. (1970). The diagnosis of the adult type of Gaucher's disease and its carrier state by demonstration of deficiency of beta-glucosidase activity in peripheral blood leucocytes. *J. Lab. Clin. Med.*, **76**, 747

138. CHILDS, B., ZINKHAM, W., BROWNE, E. A., KIMBRO, E. L. and TOBERT, J. V. (1958). A genetic study of a defect in glutathione metabolism of the erythrocyte. *Bull. Johns Hopkins Hosp.*, **102**, 21

139. GARTLER, S. H. (1961). Maintenance of genetically determined glucose-6-phosphates dehydrogenase differences in human cell culture. *Proc. 2nd Int. Con. Hum. Genet.*, *1*, 622

140. RAMOT, B., FISHER, S., SZEINBERG, A., ADAM, A., SHEBA, C. and GAFNI, D. (1959). A study of subjects with erythrocyte G-6-PD deficiency. II Investigation of leucocyte enzymes. *J. Clin. Invest.*, **38**, 2234

141. NECHELES, T. F., MALDONADO, N., BARQUET-CHEDIAK, A. and ALLEN, D. M. (1969). Homozygous erythrocyte glutathione peroxidase deficiency: clinical and bio-chemical studies. *Blood*, **33**, 164

142. MOHLER, D. N., MAJERUS, P. W., MINNICH, V., HESS, C. E. and GARRICK, M. D. (1970). Glutathione synthetase deficiency as a cause of hereditary haemolytic disease. *N. Engl. J. Med.*, **283**, 1253

143. NITOWSKY, H. M. and GRUNFELD, A. (1967). Lysosomal alpha-glucosidase in type II glycogenosis: activity in leucocytes and cell cultures in relation to genotype. *J. Lab. Clin. Med.*, **69**, 472

144. KOSTER, J. F., SLEE, R. G. and HULSMANN, W. C. (1974). The use of leucocytes as an aid in the diagnosis of glycogen storage disease type II (Pompe's disease). *Clin. Chim. Acta*, **51**, 319

145. HOWELL, R. R., KABACK, M. M. and BROWN, B. I. (1971). Type IV glycogen storage disease. Branching enzyme deficiency in skin fibroblasts and possible heterozygote detection. *J. Pediatr.*, **78**, 638

146. TARUI, S., KONO, N., NASU, T. and NISHIKAWA, M. (1969). Enzymatic basis for the coexistence of myopathy and haemolytic disease in inherited muscle phosphofructokinase deficiency. *Biochem. Biophys. Res. Commun.*, **34**, 77

147. HUIJING, F. and FERNANDES, J. (1969). X-chromosomal inheritance of liver glycogenosis with phosphorylase kinase deficiency. *Am. J. Hum. Genet.*, **21**, 275

148. KINT. J. A., DACREMONT, G. and VLIETINCK, R. (1969). Type II GM₁ gangliosidosis? *Lancet*, **ii**, 108

149. FRIEDLAND, J., SCHNECK, L., SAIFER, A., POURFAR, M. and VOLK, B. W. (1970). Identification of Tay–Sach's disease carriers by acrylamide gel electrophoresis. *Clin. Chim. Acta*, **28**, 397

150. O'BRIEN, J. S., OKADA, S., CHEN, A. and FILLERUP, D. L. (1970). Tay–Sach's disease. Detection of heterozygotes and homozygotes by serum hexosaminidase assay. *N. Engl. J. Med.*, **283**, 15

151. SUZUKI, Y., KOIZUMI, Y., TOGARI, H. and OGAWA, Y. (1973). Sandhoff disease: diagnosis of heterozygous carriers by serum hexosaminidase assay. *Clin. Chim. Acta*, **48**, 153

152. VALENTINE, W. N., OSKI, F. A., PAGLIA, D. E., BAUGHAN, M. A. and SCHNEIDER, A. S. (1967). Hereditary haemolytic anaemia with hexokinase deficiency. *N. Engl. J. Med.*, **276**, 1

153. PAGLIA, D. E., HOLLAND, P., BAUGHN, M. A. and VALENTINE, W. N. (1969). Occurence of defective hexose phosphate isomerization in human erythrocytes and leukocytes. *N. Engl. J. Med.*, **280**, 66

154. LEVIN. B., OBERHOLZER, V. G. and SINCLAIR, L. (1969). Biochemical investigations of hyperammonaemia. *Lancet*, **ii**, 170

155. HAVEL, R. J. and GORDON, R. S. (1960). Idiopathic hyperlipaemia: metabolic studies in an affected family. *J. Clin. Invest.*, **39**, 1777

156. HARRIS, H. and ROBSON, E. B. (1959). A genetical study of ethanolamine phosphate excretion in hypophosphatasia. *Ann. Hum. Genet.*, **23**, 421

157. SUZUKI, Y. and SUZUKI, K. (1971). Krabbe's globoid cell leucodystrophy.

Deficiency of galactocerebrosidase in serum, leucocytes, and fibroblasts. *Science (N.Y.)*, **171**, 73

158. DAWSON, G., MATALON, R. and STEIN, A. O. (1971). Lactosylceramidosis: lactosylceramide galactosyl hydrolase deficiency and accumulation of lactosyl-ceramide in cultured skin fibroblasts. *J. Pediatr.*, **79**, 423

159. LEROY, J. G., DUMON, J. and RADERMECKER, J. (1970). Deficiency of aryl-sulphatase A in leucocytes and skin fibroblasts in juvenile metachromatic leucodystrophy. *Nature (London)*, **226**, 553

160. BASS, N. H., WITMER, J. E. and DREIFUSS, F. E. (1970). A pedigree study of metachromatic leucodystrophy. Biochemical identification of the carrier state. *Neurology*, **20**, 52

161. SASS, M. D., CARUSO, C. J. and FARHANGI, M. (1967). TPNH-methaemoglobin reductase deficiency: a new red cell enzyme defect. *J. Lab. Clin. Med.*, **70**, 760

162. SCOTT, E. M. (1960). The relation of diaphorase of human erythrocytes to inheritance of methaemoglobinaemia. *J. Clin. Invest.*, **39**, 1176

163. VON FIGURA, K., LÖGERING, M., MERSMANN, G. and KRESSE, H. (1973). Sanfilippo B disease: serum assays for detection of homozygous and heterozygous individuals in three familes. *J. Pediatr.*, **83**, 607

164. SLY, W. S., QUINTON, B. A., McALISTER, W. H. and RIMOIN, D. L. (1973). Beta-glucuronidase deficiency: report of clinical, radiologic and biochemical features of a new mucopolysaccharidosis. *J. Pediatr.*, **82**, 249

165. LEHRER, R. I. and CLINE, M. J. (1969). Leucocyte myeloperoxidase deficiency and disseminated candidiasis: the role of myeloperoxidase in resistance to Candida infection. *J. Clin. Invest.*, **48**, 1478

166. FALLON, H. J., SMITH, L. H., GRAHAM, J. B. and BURNETT, C. H. (1964). A genetic study of hereditary orotic aciduria. *N. Engl. J. Med.*, **270**, 878

167. FOX, R. M., O'SULLIVAN, W. J. and FIRKIN, B. G. (1969). Orotic aciduria. Differing enzyme patterns. *Am. J. Med.*, **47**, 332

168. WANG, Y. M. and VAN EYS, J. (1970). The enzymatic defect in essential pento-suria. *N. Engl. J. Med.*, **282**, 892

169. VALENTINE, W. N., HSIEH, H., PAGLIA, D. E., ANDERSON, H. M., BAUGHAN, M. A., JAFFE, E. R. and GARSON, O. M. (1969). Hereditary haemolytic anaemia associated with phosphoglycerate kinase deficiency in erythrocytes and leucocytes: a probable X-chromosome linked syndrome. *N. Engl. J. Med.*, **280**, 528

170. HSIA, Y. E., SCULLY, K. J. and ROSENBERG, L. E. (1971. Inherited propionyl-CoA carboxylase deficiency in ketotic hyperglycinaemia. *J. Clin. Invest.*, **50**, 127

171. VALENTINE, W. N., FINK, K., PAGLIA, D. E., HARRIS, S. R. and ADAMS, W. S. (1974). Hereditary haemolytic anaemia with human erythrocyte pyrimidine-5'-nucleotidase deficiency. *J. Clin. Invest.*, **54**, 866.

172. HERNDON, J. H., STEINBERG, D. and UHLENDORF, B. W. (1969). Refsum's disease: defective oxidation of phytanic acid in tissue cultures derived from homozygotes and heterozygotes. *N. Engl. J. Med.*, **281**, 1034

173. LEHMANN, H. and LIDDELL, J. (1969). Human cholinesterase (pseudocholin-esterase): genetic variants and their recognition. *Br. J. Anaesth.*, **41**, 235

174. SCHNEIDER, A. S., VALENTINE, W. N., HATTORI, M. and HEINS, H. L. (1964). A new erythrocyte enzyme defect with haemolytic anaemia—triose phosphate isomerase (TPI) deficiency. *Blood*, **24**, 855

175. YOUNG, E. P. and PATRICK, A. D. (1970). Deficiency of acid esterase activity in Wolman's disease. *Arch. Dis. Child.*, **45**, 664

176. CHILDS, B., SIDBURY, J. B. and MIGEON, C. J. (1959). Glucuronic acid conjugation by patients with familial non-haemolytic jaundice and their relatives. *Paediatrics.*, **23**, 903

177. MONGEAU, J. G., HILGARTNER, M., WORTHEN, H. G. and FRIMPTER, G. W. (1966). Cystathioninuria: a study of an infant with normal mentality, throm-bocytopenia, and renal calculi. *J. Pediatr.*, **69**, 1113

178. HAGUE, R. V. and HOLTON, J. B. (1971). Intravenous histidine load test for detection of heterozygotes for histidinaemia. *Clin. Chim. Acta.*, **33**, 462

179. KOMROWER, G. M., WILSON, V., CLAMP, J. R. and WESTALL, R. G. (1964). Hydroxykynureninuria. A case of abnormal tryptophan metabolism probably due to deficiency of kinureninase. *Arch. Dis. Chld.*, **39**, 250

180. HOOFT, C., CARTON, D., SNOECK, J., TIMMERMANS, J., ANTENER, I., VAN DER HENDE, C. and TOYAERT, W. (1968). Further investigations in the methionine malabsorption syndrome. *Helv. Paediatr. Acta*, **23**, 334

181. FREEDBERG, I. M., FEINGOLD, D. S. and HIATT, H. H. (1959). Serum and urine L-xylulose in pentosuric and normal subjects and in individuals with pentosuria trait. *Biochem. Biophys. Res. Commun.*, **1**, 328

182. GERRITSEN, T. and WAISMAN, H. A. (1966). Hypersarcosinaemia: an inborn error of metabolism. *N. Engl. J. Med.*, **275**, 66

183. STERNLIEB, I., MORELL, A. G., BAUER, C. D., COMBES, B., DE BOBES-STERNBERG, S. and SCHEINBERG, I. H. (1961). Detection of the heterozygous carrier of the Wilson's disease gene. *J. Clin. Invest.*, **40**, 707

184. CORGELL, M. E., KNOWLTON, W., HALL, W. K., THEVAOS, G., WELTER, D. A., GATZ, A. J., HORTON, B. F., SISSON, B. D., LOOPER, J. W. and FARROW, R. T. (1964). A familial study of a human enzyme defect, argininosuccinic aciduria. *Biochem. Biophys. Res. Commun.*, **14**, 307

185. FRIMPTER, G. W., HAYMOVITZ, A. and HORWITH, M. (1963). Cystathioninuria. *N. Engl. J. Med.*, **268**, 333

186. SCHNEIDER, J. A., BRADLEY, K. and SEEGMILLER, J. E. (1967). Increased cystine in leucocytes from individuals homozygous and heterozygous for cystinosis. *Science (N.Y.)*, **157**, 1321

187. WALLIS, P. G., SIDBURY, J. B. and HARRIS, R. C. (1966). Hepatic phosphorylase defect. *Am. J. Dis. Child.*, **111**, 278

188. ROSENBERG, L. E., DURANT, J. L. and ELSAS, L. J. (1968). Familial iminoglycinuria: an inborn error of renal tubular transport. *N. Engl. J. Med.*, **278**, 1407

189. TELLER, W. M., ROSEVEAR, J. W. and BURKE, E. C. (1961). Identification of heterozygous carriers of gargoylism. *Proc. Soc. Exp. Biol. Med.*, **108**, 276

190. TELLER, W. M., BUSCH, C. and BODE, H. H. (1969). Re-evaluation of heterozygous carriers of mucopolysaccharidoses. *Horm. Metab. Res.*, **1**, 78

191. CARTER, C. O. and SIMPKISS, M. (1956). The carrier state in nephrogenic diabetes insipidus. *Lancet*, **ii**, 1069

192. PERRY, T. L., TISCHLER, B., HANSEN, S. and McDOUGALL, L. (1967). A simple test for heterozygosity for phenylketonuria. *Clin. Chim. Acta*, **15**, 47

193. PERRY, T. L., HARDWICK, D. F., LOWRY, R. B. qnd HANSEN, S. (1968). Hyperprolinaemia in two successive generations of a North American Indian family. *Ann. Hum. Genet.*, **31**, 401

194. KHACHADURIAN, A. K. and KHACHADURIAN, L. A. (1964). The inheritance of renal glycosuria. *Am. J. Hum. Genet.*, **16**, 189

195. WADA, Y., TADA, K., MINAGAWA, A., YOSHIDA, T., MORIKAWA, T. and OKAMURA, T. (1963). Idiopathic hypervalinaemia. Probably a new entity of inborn error of valine metabolism. *Tohoku J. Exp. Med.*, **81**, 46

196. MUDD, S. H. (170). Error of sulfur metabolism. In O. H. Muth and J. E. Oldfield (eds.), *Sulfur in Nutrition*, p.222. (Connecticut: A.V.I. Publishers)

13

Prenatal diagnosis

A. D. Patrick

Reference to successive editions of *Mendelian Inheritance in Man*[1] and *The Metabolic Basis of Inherited Disease*[2] conveys vividly the rapidly increasing rate of discovery of recessively inherited biochemical abnormalities. These advances have often been of immediate use in diagnosis and management of patients; indeed, the impetus for research has often derived from these aims. Central to this scheme for prenatal diagnosis is the fact that the diseases are characterized by a deficiency of a specific enzyme activity, the result of the genetic mutation. Until about 10 years ago, enzymic diagnosis of a metabolic disease often required biopsy of the liver or another affected organ. Now, more sensitive methods of enzyme assay allow the use of leukocytes as an alternative to surgical biopsy specimens. Tests became more convenient and effective, could be applied in early infancy and, for the first time, specific enzyme assessment was routinely extended to the investigation of family members.

The same techniques also brought cultured cells within the biochemists' field. Sustained cultures of skin fibroblasts, established for cytogenetic studies, were used to demonstrate that these cells also maintained their characteristic enzyme patterns throughout many cycles of growth and subculture. Realization that cultures of cells from amniotic fluid obtained by amniocentesis had similar properties allowed the use of such cultures for intrauterine diagnosis of enzyme deficiencies and other metabolic abnormalities. With these developments a number of laboratories have gained experience of methods and diagnostic interpretation, and now collaborate closely with cytogeneticists, and obstetricians in performing prenatal diagnosis. Over the past few years, considerable success has been achieved with consequent benefit to families affected by inborn errors of metabolism.

In this chapter current experience of the practical aspects of prenatal diagnosis is described and the limitations and pitfalls that impose the need for the utmost care in its performance are discussed.

Biochemical indications for prenatal diagnosis

Prenatal diagnosis is indicated for inherited metabolic diseases that result in serious handicap to the child. An obvious requirement, but one that is often not fully appreciated, is that the specific enzyme deficiency or characteristic metabolic abnormality for which the fetus is at risk is known with certainty. It also follows that methods must be available for the reliable detection of the abnormality in amniotic fluid or amniotic fluid cells in a time that will allow therapeutic termination of the pregnancy.

Usually, only after the birth of an affected infant is the specific genetic risk in a family recognized so that, in most cases, prenatal diagnosis is undertaken to prevent recurrence of the abnormality in subsequent pregnancies. It must be emphasized that the presumptive diagnosis of an index case, based solely on clinical or histopathological findings or even on both, cannot be accepted as sufficiently firm evidence on which to attempt a prenatal diagnosis; closely similar clinical phenotypes may result from entirely different enzyme deficiencies. For this reason, every effort must be made to establish the specific biochemical diagnosis in the index case. This may not be possible if the affected child is no longer alive and the possible need for further investigation should always be considered, and tissue taken at autopsy and biopsy properly frozen and stored. The establishment of cultures of skin fibroblasts from patients and parents is also useful as it allows future comparison of enzymic activity with that of amniotic fluid cells obtained from subsequent pregnancies.

Determination of enzymic activity in leukocytes, serum or skin fibroblasts of parents, may be diagnostic if the appropriate test differentiates reliably between heterozygous and normal levels of activity. In certain circumstances, heterozygote recognition may prevent the birth of even the first affected infant in a family. For an X-linked disorder, this might arise because an affected male has caused the female members, including the mother's sisters and cousins to be examined and the carriers identified. Sometimes, the female carrier will show clinical manifestations of the disorder (as in Fabry's disease) which prompt confirmatory tests for a heterozygous level of enzymic activity. Heterozygosity for an autosomal recessive disorder in a couple is rarely recognized before the birth of an affected infant, although the confirmed carriers within that family and its relatives may then wish to determine whether their existent or future spouses are similarly affected.

Mass screening of a population for carriers will not be practical except for those conditions in which the carrier frequency is high and can be determined by simple and reliable tests. Future developments will, hopefully, permit the realization of this goal for cystic fibrosis, the commonest inherited disease in our population with a carrier frequency approaching 1 in 20. A defined high-risk population for which some success and valuable experience in mass-screening has been gained is the Ashkenazi-Jewish community, in which the carrier frequency for Tay–Sachs disease is approximately 1 in 30. The Baltimore study of Kaback and colleagues,[3] employing an automated method for the determination of hexosaminidase A in serum, screened 7000 volunteer Jewish subjects in one year and detected 300 carriers, including 11 married couples who had not at that time had an affected child.

Genetic counselling

The purpose of genetic counselling is to provide all necessary information and support to prospective parents at serious genetic risk, in order that they can decide on family planning in accordance with their wishes and circumstances. In most cases involving a metabolic disorder, informed genetic counselling must begin with the diagnosis of an affected child and a knowledge of the attendant risk of recurrence in subsequent pregnancies. The diagnosis must be accurate and the genetic implications must be fully understood. These conditions demand considerable experience of both the biochemist, who performs the specific diagnostic tests, and of the clinician, who uses this information as the basis for genetic counselling.

The counsellor will inform parents of the severity of the disease and prognosis for the child, the impact of which they may already be tragically aware, and of the management and possible means of treating the disease. He will also discuss the possible alternatives to not having any more children, or running the risk of having further affected children. Traditionally, the main alternative has been that of adoption, but in recent years, the prospect of planned pregnancies resulting in the birth only of unaffected infants, has been realized through the prenatal diagnosis of a steadily increasing number of recessive diseases. This has added a hopeful new aspect to genetic counselling. At the same time, these measures have placed new burdens of responsibility on all those concerned with prenatal diagnosis. Not least is the responsibility of the genetic counsellor, who has the task of explaining to the couple concerned, not only the manner of performance of prenatal diagnosis, but also the limitations and risks of the procedures, including those of possible technical failure or misinterpretation of data.

In many cases, it will be the counsellor who also makes the necessary arrangements following a parental decision to submit to an attempt at prenatal diagnosis. Effective collaboration with an obstetric unit experienced in amniocentesis, and with a cell culture laboratory, may already have been established for the prenatal detection of chromosomal abnormalities. Provision of the biochemical service required for the diagnosis of a metabolic disease, and an assessment of the reliability of the service available may, however, present some problems. Only a small number of laboratories are adequately equipped to engage in this work, and at this early stage of development, few can claim substantial experience in the prenatal diagnosis of particular diseases. It is important, therefore, that some means of assessing this experience should be available to the clinician seeking this service. At the present time, a simple, regularly up-dated register of names and addresses of participating laboratories, listing for each the numbers of pregnancies tested for specific diseases, the biochemical diagnoses made and their proven accuracy would appear to be adequate. Such a register of United Kingdom laboratories has been compiled by the Clinical Genetics Society. Similar lists have also been compiled for Germany and Scandinavia, and efforts are currently being made to organize a co-operative system between most European countries.

Amniocentesis

Prenatal diagnosis of an inborn error of metabolism requires material of fetal origin to which specific biochemical tests can be applied for the detection of the abnormality. Such material is obtained by amniocentesis, the technique of removal of a specimen of fluid from the amniotic sac by needle aspiration.[4] The method has been widely used for many years in monitoring late pregnancy for fetal haemolytic disease due to Rh incompatibility, and with technical improvements and a greater knowledge of its risks and complications, is now being applied routinely as an outpatient procedure in the earlier stages of pregnancy.

Much of this experience has been gained from investigations of possible chromosomal abnormalities, particularly where the mother's age is 40 or over. Now, with the important advances of the past 5 years in the detection of metabolic disorders in amniotic fluid cells, 2nd trimester amniocentesis is indicated for a steadily expanding number of recessive diseases.

The timing of amniocentesis is obviously of the utmost importance to the success of these investigations, since it must allow sufficient time for the appropriate diagnostic tests to be completed satisfactorily and for abortion to be performed if this is indicated by the results of these tests. It is generally accepted that transabdominal amniocentesis should not be carried out earlier than the 14th week after the 1st day of the last menstruation. Before that time, both the volume of amniotic fluid and the number of viable cells it contains are small, and attempts to obtain a specimen might incur serious risk to the pregnancy. It would appear that most centres now accept that 14–16 weeks is the optimum gestational age at which to perform amniocentesis. The volume of fluid is then increasing rapidly and, with placental localization by ultrasonography, it is usually possible to obtain 10–20 ml of clear fluid at the first attempt. The number of viable cells contained in the fluid is also increasing at that time, and, in most cases is adequate to establish successful cell cultures.

The risk to the mother and fetus of trauma, haemorrhage or infection due to amniocentesis before 20 weeks gestation has not been fully evaluated, but appears to be very low. Nadler and Gerbie[5] considered the overall risk to be less than 1%, while Scrimgeour[4] in a review of 529 cases found no reports of fetal trauma, or maternal or fetal deaths. Jacobson[6] reported a spontaneous abortion 1 month after amniocentesis as the only abnormal event in a series of 300 pregnancies, but Milunsky[7] recorded complications, which included a fetal death, in 11 cases in a series of 298 amniocenteses. However, the most recent survey found that the overall fetal loss in 1000 pregnancies with amniocentesis was not significantly different from that in an equal number of age-matched controls without amniocentesis.[8]

The incidence of grossly bloody specimens of amniotic fluid appears to be less than 10%. The overall rate for failed and bloody taps in the series reviewed by Scrimgeour[4] was 3.6%, while Jacobson[6] mentioned a rate of 8% for gross contamination by maternal blood in his own series of 350 cases and in 2500 cases carried to term by other investigators. While there was no evidence of placental haemorrhage in these cases, transplacental haemorrhage leading to Rh-immunization is a potential risk requiring evaluation.

Cell culture

The specimen of amniotic fluid obtained by amniocentesis has only limited, though important (see later), immediate diagnostic use. For most purposes, both in chromosomal and biochemical investigations, the viable cells contained in the fluid need to be cultured; that is, placed in a nutrient medium in which they will continue to grow and multiply until they provide sufficient material for the test required. Cell culture methods have been in use for more than 60 years, during which time numerous types and modifications of culture media have been developed. For the maintenance of cells for several weeks in culture, as required for biochemical prenatal diagonsis, media generally contain a balanced solution of salts, all the essential amino acids, vitamin supplements and serum protein, usually that provided by fetal calf serum. Antibiotics are also included to minimize infection.

Based on practical experience, different laboratories have their individual preferences for one or other of the available types of medium. While it would perhaps be an advantage if some measure of standardization of culture conditions could be introduced, the main consideration at this time is that laboratories intending to engage in the culture of amniotic fluid cells for the purpose of prenatal diagnosis, should have considerable experience of cell culture. A good record of successful growth of human diploid cells, particularly in the maintenance of skin fibroblast cultures, is essential. Such success will only have been achieved by an awareness and careful practice of the strict control of technique that is required.

The definition of successful culture will depend on the use to which the culture is to be put. For chromosomal analysis, the number of cells required is relatively small, and these can usually be obtained from a primary culture. Such cultures are exposed to minimum risk of degeneration, and most experienced cytogenetics laboratories achieve a karyotype report in at least 90% of cases after a mean culture period of 13–28 days.[7-9] But for conventional biochemical tests, the present needs are for much higher numbers of cells, perhaps several millions, and to obtain these it is necessary to detach the cells of the primary culture from the original dish and reseed these into fresh dishes for continued growth. This process of subculture is repeated until the required number of cells is obtained. As might be expected, this requirement incurs increased risks of degeneration that may seriously reduce the overall success rate for biochemical diagnosis.

In addition to the possibility of culture failure that may occur too late to consider repeat amniocentesis, there is the over-riding need to produce sufficient cells for satisfactory biochemical assay within a time limit compatible with therapeutic abortion. This difficulty is well-illustrated by the report of Sutherland and Bain[10] who obtained 100% initial cell growth from 62 amniotic fluids, and sufficient cells for biochemical assay in 90% of these. However, if a time limit of 6 weeks for the production of a biochemical report had been imposed, this success rate would have been reduced to 58%; the mean period from amniocentesis to biochemical result was 39.5 days. Thus far, attempts to resolve these difficulties by inducing a more rapid growth rate of amniotic fluid cells have not been successful, and it appears more likely that a solution to these problems will be provided by the development of histochemical and microbiochemical techniques applied to much smaller numbers of cells.[11-13]

Certain other considerations are important to an assessment of the reliability of prenatal biochemical diagnosis, not least being the possible contamination of cultures by maternal cells. It was mentioned earlier that a small proportion of amniotic fluid specimens are grossly contaminated by blood; it is also found that the majority of specimens contain microscopic amounts. In almost all cases this blood proves to be of maternal origin. While its presence does not appear to have an adverse effect on the establishment of cell cultures, the possibility that cultures might contain maternal cells from which a mistaken diagnosis could be derived, has to be considered. Fortunately, leukocytes do not persist in amniotic fluid cell cultures, so that their presence at the time of karyotype or conventional biochemical analysis can be largely discounted. Another possible source of contamination is maternal skin introduced at abdominal puncture, although admixture of fetal and maternal cells in amniotic fluid cell cultures is an uncommon finding, and total overgrowth by maternal cells a very rare occurrence. Nevertheless, these possibilities should be considered, and the karyotype and other characteristics, including cell morphology, of the cultures should be determined in all cases by an experienced cytogeneticist.

Laboratories performing cell culture for prenatal biochemical diagnosis, also have the task of providing the necessary control cultures for use whenever a pregnancy is being monitored for a specific disease. In addition to normal amniotic fluid cells, cultures of skin fibroblasts from an affected child and from heterozygous carriers should also be available for comparison with amniotic fluid cells from the pregnancy at risk. For this purpose, many laboratories now maintain extensive frozen banks of such control cultures for regrowth when the need arises, and an admirable measure of collaboration in the donation of cultures has developed between diagnostic centres. With proper care, cell cultures or specimens of amniotic fluid usually survive for up to a week in transit and can be cultured successfully by the receiving laboratory. In this way, referral of specimens to diagnostic centres having the appropriate biochemical experience has become an established practice at both national and international levels, and will provide an increasing service as more diseases become amenable to prenatal diagnosis. It is essential that these developments should be incorporated into the general scheme of health care of affected families and be secured by firm financial and organizational support.

Biochemical investigation

The use of cultured amniotic fluid cells for the prenatal diagnosis of a metabolic disease, requires that manifestations of the primary genetic defect will be expressed in these cells and can be detected reliably by specific techniques. Although different types of cells may perform diverse functions, they depend for their integrity on a relatively constant set of basic metabolic processes governed by a common array of enzymes. Cultured human skin fibroblasts are a convenient source of cellular material for the investigation of abnormalities in this basic pattern, and have been used extensively both for the detection of specific enzyme deficiencies and also the resultant metabolic defects. The basic biochemistry of cultured amniotic fluid cells would be expected to be qualitatively similar to that of fibroblasts and, therefore, to be equally applicable to the purpose of detecting abnormality. This premise has been confirmed in all cases of metabolic disease for which prenatal diagnosis has been indicated. Nevertheless, the biochemistry of normal amniotic fluid cells is at present poorly understood, and requires active investigation in order to provide the comparative and control data necessary for reliable prenatal diagnosis.

It is known, for example, that the enzymic activities of cultured cells may show wide variations, even when the conditions and technique of cell culture conform to the strictest standard practice. The type of culture medium,[14,15] concentration of fetal calf serum,[16] and the pH·of the medium[17] have all been shown to influence the levels of enzymic activity. The state of the culture at the time the cells are harvested for enzyme assays is also important, particularly with respect to the stage of subculture,[18] cell density,[15,19] time after feeding,[15] or subculture,[20,21] phase of cell growth,[22] and the age of the culture.[23,24]

The endocytotic uptake by cultured cells of proteins and other substances present in culture media might also introduce artefactual error into the subsequent biochemical analysis. For example, as pointed out by Brock,[25] the possibility of endocytosis of lysosomal hydrolases present in the serum constituents of culture media needs to be borne in mind when cultured cells are examined for lysosomal storage diseases, especially the mucopolysaccharidoses. Similarly, intracellular infection, particularly by mycoplasma, might lead to spurious biochemical findings.

Any laboratory intending to engage in the prenatal diagnosis of metabolic disorders should be aware of these many considerations, and of the consequent experience of technique and interpretation required to provide a reliable prediction of fetal status. The importance of each laboratory establishing control ranges of test values relevant to the particular conditions of cell culture and biochemical assay employed, cannot be overstated. To this end, many centres now hold and are prepared to donate specimens of homozygous and heterozygous fibroblasts covering a wide range of diseases. However, it must be emphasized that data for fibroblasts alone do not provide a satisfactory measure of control. There may be marked differences between the enzymic activities of cultured fibroblasts and cultured amniotic fluid cells[26] such that heterozygous and homozygous affected states, while being clearly differentiated for fibroblasts, are difficult to resolve for amniotic fluid cells. In these cases expression of the activity of an enzyme relative to that of another marker enzyme often aids interpretation and reduces the risk of mistaken diagnosis.[18] A prenatal diagnosis must, of course, always be controlled by simultaneous tests on cultures of normal amniotic fluid cells.

All of these considerations have rightly led to a careful, systematic approach to the development of prenatal biochemical diagnosis. Nevertheless, the number of diseases for which prenatal diagnoses have been made is already considerable and will no doubt increase steadily and become consolidated into routine service in the future. Ideally, cultured amniotic fluid cells will be employed for biochemical evaluation, preferably by means of specific assay for the deficient enzyme. But in the fullest use of amniotic fluid and its contained cells for prenatal diagnosis, both uncultured cells and cell-free fluid may also yield valuable corroborative information.

Cultured amniotic fluid cells

A list of inherited metabolic diseases for which prenatal diagnoses have already been made is given in Table 13.1. Further diseases, for

Table 13.1   Prenatal diagnosis of inherited metabolic diseases

Disorder	Enzyme deficiency or metabolic abnormality
Lysosomal diseases	
GM2 gangliosidosis	
type 1, Tay–Sachs	hexosaminidase A[27–29]
type 2, Sandhoff	hexosaminidases A and B[30]
GM1 gangliosidosis	
type 1	β-galactosidase[31,32]
type 2	β-galactosidase[33]
Gaucher disease, infantile	glucocerebroside β-glucosidase[34]
Niemann–Pick disease,	
type A	sphingomyelinase[35]
Metachromatic leukodys-trophy	cerebroside sulphate sulphatase (arylsulphatase A)[36,37]
Krabbe disease	galactocerebroside β-galactosidase[38]
Fabry's disease	ceramide trihexoside α-galactosidase[39]
Wolman disease	cholesteryl ester/triglyceride esterase[40]
I-cell disease (Muco-lipidosis 2)	loss of lysosomal hydrolases[41]
Acid phosphatase deficiency	lysosomal acid phosphatase[42]
Glycogen storage disease,	
type 2	α-1, 4-glucosidase[43]
Cystinosis	cystine storage[44,45]

Disorder	Enzyme deficiency or metabolic abnormality
Mucopolysaccharidosis :*	accumulation of glycosaminoglycans[46]
type 1H, Hurler	α-L-iduronidase[47]
type 1S, Scheie	α-L-iduronidase[47]
type 2, Hunter	iduronate sulphatase[48]
type 3A, Sanfilippo A	heparan *N*-sulphatase[49]
type 3B, Sanfilippo B	*N*-acetyl-α-glucosaminidase[50]
type 6, Maroteaux-Lamy	arylsulphatase B[51]
type 7	β glucuronidase[52]
Other diseases	
Galactosaemia	galactose 1-phosphate uridy transferase[53]
Maple syrup urine disease	branched-chain ketoacid decarboxylase[54,55]
Homocystinuria	cystathionine synthase[56]
Argininosuccinic aciduria	argininosuccinase[57]
Citrullinaemia	argininosuccinate synthase[58]
Propionic acidaemia	propionyl-CoA carboxylase[59]
Methylmalonic aciduria	
B_{12}-sensitive	deoxyadenosyl-B_{12} synthesis[60]
B_{12}-insensitive	methylmalonyl-CoA mutase[60,61]
Lesch–Nyhan syndrome	hypoxanthine-guanine phosphoribosyl transferase[62–64]
Severe combined immunodeficiency	adenosine deaminase[65]
Xeroderma pigmentosum	DNA repair[66]

* A number of laboratories are now performing specific enzymic diagnosis, in addition to the measurement of $^{35}SO_4$ incorporation

which the appropriate enzyme tests have been applied to cultured skin fibroblasts or amniotic fluid cells, are given in Table 13.2.

It can be seen that the lysosomal storage diseases, notably the sphingolipidoses, comprise a prominent general group for which particular success has been achieved. The concept that the intralysosomal storage of macromolecules was due to deficiencies of specific hydrolytic enzymes responsible for the normal intracellular digestion of these substances,[74] had led to the rapid elucidation of these enzyme deficiencies

Table 13.2 Further diseases for which prenatal diagnosis is possible

Disorder	Enzyme deficiency
Fucosidosis	α-L-fucosidase[67]
Mannosidosis	α-D-mannosidase[52]
Aspartylglucosaminuria	aspartylglucosaminidase[68]
Galactokinase deficiency	galactokinase[69]
Glycogen storage disease, type 4	α-1, 4-glucan : α-1, 4-glucan 6-glucosyl transferase[70]
Pyruvate decarboxylase deficiency	pyruvate decarboxylase[71]
Hyperlysinaemia	lysine : ketoglutarate reductase[72]
Refsum disease	phytanic acid α-oxidase[73]

and the development of assays for their detection. In many cases, these tests were simple and highly sensitive, particularly where artificial chromogenic or fluorogenic substrates could be used, and were readily adapted to the microscale required when testing homogenates or extracts of the small amounts of cellular material obtained from amniotic fluid cell cultures. But while Table 13.1 conveys a measure of the feasibility and potential of prenatal diagnosis, it may be misleading in that only for a few of these diseases can it be said that feasibility has been adequately confirmed by the performance of appreciable numbers of diagnoses. By far the greatest experience relates to the detection of Tay–Sachs disease,[28,29] for which approximately 400 pregnancies have to date been monitored worldwide; but significant numbers of cases of glycogen storage disease, type 2, and mucopolysaccharidosis have also been tested.

Detection of a mucopolysaccharidosis, although now possible by direct examination for the specific enzyme deficiencies in most of the individual diseases, has been achieved mainly by the demonstration of an abnormal accumulation of glycosaminoglycans in cultured amniotic fluid cells. Uptake of $^{35}SO_4$ by the cells and its retention in the sulphated polysaccharides that accumulate gives an easily measured index of abnormality.[46] Cystinosis is a further example for which the storage of a metabolite can be used as a reliable test for affected cells. Here, the excessive incorporation of ^{35}S-cystine into cultured amniotic fluid cells is revealed by suitable analytical techniques applied to the cell extracts.[44,45,75] Prenatal diagnosis of the Lesch–Nyhan syndrome, and detection of the heterozygous state are elegantly demonstrated by the level of incorporation of tritiated hypoxanthine into the nucleic acids of cultured cells. Two cell populations, one positive and one negative for hypoxanthine-guanine phosphoribosyl transferase (HGPRT) activity are clearly differentiated in the autoradiographs of labelled heterozygous cell cultures.[62]

Tests such as that employed for the detection of HGPRT deficiency are particularly valuable in that they require relatively small numbers of cultured cells. But, as mentioned earlier, the use of cultured cells for most types of conventional biochemical test incurs the serious limitation that periods of culture of up to 8 weeks may be required before sufficient cells (perhaps 1–2 million) are available for testing. This long delay may be psychologically damaging to the mother and is clearly undesirable where elective abortion is indicated. Consequently, attempts have been made to reduce this waiting period by the use of micro-methods of enzyme assay which require only a few thousand cells, and have achieved notable success. Thus, prenatal diagnosis of Fabry's disease has been completed 11 days after amniocentesis,[76] type 2 glycogen storage disease after 11–22 days,[77] GM1 gangliosidosis after 9 and 12 days, metachromatic leukodystrophy after 16 and 18 days, and maple syrup urine disease after 11 days.[78] These techniques are capable of further refinement to an ultramicro level, whereby colonies of cells in primary cultures are isolated, freeze-dried and assayed in volumes of 1–5 μl.[12] In this manner, it has been reported that more than 20 metabolic diseases can be diagnosed using 25, or less, amniotic fluid cells after periods of culture as short as 7 days.[11]

However, Brock[79] has drawn attention to a potential pitfall inherent in the use of short-term cultures in these microtechniques. A number of morphologically distinct cell types occur in amniotic fluid, the two main forms being epithelial and fibroblast-types. Whereas long-term cultures appear to consist only of fibroblasts, early cultures may be predominantly either epithelioid or fibroblast-like, or may contain mixtures of several cell types. Since the different cells may show marked qualitative and quantitative differences in their enzymology, it is essential that early cultures used for rapid diagnosis should be characterized morphologically, in order that biochemical control data relevant to the particular cell type may be applied.

Amniotic fluid and uncultured cells

The inherent problems of delay in arriving at a diagnosis requiring cultured cells, and the possible loss of specimens, would, of course, be avoided if amniotic fluid and its contained cells could be used immediately for reliable biochemical assessment. This approach might have particular application to those disorders in which the metabolic abnormality is reflected by characteristic changes in the composition of urine, since the formation of amniotic fluid depends in part on contributions from the fetal urine. However, it seems likely that placental function would effect the rapid turnover of many metabolites tending to increase in the fetal circulation. Furthermore, at least for constituent amino acids, it is known that the composition of normal amniotic fluid undergoes dynamic change throughout pregnancy,[80] so that control data carefully matched for gestational age would be required for valid comparison. Much further investigation of these problems is required. Variability in the constitution of amniotic fluid is also derived from the breakdown of its contained cells and macromolecular components (perhaps including maternal cells introduced at amniocentesis). As mentioned earlier, the majority of amniotic fluid cells are in varying states of decay, judging by their non-viability, and as such are found to express wide variation in any index of direct metabolic assessment, including enzymic activity.

In spite of these limitations, the analysis of amniotic fluid and uncultured amniotic fluid cells has certain valuable applications. In late pregnancy, measurement of increasing bilirubin levels in amniotic fluid has long been used in the diagnosis of erythroblastosis fetalis, and congenital adrenal hyperplasia has been indicated by increased concentrations of pregnanetriol and 17-ketosteroids.[81,82] A finding with greater bearing on the prospects for early diagnosis was the detection of methylmalonic acid in amniotic fluid at the 17th week of a pregnancy which resulted in the birth of an infant affected with methylmalonic aciduria.[61] Interestingly, the levels of methylmalonic acid in the maternal urine were also elevated during the 3rd trimester of pregnancy. But the prospect of reliable detection of mucopolysaccharidosis by the measurement of glycosaminoglycans in amniotic fluid, based on the initial report[83] of raised levels in the 14th week of a pregnancy which resulted in the birth of an infant with Hurler disease, has not been realized. Indeed, Matalon *et al.*[84] later cautioned against the use of such analyses, and Brock *et al.*[85] reported finding no quantitative or qualitative abnormality of glycosaminoglycans in the 18th week of a pregnancy resulting in an infant with Hurler disease. However, the method of two-dimensional electrophoresis of glycosaminoglycans isolated from amniotic fluid as complexes with Alcian Blue,[86] appears to be a useful ancillary means of investigating this group of disorders. A further cautionary example of the use of amniotic fluid analysis in prenatal diagnosis is that of α-glucosidase assay for the detection of type 2 glycogen storage disease,[43] a method later shown to be inappropriate by the demonstration that the α-glucosidase activities of amniotic fluid and cultured amniotic fluid cells were due to different enzymes.[87,88]

But for several other lysosomal diseases, notably Tay–Sachs disease, the determination of the appropriate enzymic activity in both amniotic fluid and uncultured amniotic fluid cells adds useful confirmatory data to the results obtained from cultured cells, particularly those predicting a normal fetus.[28,30,31,89] For the prenatal diagnosis of Tay–Sachs disease, it is the customary practice of this laboratory to test amniotic fluid, uncultured and cultured cells for the activity of hexosaminidase A by an automated method of assay linked to DEAE-cellulose chromatography on microcolumns.[90] In two cases out of a total 25 pregnancies monitored, amniotic cells failed to grow in culture, despite the normal precaution of using two different culture laboratories. In each case, a prediction that the fetus would be unaffected was confidently made and subsequently confirmed when hexosaminidase A was shown to be present in the cell-free fluids and uncultured cells. In all the other cases, there was close agreement between results obtained with amniotic fluid, and cultured and uncultured cells.

With due regard to the limitations and present uncertainties in the use of amniotic fluid and uncultured cells for the prenatal diagnosis of metabolic disease, it is nevertheless essential that a critical appraisal of the possible applications of such tests should continue, with the aim of providing ancillary methods which add to the overall certainty of diagnosis.

Follow-up studies

The immediate biochemical follow-up to prenatal diagnosis is the presentation of unambiguous results to the person, ideally the clinician involved in the initial genetic counselling, who is to convey this information to the parents. The second requirement, which provides an ongoing assessment of the reliability of the tests employed, is the subsequent confirmation of predicted abnormality by the examination of tissues of the aborted fetus, or of predicted normality by appropriate tests on the newborn infant. Provision of normal fetal tissues for purposes of comparison may present some difficulty, a possible solution to which would be the establishment of banked cultures of fetal tissue cells in the same manner as for the preservation of skin fibroblast cultures.

The wider aspects of follow-up studies are mainly concerned with determining the safety to mother and fetus of early amniocentesis. Large-scale controlled studies, now being conducted in the UK and USA, include not only the question of incidence of pregnancy complications, such as induced abortion, haemorrhage, isoimmunization and infection, but also the long-term follow-up of the health and development of children born after amniocentesis. Preliminary data indicate that the overall rate of complication is low.

REFERENCES

1. McKusick, V. A. (1971). *Mendelian Inheritance in Man*, 3rd ed. (Baltimore: Johns Hopkins Press)
2. Stanbury, J. B., Wyngaarden, J. B. and Fredrickson, D. S. (1972). *The Metabolic Basis of Inherited Disease* 3rd ed. (New York: McGraw-Hill)
3. Kaback, M. M., Zeiger, R. S., Reynolds, L. W. and Sonneborn, M. (1974). Approaches to the control and prevention of Tay–Sachs disease. *Prog. Med. Genet.*, **10**, 103
4. Scrimgeour, J. B. (1973). In A. E. H. Emery (ed.), *Antenatal Diagnosis of Genetic Disease*, pp. 11–39. (Edinburgh and London: Churchill Livingstone)
5. Nadler, H. L. and Gerbie, A. B. (1970). Role of amniocentesis in the intrauterine detection of genetic disorders. *N. Engl. J. Med.*, **282**, 596
6. Jacobson, C. B. (1972). In A. Dorfman (ed.), *Antenatal Diagnosis*, pp. 29–32. (Chicago: University of Chicago Press)
7. Milunsky, A. (1973). *The Prenatal Diagnosis of Hereditary Disorders*. (Springfield, Illinois: Thomas)
8. Amniocentesis Registry Project, Nat. Inst. of Child Health and Human Development. Presented at a meeting of the American Academy of Pediatrics, Washington, D.C. Oct. 20th, 1975
9. Butler, L. J. and Reiss, H. E. (1970). Antenatal detection of chromosome abnormalities. *J. Obstet. Gynaecol. Br. Cwlth.*, **77**, 902
10. Sutherland, G. R. and Bain, A. D. (1973). Antenatal diagnosis of inborn errors of metabolism: tissue culture aspects. *Humangenetik*, **20**, 251
11. Hosli, P. (1973). In *Proc. 4th Int. Conf. on Birth Defects*, Vienna: Excerpta Medica Int. Congr. Ser. No. 297, pp. 13–14
12. Galjaard, H., Mekes, M., de Josselin de Jong, J. E. and Niermeijer, M. F. (1973). A method for rapid prenatal diagnosis of glycogenosis II. (Pompe's disease). *Clin. Chim. Acta*, **49**, 361
13. Galjaard, H., van Hoogstraaten, J. J., de Josselin de Jong, J. E. and Mulder, M. P. (1974). Methodology of the quantitative cytochemical analysis of single or small numbers of cultured cells. *Histochem. J.*, **6**, 409
14. Beutler, E., Kuhl, W., Trinidad, F., Teplitz, R. and Nadler, H. (1971). β-Glucosidase activity in fibroblasts from homozygotes and heterozygotes for Gaucher's disease. *Am. J. Hum. Genet.*, **23**, 62

15. RYAN, C. A., LEE, S. Y. and NADLER, H. L. (1972). Effect of culture conditions on enzyme activities in cultivated human fibroblasts. *Exp. Cell Res.*, **71**, 388

16. KITTLICK, P. D., NEUPERT, G. and LUMKEMAN, U. (1973). Effect of the different sera on mucopolysaccharide synthesis in fibroblast cultures. *Exp. Pathol.*, **8**, 194

17. BUTTERWORTH, J., SUTHERLAND, G. R., BROADHEAD, D. M. and BAIN, A. D. (1974). Effect of serum concentration, type of culture medium and pH on the lysosomal enzyme activity of cultured human amniotic fluid cells. *Clin. Chim. Acta*, **53**, 239

18. YOUNG, E., WILLCOX, P., WHITFIELD, A. E. and PATRICK, A. D. (1975). Variability of acid hydrolase activities in cultured skin fibroblasts and amniotic fluid cells. *J. Med. Genet.*, **12**, 224

19. LEROY, J. G., DUMON, J. and RADERMECKER, J. (1970). Deficiency of arylsulphatase A in leucocytes and skin fibroblasts in juvenile metachromatic leucodystrophy. *Nature (London)*, **226**, 553

20. CRISTOFALO, V. J., PARRIS, N. and KRITCHEVSKY, D. (1967). Enzyme activity during the growth and ageing of human cells *in vitro*. *J. Cell Physiol.*, **69**, 263

21. OKADA, S., VEATH, M. L., LEROY, J. and O'BRIEN, J. S. (1971). Ganglioside GM2 storage diseases: Hexosaminidase deficiencies in cultured fibroblasts. *Am. J. Hum. Genet.*, **23**, 55

22. PAN, Y. L. and KROOTH, R. S. (1968). The influence of progressive growth on specific catalase activity of human diploid cell strains. I. Effect of cellular genotype: homozygous strain. *J. Cell Physiol.*, **71**, 151

23. HOLLIDAY, R. (1972). Ageing of human fibroblasts in culture: Studies on enzymes and mutation. *Humangenetik*, **16**, 83

24. BUTTERWORTH, J., SUTHERLAND, G. R., BROADHEAD, D. M. and BAIN, A. D. (1973). Lysosomal enzyme levels in human amniotic fluid cells in tissue culture. I. α-Glucosidase and β-glucosidase. *Life Sci.*, **13**, 713

25. BROCK, D. J. H. (1973). In A. E. H. Emery (ed.), *Antenatal Diagnosis of Genetic Disease*, pp. 82–112

26. KABACK, M. K., LEONARD, C. O. and PARMLEY, T. H. (1971). Intrauterine diagnosis: Comparative enzymology of cells cultivated from maternal skin, fetal skin and amniotic fluid cells. *Pediatr. Res.*, **5**, 366

27. SCHNECK, L., FRIEDLAND, J., VALENTI, C., ADACHI, M., AMSTERDAM, D. and VOLK, B. W. (1970). Prenatal diagnosis of Tay–Sachs disease. *Lancet*, **i**, 582

28. O'BRIEN, J. S., OKADA, S., FILLERUP, D. L., VEATH, M. L., ADORNATO, B., BRENNER, P. H. and LEROY, J. G. (1971). Tay–Sachs disease: Prenatal diagnosis. *Science (N.Y.)*, **172**, 61

29. ELLIS, R. B., IKONNE, J. U., PATRICK, A. D., STEPHENS, R. and WILLCOX, P. (1973). Prenatal diagnosis of Tay–Sachs disease. *Lancet*, **ii**, 1144

30. DESNICK, R. J., KRIVIT, W. and SHARP, H. L. (1973). *In utero* diagnosis of Sandhoff's disease. *Biochem. Biophys. Res. Commun.*, **51**, 20

31. LOWDEN, J. A., CUTZ, E., CONEN, P. E., RUDD, N. and DORAN, T. A. (1973). Prenatal diagnosis of GM1-gangliosidosis. *N. Engl. J. Med.*, **288**, 225

32. KABACK, M. M., SLOAN, H. R., SONNEBORN, M., HERNDON, R. M. and PERCY, A. K. (1973). GM1-gangliosidosis type I: *in utero* detection and fetal manifestations. *J. Pediatr.*, **82**, 1037

33. BOOTH, C. W., GERBIE, A. B. and NADLER, H. L. (1973). Intrauterine detection of GM1-gangliosidosis, type 2. *Pediatrics*, **52**, 521

34. SCHNEIDER, E. L., ELLIS, W. G., BRADY, R. O., McCULLOCH, J. R. and EPSTEIN, C. J. (1972). Infantile (type II) Gaucher's disease: *in utero* diagnosis and fetal pathology. *J. Pediatr.*, **81**, 1134

35. EPSTEIN, C. J., BRADY, R. O., SCHNEIDER, E. L., BRADLEY, R. M. and SHAPIRO, D. (1971). *In utero* diagnosis of Niemann–Pick disease. *Am. J. Hum. Genet.*, **23**, 533

36. VAN DER HAGEN, C. B., BORRESEN, A. L., MOLNE, K., OFTEDAL, G., BJORO, K. and BERG, K. (1973). Metachromatic leukodystrophy: I. Prenatal detection of arylsulphatase A deficiency. *Clin. Genet.*, **4**, 256

37. LEROY, J. G., VAN ELSEN, A. F., MARTIN, J. J., DUMON, J. E., HULET, A. E., OKADA, S. and NAVARRO, C. (1973). Infantile metachromatic leukodystrophy. Confirmation of a prenatal diagnosis. *N. Engl. J. Med.*, **288**, 1365

38. SUZUKI, K., SCHNEIDER, E. L. and EPSTEIN, C. J. (1971). *In utero* diagnosis of globoid cell leukodystrophy (Krabbe's disease). *Biochem. Biophys. Res. Commun.*, **45**, 1363

39. BRADY, R. O., UHLENDORF, B. W. and JACOBSON, C. B. (1971). Fabry's disease: Antenatal detection. *Science (N.Y.)*, **172**, 174

40. PATRICK, A. D., WILLCOX, P., STEPHENS, R. and KENYON, V. G. (1976). Prenatal diagnosis of Wolman's disease. *J. Med. Genet.*, **13**, 49
41. HUIJING, F., WARREN, R. J. and McLEOD, A. G. W. (1973). Elevated activity of lysosomal enzymes in amniotic fluid of fetus with mucolipidosis II (I-cell disease). *Clin. Chim. Acta*, **44**, 453
42. NADLER, H. L. and EGAN, T. J. (1970). Deficiency of lysosomal acid phosphatase; A new familial metabolic disorder. *N. Engl. J. Med.*, **282**, 302
43. NADLER, H. L. and MESSINA, A. M. (1969). *In utero* detection of type II glycogenosis (Pompe's disease). *Lancet*, **ii**, 1277
44. SCHULMAN, J. D., FUJIMOTO, W. Y., BRADLEY, K. H. and SEEGMILLER, J. E. (1970). Identification of heterozygous genotype for cystinosis *in utero* by a new pulse-labelling technique: Preliminary report. *J. Pediatr.*, **77**, 468
45. SCHNEIDER, J. A., VERROUST, F. M., KROLL, W. A., GARVIN, A. J., HORGER, E. O., WONG, V. G., SPEAR, G. S., JACOBSON, C., PELLETT, O. L. and BECKER, F. L. A. (1974). Prenatal diagnosis of cystinosis. *N. Engl. J. Med.*, **290**, 878
46. FRATANTONI, J. C., NEUFELD, E. F., UHLENDORF, B. W. and JACOBSON, C. B. (1969). Intrauterine diagnosis of the Hurler and Hunter syndromes. *N. Engl. J. Med.*, **280**, 686
47. HALL, C. W. and NEUFELD, E. F. (1973). α-L-iduronidase activity in cultured skin fibroblasts and amniotic fluid cells. *Arch. Biochem. Biophys.*, **158**, 817
48. LIM, T. W., LEDER, I. G., BACH, G. and NEUFELD, E. F. (1974). An assay for iduronate sulfatase (Hunter corrective factor). *Carbohydr. Res.*, **37**, 103
49. KRESSE, H. (1973). Mucopolysaccharidosis IIIA (Sanfilippo A disease): Deficiency of a heparin sulfamidase in skin fibroblasts and leucocytes. *Biochem. Biophys. Res. Commun.*, **54**, 1111
50. O'BRIEN, J. S. (1972). Sanfilippo syndrome: Profound deficiency of alpha-acetyl-glucosaminidase activity in organs and skin fibroblasts from type B patients. *Proc. Natl. Acad. Sci. U.S.A.*, **69**, 1720
51. BERATIS, N. G., TURNER, B. M., WEISS, R. and HIRSCHHORN, K. (1975). Aryl-sulfatase B deficiency in Maroteaux–Lamy syndrome: Cellular studies and carrier identification. *Pediatr. Res.*, **9**, 475
52. BUTTERWORTH, J., SCOTT, F., McCRAE, W. M. and BAIN, A. D. (1972). Lysosomal enzymes of cultured fibroblasts of cystic fibrosis patients. *Clin. Chim. Acta*, **40**, 139
53. FENSOM, A. H., BENSON, P. F. and BLUNT, S. (1974). Prenatal diagnosis of galactosaemia. *Br. Med. J.*, **4**, 386
54. HOO, J. J., LATTA, E. and SCHAUMLOFFEL, E. (1974). Antenatal diagnosis of maple syrup urine disease. *Z. Kinderheilkd.*, **118**, 225
55. ELSAS, L. J., PRIEST, J. H., WHEELER, F. B., DANNER, D. J. and PASK, B. A. (1974). Maple syrup urine disease: Coenzyme function and prenatal monitoring. *Metabolism*, **23**, 569
56. UHLENDORF, B. W. (1970). In M. Harris (ed.), *Early Diagnosis of Human Genetic Defects*. Fogarty, Int. Centre Proc., No. 6, pp. 149–68
57. GOODMAN, S. I., MACE, J. W., TURNER, B. and GARRETT, W. J. (1973). Antenatal diagnosis of argininosuccinic aciduria. *Clin. Genet.*, **4**, 236
58. ROERDINK, F. H., GOUW, W. L. M., OKKEN, A., VAN DER BLIJ, J. F., LUIT-DE HAAN, G. and HOMMES, F. A. (1973). Citrullinemia; Report of a case, with studies on antenatal diagnosis. *Pediatr. Res.*, **7**, 863
59. GOMPERTZ, D., GOODEY, P. A., THOM, H., RUSSELL, G., MacLEAN, M. W., FERGUSON-SMITH, M. E. and FERGUSON-SMITH, M. A. (1973). Antenatal diagnosis of propionic-acidaemia. *Lancet*, **i**, 1009, (Letter)
60. MAHONEY, M. J., ROSENBERG, L. E., LINDBLAD, B., WALDENSTROM, J. and ZETTERSTROM, R. (1975). Prenatal diagnosis of methylmalonic aciduria. *Acta Paediatr. Scand.*, **64**, 44
61. MORROW, G., SCHWARZ, R. H., HALLOCK, J. A. and BARNESS, L. A. (1970). Prenatal detection of methylmalonic aciduria. *J. Pediatr.*, **77**, 120
62. FUJIMOTO, W. Y., SEEGMILLER, J. E., UHLENDORF, B. W. and JACOBSON, C. B. (1968). Biochemical diagnosis of X-linked disease *in utero*. *Lancet*, **ii**, 511
63. DE MARS, R., SARTO, G., FELIX, J. S. and BENKE, P. (1969). Lesch–Nyhan mutation: Prenatal detection with amniotic fluid cells. *Science* (*N.Y.*), **164**, 1303
64. BOYLE, J. A., RAIVIO, K. A., AUSTIN, K. H., SCHULMAN, J. D., GRAF, M. L., SEEGMILLER, J. E. and JACOBSON, C. B. (1970). Lesch–Nyhan syndrome: Preventive control by prenatal diagnosis. *Science* (*N.Y.*), **169**, 688
65. HIRSCHHORN, R., BERATIS, N., ROSEN, F. S., PARKMAN, R., STERN, R. and POLMER,

S. (1975). Adenosine deaminase deficiency in a child diagnosed prenatally. *Lancet*, **i**, 73

66. RAMSAY, C. A., COLTART, T. M., BLUNT, S., PAWSEY, S. A. and GIANNELLI, F. (1974). Prenatal diagnosis of xeroderma pigmentosum. *Lancet*, **ii**, 1109.

67. ZIELKE, K., VEATH, M. L. and O'BRIEN, J. S. (1972). Fucocidosis: deficiency of α-L-fucosidase in cultured skin fibroblasts. *J. Exp. Med.*, **136**, 197.

68. AULA, P., NANTO, V., LAIPIO, M. L. and AUTIO, S. (1973). Aspartylglucosaminuria: deficiency of aspartyl-glucosaminidase in cultured fibroblasts of patients and their heterozygous parents. *Clin. Genet.*, **4**, 297

69. BENSON, P. F., BLUNT, S. and BROWN, S. P. (1973). Amniotic-cell galactokinase activity: stimulation by galactose. *Lancet*, **i**, 106

70. HOWELL, R. R., KABACK, M. M. and BROWN, B. I. (1971). Type IV glycogen storage disease: branching enzyme deficiency in skin fibroblasts and possible heterozygote detection. *J. Pediatr.*, **78**, 638

71. BLASS, J. P., AVIGAN, J. and UHLENDORF, B. W. (1970). A defect in pyruvate decarboxylase in a child with an intermittent movement disorder. *J. Clin. Invest.*, **49**, 423

72. DANCIS, J., HUTZLER, J., COX, R. P. and WOODY, N. L. (1969). Familial hyperlysinemia with lysine-ketoglutarate reductase insufficiency. *J. Clin. Invest.*, **48**, 1447

73. HERNDON, J. H., STEINBERG, D. and UHLENDORF, B. D. (1969). Refsum's disease: Defective oxidation of phytanic acid in tissue cultures derived from homozygotes and heterozygotes. *N. Engl. J. Med.*, **281**, 1034

74. HERS, H. G. (1965). Inborn lysosomal diseases. *Gastroenterology*, **48**, 625

75. WILLCOX, P. and PATRICK, A. D. (1974). Biochemical diagnosis of cystinosis using cultured cells. *Arch. Dis. Child.*, **49**, 209

76. GALJAARD, H., NIERMEIJER, M. F., HAHNEMANN, N., MOHR, J. and SORENSEN, S. A. (1974). An example of rapid prenatal diagnosis of Fabry's disease using micro techniques. *Clin. Genet.*, **5**, 368

77. NIERMEIJER, M. F., KOSTER, J. F., JAHODOVA, M., FERNANDES, J., HEUKELS-DULLY, M. J. and GALJAARD, H. (1975). Prenatal diagnosis of Type II glycogenosis (Pompe's disease) using microchemical analyses. *Pediatr. Res.*, **9**, 498

78. NIERMEIJER, M. F., SACHS, E. S., JAHODOVA, M., TICHELAAR-KLEPPER, W. J., KLEIJER, W. J. and GALJAARD, H. (1976). Prenatal diagnosis of genetic disorders in 350 pregnancies. *J. Med. Genet.* (In press)

79. BROCK, D. J. H. (1974). Prenatal diagnosis and genetic counselling. *J. Clin. Pathol.* **27** (Suppl.) (Roy. Coll. Pathol.), **8**, 150

80. EMERY, A. E. H., BURT, D., NELSON, M. M. and SCRIMGEOUR, J. B. (1970). Antenatal diagnosis and aminoacid composition of amniotic fluid. *Lancet*, **i**, 1307

81. JEFFCOATE, T. N. A., FLIEGNER, J. R. H., RUSSELL, S. H., DAVIS, J. C. and WADE, A. P. (1965). Diagnosis of the adreno-genital syndrome before birth. *Lancet*, **ii**, 553

82. MERKATZ, I. R., NEW, M. I., PETERSON, R. E. and SEAMAN, M. P. (1969). Prenatal diagnosis of adrenogenital syndrome by amniocentesis. *J. Pediatr.*, **75**, 977

83. MATALON, R., DORFMAN, A., NADLER, H. L. and JACOBSON, C. B. (1970). A chemical method for the antenatal diagnosis of mucopolysaccharidoses. *Lancet*, **i**, 83

84. MATALON, R., DORFMAN, A. and NADLER, H. L. (1972). A chemical method for the antenatal diagnosis of mucopolysaccharidosis. *Lancet*, **i**, 798

85. BROCK, D. J. H., GORDON, H., SELIGMAN, S. and LOBO, E. (1971). Antenatal detection of Hurler's syndrome. *Lancet*, **ii**, 1324

86. WHITEMAN, P. (1973). Prenatal diagnosis of mucopolysaccharidosis. *Lancet*, **i**, 1249, (Letter)

87. SALAFSKY, I. and NADLER, H. L. (1971). Alpha-1, 4-glucosidase activity in Pompe's disease. *J. Pediatr.*, **79**, 794

88. SUTCLIFFE, R. G. and BROCK, D. J. H. (1972). Observation on the origin of amniotic fluid enzymes. *J. Obstet. Gynaecol. Br. Cwlth.*, **79**, 902

89. BORRESEN, A. L. and VAN DER HAGEN, C. B. (1973). Metachromatic leukodystrophy: II. Direct determination of arylsulphatase A activity in amniotic fluid. *Clin. Genet.*, **4**, 442

90. ELLIS, R. B., IKONNE, J. U. and MASSON, P. K. (1975). DEAE-cellulose microcolumn chromatography coupled with automated assay: application to resolution of N-acetyl-β-D-hexosaminidase components. *Analyt. Biochem.*, **63**, 5

14

The phenylketonuria register for the United Kingdom

F. P. Hudson* and Janet Hawcroft

After a series of meetings held at the headquarters of the Medical Research Council in 1962 and 1963 a committee, under the chairmanship of the late Sir Alan Moncrieff, decided to collect information relating to the diagnosis and progress of all phenylketonuric patients born in the United Kingdom on and after January 1st 1964. Out of this project has developed the Phenylketonuria Register for the United Kingdom, now maintained at Alder Hey Children's Hospital in Liverpool. The original committee has been replaced by a small steering committee which meets about once a year.

It seems strange to recall that only 11 years ago some people were sceptical of the benefits claimed for the dietary treatment of phenylketonuria,[1] and many considered screening for this disorder to be a waste of time and money. At the outset the register was designed simply to collect as many facts as possible relating to the diagnosis and progress of each patient. The objectives were to assess the efficiency of the screening programme, which was then in its infancy and based mainly on modifications of the ferric chloride test on urine, and also to determine whether early treatment really produced the benefits being claimed.

No attempts were made to initiate a controlled trial, to centralize treatment in a few clinics, or to recommend standards for biochemical control. This of course fitted in with the British medical tradition of complete freedom for the individual clinician. With passing years, and rapidly increasing knowledge of the subject, changes became necessary in the type of information collected. For example, rather crude methods for estimating eye and hair colour have been discontinued, and a request for biochemical details which might help to distinguish variant forms of the disease has been added.

Interest is now centred almost entirely on patients who have been

* Dr Hudson died on 2nd June 1976.

diagnosed early, usually as a result of a screening test. Of patients born in the first 2 years of the register (1964 and 1965) nearly half were mentally retarded at the time of diagnosis. By June 1975, of the 760 cases on the register, nearly 600 were diagnosed before the age of 4 months. Today phenylketonuria as a cause of mental retardation is a rarity. The steady fall to almost complete elimination of cases detected after the age of 3 months is shown in Figure 14.1.

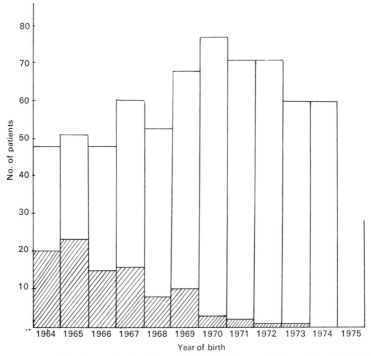

FIGURE 14.1 Numbers of phenylketonuric patients notified to the MRC/DHSS Register according to year of birth and whether the diagnosis was made early (less than 4 months of age) or late (4 months of age or more). Open columns represent early diagnosed cases and shaded columns those diagnosed late (after 4 months)

Organization of the register

Notification of cases is entirely voluntary. Some disease registers offer treatment or expert diagnostic services in return for notification. The British Diabetic Association offers doctors the sum of £1 for each new juvenile diabetic notified. The Phenylketonuria Register relies solely on goodwill for notification of patients.

Information about newly diagnosed patients may reach the office from a Community Physician (formerly Medical Officer of Health) or from a paediatrician, or more recently from a screening laboratory. When the initial notification is received a request is sent to the paediatrician in charge of the patient asking for certain data relating to the diagnosis, clinical and biochemical findings, and perinatal history, together with a request for future cooperation in the completion of an annual progress report. This cooperation has always been given, though reminders that forms await completion are sometimes needed. The annual progress report includes data on the child's growth, general health, changes in social circumstances and all serum phenylalanine results. At the outset a development quotient measured by the Griffiths scale was requested every 3 months in the 1st year, and then every 6 months until the child was old enough to undertake a Merrill–Palmer or Stanford–Binet test. It soon became clear that this exercise was neither practicable nor useful. Measurement of the IQ on a Stanford–Binet form at age 4 years and on the Wechsler Intelligence Scale for Children at age 8 is now considered adequate. At the age of 8 a request is also made for the completion of standardized questionnaires relating to behaviour.[2,3] One form is completed by a parent, and a slightly different one by the child's school teacher, who also completes forms for two control children from the same class.

The staff of the Register office never make contact with patients or parents directly, the majority of whom are probably unaware of the existence of this register. Most people quite rightly feel that disease should be a private affair between patient and doctor. Forms for IQ testing and the parents section of the behaviour test are sent from the office to the clinician in charge who personally arranges for their completion. When IQ forms have been completed by the local psychologist they are sent to the principal psychologist at the Hospital for Sick Children in London for review. The parents' behaviour form includes a request for permission to send a similar form to the child's school. When this permission reaches the office the relevant forms and explanatory letter are sent to the Area Community Physician so that the approach to the school may be made through the local school medical department.

All the records for each child and any special correspondence are stored in lever arch files. Essential data is extracted from the forms and entered on specially designed cards for easy access and analysis. These are filed by sex and year of birth. A call forward system, used to identify patients due for completion of the annual follow-up form, consists of a card for each child filed by month of birth. Identifying colour tags, which can be attached to these cards, show the clerk which patient is due for special investigation, such as IQ testing, or for which patient return of the form is long overdue. Altogether each patient's name is recorded in five places: (1) a book containing a nominal roll in numerical order, (2) an alphabetical card index for which the initial notification card is used, (3) a card index filed by month of birth which forms the call forward system, (4) detailed annual reports completed by the clinician filed in lever arch files, (5) the analysis card. This system may sound cumbersome but the part-time staff in the office find it works smoothly. If for example the records are required of all early-treated cases with an IQ of less than 70 the relevant analysis cards can be quickly extracted. Certain data about these patients will then either be instantly available, or the card will indicate that fuller information (e.g. details of perinatal abnormality or an unusual social history) should be obtained from the initial or annual report.

The state of the register is constantly changing. Each month some 50 or 60 annual follow-up forms arrive in the office, and notification of five or six new cases is received. No doubt computerization would allow speedy retrieval of some data but the expense would be considerable and staff would have to travel to and from the computer site. However, when computerized methods of analysis are required, these are undertaken on our behalf by Dr Ian Sutherland of the MRC Statistical Research Unit.

The identification of each patient is ensured by recording the name, the date of birth and the case record number from the hospital where the patient is being treated. The National Health Service number is also requested but seldom obtained. In the register each patient is also identified by a serial number, followed by the year of birth, followed by the letter A, B, or C. A indicates that the diagnosis was made in the first 3 months of life, B that the diagnosis was made between the age of 4 and 12 months, and C that the diagnosis was made after the age of 12 months.

All patient records are, of course, received and maintained in strict confidence, but can, with the approval of the steering committee, be made available to research workers both in this country and overseas.

The annual running cost includes salaries based on National Health Service scales for one part-time medical research assistant (five sessions in Senior Registrar grade), one part-time secretary (three sessions) and one part-time filing clerk (two sessions). In addition there is the cost of postage, telephone, stationery and travelling expenses. The cost is met jointly by the Department of Health and Social Security and the Medical Research Council.

To know about every phenylketonuric patient in the United Kingdom born since January 1st 1964, has required goodwill and cooperation from many paediatricians. An attempt was made 2 years ago to find out how many patients had been overlooked. The chairman of the steering committee, Professor O. H. Wolff, sent a letter to all paediatricians asking for information about cases not known to be registered. As a result of this request, followed where necessary by a reminder letter from the Phenylketonuria Office (which also asked for nil returns) a reply was received from almost every paediatrician in the country, adding 114 names, an addition of about 20%, to the register. It is hoped that ascertainment of new cases will be complete in the future because screening laboratory directors notify the office of all positive tests, either at the time of testing or in an annual report.

Liaison with screening laboratories

The staff of the Phenylketonuria Office has established and maintains contact with all screening laboratories by telephone, letter, or in many cases by a personal visit. This aspect of the work started soon after 1969 when the Department of Health and Social Security recommended the use of a blood test in preference to a urine test for early detection of phenylketonuria.[4] At that time the Guthrie test was already being used extensively in Scotland. In England, a few laboratories were using blood screening, but only for limited areas, and usually financed by research monies. Following the Department's recommendation many other laboratories set up a screening unit. The location of these was not determined by central planning, but rather by the existence of local enthusiasm. The result was the establishment of 34 screening centres in England alone. All directors of screening laboratories kindly supply the Register Office with annual statistics relating to number of babies tested and cases of phenylketonuria (Table 14.1). It is thus possible to estimate the percentage of babies tested. The number of births, kindly supplied by the Office of Population Censuses and Surveys does of course include early neonatal deaths where testing will not have been possible.

Table 14.1   Screening   for   phenylketonuria   in   the   United Kingdom.

Year	Estimated births	Babies tested	Percentage tested	Phenylketonuric patients diagnosed by screening
1972	846 058	803 492	94	70
1973	780 729	772 971	99	58
1974	755 592	732 167	96	60

It is hoped that this valuable liaison will continue to be maintained on a personal and unofficial basis. It should serve as an early warning system if enthusiasm for screening were to decline in any part of the country, in addition to providing the Health Service administrators with information showing that financial investment in screening for phenylketonuria is both efficient and productive.

In the past 3 years an annual newsletter has been prepared and sent to all directors of screening laboratories, all members of the British Paediatric Association, and to a number of other interested persons in this country and abroad. These notes provide information regarding the numerical state of the Register, and give some account of the use made by the Register office of the details supplied about patients. They also serve as a reminder that notification of every case is still requested.

Benefits of the register

In 1968 information from the register was used in the preparation of a report to the Medical Research Council on the availability and efficiency of screening tests for phenylketonuria in the United Kingdom.[5] Following this report the Department of Health and Social Security recommended the use of a blood test for screening,[4] and this was rapidly followed by great improvement in early diagnosis. On the same theme the Register provides the yearly report on the percentage of babies tested and the number of cases detected. Should there be an unexpected fall the area in which this occurred could probably be promptly identified.

In 1970 concern was expressed in America about some unexpected figures regarding the sex incidence of phenylketonuria and possible danger that early screening failed to detect some female cases.[6] Rapid retrieval of information from the Phenylketonuria Register showed that the timing of the test in the United Kingdom made it unlikely that cases would be missed, even should the rise in phenylalanine be delayed in girls, and also that the sex incidence was equal for cases detected by screening.[7] This information was made available in greater detail to Drs Starfield and Holtzman who recently published their observations on the relative efficiency of screening and confirmatory diagnosis in the United Kingdom, Eire and the USA.[8]

To some questions there can be no quick return of an answer. An adequate number of patients must be followed for a sufficiently long period. Adequate data is now available on 226 patients followed from birth to the time of the first IQ test at 4 years. This material is at present being analysed by Dr Ian Sutherland, with particular reference to the factors influencing the intelligence quotient, but detailed findings are not yet available. By the end of 1976, 178 children will have been followed from birth to the age of 8, when the second IQ test is performed. Review of these children will probably give some information about the effect of terminating or relaxing dietary treatment.

Measurements of intelligence quotient and behaviour in childhood are of considerable interest, but the steering committee is now considering the problems of follow-up extending into adult life. It will not be easy for the Register office to keep in touch, indirectly and without any personal approach, when the patients leave school, leave paediatric clinics, and if dietary treatment has ended, do not feel the need for regular hospital supervision.

Assistance in keeping track of patients, particularly those who change their name or address, will probably be possible through collaboration with the Office of Population Censuses and Surveys and the National Health Service Central Register. Time may show that this part of the work is even more important than all that precedes it, for eventually the success or failure of screening programmes and dietary treatment will be judged by the ability of the patients to play a useful role in society.

REFERENCES

1. BIRCH, H. G. and TIZARD, J. (1967). The dietary treatment of phenylketonuria: not proven? *Dev. Med. Child. Neurol.*, **9**, 9
2. RUTTER, M. (1967). A children's behaviour questionnaire for completion by teachers: preliminary findings. *J. Child Psychol. Psychiat.*, **8**, 1
3. RUTTER, M., TIZARD, J. and WHITMORE, K. (1970). *Education, Health and Behaviour*. (London: Longman)

4. Department of Health and Social Security (1969). Screening for early detection of phenylketonuria. (HM(69)72)
5. Present status of different mass screening procedures for phenylketonuria. (1968). *Br. Med. J.*, **4**, 7
6. KOCH, R., DOBSON, J., HSIA, D. Y. Y. and WOOLF, L. I. (1971). Conference on sex ratio in phenylketonuria. *J. Pediatr.*, **78**, 157
7. HAWCROFT, J. and HUDSON, F. P. (1973). Sex ratio among phenylketonuric infants in the United Kingdom. *Lancet*, **ii**, 702
8. STARFIELD, B. and HOLTZMAN, N. A. (1975). A comparison of effectiveness of screening for phenylketonuria in the United States, United Kingdom and Ireland. *N. Engl. J. Med.*, **293**, 118

15

Computerized central registers

A. J. Hedley

The title of this chapter embraces a large number of medical, social, administrative and economic issues so that, in the space available, no more can be done than introduce some of the important topics and provide the basis for more detailed planning of specific applications. The problem of maintaining long-term contact with patients is not a new one. In 1916, writing a report on the natural history of retinal changes in arteriosclerosis, R. F. Q. Moore[1] commented: 'The difficulty of keeping in touch with patients owing to their migratory habits is notorious . . . I have always from the first observed the precaution of taking in addition to the patient's address . . . the address of one or more of their relatives.' A statement which epitomizes the difficulties which professional health workers continue to experience in their attempts to maintain contact with patients over long periods—including the entire life span of some individuals. The register is one device which has been used to achieve this particular objective within the framework of a health service which aims to provide continuous and comprehensive health care.

Registers: some definitions

It will assist our discussion if we first define the structure and functions of registers. In its most basic form a register may simply consist of a list of items or names, each of which can be individually identified. Even in the simplest register, however, more information is usually collected in addition to that actually needed to identify the individual or provide basic medical care. Both the opportunity and the need to study the various epidemiological aspects of the disease under surveillance will determine the quantity of additional information which is collected. Death registration, for example, includes *causes* of death because of the utility of this information in studying the natural history of diseases and their response to treatment.

A register may be a file or series of files of documents on individuals—

the contents of which are compiled by a standard method so that information obtained from the whole population is uniform in nature. This
demands adherence to a systematic and comprehensive approach to data
collection.[2] From the point of view of effectiveness, value for money and
not least, motivation, there should be a predetermined purpose for the
use of the information collected. Finally under definitions, there is a
helpful statement by an expert committee of WHO (1967).[3] 'The term
registration implies something more than notification. A register
requires that a permanent record be established, that cases be followed
up and that basic statistical tabulations be prepared both on frequency
and survival. In addition, patients on a register should frequently be the
subjects of special studies.'

For the follow-up of chronic disease a systems approach to the
development of continuous and comprehensive patient care is required,
even if the primary task is only the most basic one of maintaining contact with patients. In its most elementary form it must include most of
the following components (Figure 15.1):

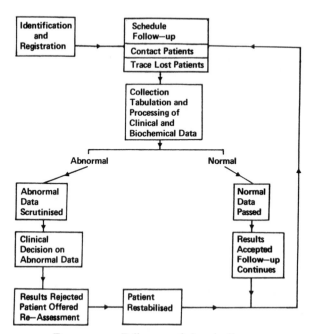

FIGURE 15.1   Follow-up of chronic disease

1. A system of patient identification and a reliable method of registration. If patient data is liable to be amended or updated for any reason then a system of scheduling and contacting patients and tracing lost individuals is required.

2. If physiological variables are to be measured and used to discriminate between normal and abnormal states then subroutines which will classify normal and abnormal results are needed.

3. If the follow-up data satisfy predetermined criteria and patients are graded as normal then records may be updated and follow-up continued without interruption. However if any information received is classified as abnormal or inconsistent provision must be made for suspension of follow-up, further scrutiny of results and decision by a trained observer.

4. If necessary further contact with the patient must be made by general practitioner or other professional health worker; this may involve a clinical assessment, additional treatment and re-stabilization before re-registration in the system.

Registers for chronic disease

The problems in iatrogenic disease which stimulated our interest in registers lead to the design of the Scottish Automated Thyroid Register (SAFUR), which has now been operating for 6 years. It has been fully documented elsewhere,[4,5] but some aspects of its organization exemplify important problems and pitfalls which accompany the establishment and maintenance of registers, particularly those with potential for development on a large scale.

One of these problems concerns large groups of patients receiving long-term treatment or replacement therapy for chronic disease. Several authors, in different clinical specialities, between 1957 and 1969 demonstrated by objective tests that default on treatment and replacement therapy ranged from 32% up to 65%, averaging around half of all patients treated.[6-9] In our own endocrine clinic we found that 70% of all patients who had been prescribed lifelong thyroxine replacement therapy were inadequately treated for one reason or another, including patient non-compliance, errors in prescribing or dispensing or a real change in patient requirements.[10] Another aspect of this problem concerns late onset complications following certain types of empirical treatment. A review of the journals shows that an evaluation of the outcome of treatment has obviously been of special interest to some workers for the best part of 50 years but our performance in maintaining contact with patients over long periods has been erratic to say the least and certainly has not noticeably improved.[11,12] Similarly in our endocrine clinic we found that 40% of a group of about 1000 patients treated for thyrotoxicosis over a 20-year period could not be identified or traced. Previously undetected morbidity was 40% in those who were traced and we must conclude that it reached at least this level in those we could not find.[13]

This is an extremely unsatisfactory method of managing long-term health problems, of assessing the outcome of particular forms of treatment and may be seriously misleading when used in the evaluation of health care.

SCOTTISH AUTOMATED FOLLOW-UP REGISTER (SAFUR)

The general approach described above has been the basis for the design of the Automated Register in Scotland which provides a follow-up facility for general practitioners and their patients who have been treated in several different ways for various forms of thyroid disease. Since its inception SAFUR has been extended from Aberdeen in the north-east of Scotland to four other centres including Inverness, Dundee, Edinburgh and Glasgow. The system provides a series of links between hospital records departments, endocrine clinics, clinical chemistry laboratories, general practitioners, patients and appropriate information handling and processing facilities. All these activities are coordinated by a central registry which provides a service with both secretarial and medical components. The registry provides for automatic registration of patients who receive certain forms of treatment in a hospital clinic. For example, treatment with radioactive iodine therapy will not be dispensed within the Grampian Area Health Board unless registration is carried out. The order form for the isotope and initial registration procedure are enjoined in the same document.[4] The register was converted from a manual to an automated system in 1969 and by the end of this year will hold records on over 4000 patients who are under the care of more than 1000 general practitioners.

LARGE-SCALE REGISTERS

The thyroid register has been mentioned as an example of a regional system which was capable of development into a national network using the original central computer-assisted registry facilities. Further examples of early work in this field include registers for psychiatric illness and mental handicap in Nottingham, Salford, Camberwell, Aberdeen and other centres holding files on between 4000 and 40 000 patients.[2,14]

However it has been suggested that those working in the field of inborn errors of metabolism might ultimately be projecting plans for a register with a file holding records on several million persons. Experience of that kind of operation does not exist in the field of registers for specific diseases. So to examine the kind of problems which would be encountered we must extrapolate from existing registers or alternatively look at large applications which are either not directly concerned with patient care or situated outside the health service. Systems of particular interest would be those in which the total volume of information handled, the level of transactions, and the method of identification will provide useful illustrations of the kind of problem solving exercises likely to be met.

For example, there are 21 government departments using computing techniques in approximately 200 tasks. Most of these deal with between 10 000 and 1 million persons each, but some are much bigger. One of these, the Driver Vehicle Licence Centre in Swansea, maintains files on several million drivers and vehicles. The size of the main file for driver licencing in mid-January 1976 was 18.5 million records, with a predicted increase to 24 million records by October 1976.[15] Some additional details from this operation are provided below to illustrate potential problems in large-scale systems.

Finally, a study of certain manual operations should also be compulsory for those interested in the construction of large registers. For example, the United States Social Security Administration operates a system which holds 272 million records and in Britain the Central National Health Service (NHS) Registers maintain between 50 and 60 million records. Both systems were developed on an index card basis with all operations conducted manually, including, in the latter, incoming notifications of 30 000 births and deaths each week.[16]

Registers: ideal conditions

SETTING OBJECTIVES

Any plan for the design of a register which will collect and record patient information in cumulative files must be accompanied by a clear statement of all principal and secondary objectives which is understood and accepted by all members of the group. The relationship between purely service functions, such as the intention to provide specific forms of patient care, must be recognized as a separate objective from say the utilization of patient data for socio-medical research. It may be insufficiently recognized that very often the information needed for the maintenance of patient care and the evaluation of this process is only a very small part of that which *may* be collected for research purposes. As much of this information is likely to be 'sensitive', scrutiny of any proposal for setting up a register is likely to be subject to such questions as:

1. For what purpose is the information being collected?
2. For how long will the information be kept?
3. How would patients be affected if the information was incomplete or inaccurate?
4. How would the patient's life be affected if sensitive information was obtained by unauthorized persons?

In a register for patients with inborn errors of metabolism the main objectives might be:

Prevention
1. Improved scope for prevention; identification, counselling and prevention of (unwanted) pregnancy in high risk couples
2. Improved records for research, better opportunities to study social, medical and environmental factors in the search for causal associations; use of the register as a sampling frame from which to obtain comparable groups of patients in randomized controlled trials.

Patient care
Certain and rapid contact with patients; standardization of and better access to patient records; monitoring of substitution therapy; prevention or early detection of complications.

RESOURCES

Even when all conditions for setting-up have been fulfilled, because of the complexity and cost of establishing and maintaining large registers, the final step should only be undertaken when the information to be obtained and objectives to be met cannot be achieved as efficiently by some other means. For example, the use of other health care agents such as general practice units or out-patient clinics should be considered. We cannot escape this clause particularly at a time of severe and increasing economic constraints and diminishing funds for new enterprises. Where would a computer-assisted central register, in your *own* sphere of interest rank in the list of priorities for health care development if it had to compete for limited resources?

The availability of secretarial and clerical staff to administer the system is a vital issue. The work of supervising central and sub-registries can be tedious and the necessary qualities of patience and tenacity, in fact total commitment, for solving problems are becoming less easy to find at the level of remuneration which normally accompanies these posts.

FIRST CONTACT WITH PATIENTS

One problem which merits emphasis concerns the initial decision on what is to be the sampling frame for the register population. There are at least three options:

1. The register population may be identified by some form of well-population screening.

2. Use may be made of the existing lines of communication with health care agents (e.g. out-patient departments and general practice units) as a means of case-finding.

3. The third option for a system of registration utilizes both the routine medical record and also the act of treatment and has to be actively contracted out of by the patient or the general practitioner if it is to be stopped.

Well-population screening may be an attractive proposition for comprehensive coverage, or even to obtain a population size which would justify the establishment of a register. However, ethical problems and the validation of screening for all the conditions to be followed-up would first have to be resolved (see the contribution in the present volume by Dr T. W. Meade). Case finding, the method used by the psychiatric register, avoids these problems and in the thyroid register, registration for lifelong follow-up is part of the treatment plan offered to patients.

PATIENT IDENTIFICATION

Some of the options open to us for accurate and reliable identification of patients are summarized in Table 15.1.

Table 15.1   Some requirements for patient identification

Personal numbers	*Nominal identifying data*
Hospital or regional unit numbers	Initials
National health service number	Forename
National insurance number	Birth name (maiden name)
Special operational numbers	Date of birth
Numbers derived from nominal data	Sex
Self-checking numbers	

Personal numbers

These may already exist on an institutional or regional basis, such as unit numbers, or a national basis such as the NHS number or National Insurance (NI) number. Alternatively, a personal number may be specially formulated and allocated as an operational number for a particular register and could be cross-indexed with another established number or with other nominal identifying data such as name, sex and date of birth. Numbers actually derived from nominal identifying data such as the Hogben number[17] (Midland Personnel Number) did not enjoy much success in medical information systems. However, in the United Kingdom the new driving licence provides a more recent example of a unique code derived from surname, initials, sex and date of birth by a technique known as 'hash coding',[18] often used in computer systems.

In addition to an allocated number such as a unit number, one or more characters which are derived by performing certain calculations on it, can be helpful in detecting errors. The additional character, which may be alphabetic or numerical depending on the method used, is called a check digit, the complete set being known as a self-checking number. This system is used for both the thyroid and psychiatric registers. It is eminently suitable for the psychiatric register which is a regional system but in the thyroid register it will not prevent transposition of a patient between the files of any of the five centres, all of which use their own local series of six digit unit numbers running from one to 999 999.

A register could be established and record linkage achieved by using data other than personal numbers. A large number of items, of nominal data such as surname, maiden name and mother's maiden name, date of birth, place of birth and sometimes geographical location or address are available for this purpose. Experience has shown that this type of information is not as standard or predictable as might be expected. There may be considerable variation in items such as date of birth when recorded by patients on different occasions.[16] Immigrants may not easily fit into a system designed for the majority of British names and information such as post codes is not readily supplied by the public.[15] It is, however, at best regarded as a supplementary rather than principal method of identification.

A system of personal, unique and universal (or nearly so) numbers does exist in several countries. For example, in the United Kingdom it is the NHS number and in the United States the Social Security Number. Unfortunately, the composition of the NHS number and its availability have not only deterred but prevented its use to index, sort and update personal cumulative records in a computer-assisted register. As a result manual files must be maintained and cross-indexed with another computer compatible number. In Scotland there are no less than 14 different formats for this number, and one of these has three variants. All of them consist of different subsets of alphabetic and numerical characters. In England and Wales there are several further forms. Discussions between the offices of the Registrars General have not yet resulted in agreement on a single format for the United Kingdom. However during the last 2 years Scotland has standardized on an eight digit all-numerical code comprising three subsets which identify registration district, year of entry and a serial number.

When the SAFUR registry was first established we chose to identify patients solely by their regional unit number and did not embark on routine collection of NHS numbers. It is a decision we have since regretted, particularly because it has not proved possible to identify all dead patients and tabulate causes of death without 'flagging' our register population in the central NHS Register. The portents for obtaining this number in retrospect were not good. For example, in the Oxford Record Linkage Study[16] it was found that even special efforts by the hospital admission offices only resulted in a yield of 40%. Indeed, how many professional health workers know their number or even where to find it? One thing is certain, if it was used to identify our pay packets, impressive progress in medical record linkage would be made. The issue and use of a universal number in several activities which are sponsored or monitored by the state is likely to remain a contentious political issue for some time.

Availability of NHS numbers

In 1974–75, a survey of patients on the register files of Aberdeen, Dundee, Edinburgh and Glasgow was carried out.[19] The main objective was to obtain a record of the NHS number. Out of 2989 information forms sent to patients, 2673 were returned completed. The non-response rate running at 9–13%, of which 4% could be attributed to incorrect identification by name or address which resulted in the form being returned undelivered.

In the 90% sample returned, between 65% and 75% of patients provided a NHS number which matched one of the 14 Scottish formats or one of the English numbers. Most of the remaining 30% provided either place of birth and/or another number, usually the NI number (Table 15.2).

The response, which is more encouraging than might have been anticipated, is remarkably uniform throughout the country. From a practical point of view we are now able to 'flag' all our patients, using either NHS number or place of birth to locate them in the NHS central register. NHS numbers for all new registrations are now routinely obtained from patients, general practice units or from the records of the primary care administrators for the appropriate area health board.

Table 15.2   SAFUR NHS numbers survey: correct returns

	No. of forms issued	Total returned (%)	Correct NHS number (%)	Incorrect information
Aberdeen	1637	1480 (90.4)	1112 (75.1)	368 (24.9)
Dundee	296	271 (91.5)	169 (62.4)	102 (37.6)
Edinburgh	207	184 (88.9)	124 (67.4)	60 (32.6)
Glasgow	849	738 (86.9)	483 (65.5)	255 (35.0)
Totals	2989	2673 (89.4)	1888 (70.6)	785 (29.4)

On the question of criteria it is rewarding to read Thomas's[20] discussion on the registration of children 'at risk' of handicap and also Richards and Roberts[21] critical article on the same subject. The latter wrote:

'the widespread adoption of the idea of an *at risk* register for the detection of handicapping disorders in infancy has led to a situation in which an undefined population is being screened for undefined conditions by people who, for the most part, are untrained to detect the conditions for which they arc looking.'

The first requirement is that the disease or conditions to be registered can be diagnosed with certainty. If there are difficulties in either establishing criteria for diagnosis or in standardizing laboratory techniques, which often appear for the first time when an exercise such as this is undertaken, or if the condition is one of multiple aetiology, then registration data may be heterogeneous and misleading. We have found that this is especially true if several different centres are involved. It is important to recognize that the detailed classification of the characteristics of patients and their diseases is frequently an entirely separate objective from that of maintaining long-term follow-up and providing appropriate specific care when required. In the thyroid register we need only identify two groups of patients, those receiving or not receiving thyroxine replacement therapy respectively, in order to monitor thyroid status and ensure the maintenance of a euthyroid state. However, the system was created with nine separate registration categories to identify variations in treatment and pathology.[4] One of these categories is allocated to the patient at the initial (first) registration procedure. A further series of re-registration categories enables changes in the patient's follow-up status to be recorded. In the 6 years since the register was converted from a manual to an automated system the initial registration categories have increased to 20 (with further additions being requested) and 14 separate re-registration options. However, because each registration category requires a certain number of re-registration options the registration form must carry a total of 79 entries in the re-registration columns (Figure 15.2).

The objective of collecting and processing these data is a perfectly legitimate and in many ways desirable one. It creates additional opportunities for the derivation of unique information about the natural

| COL. A – CONDITION FOR FIRST REGISTRATION | | | |
| COL. B – CONDITION FOR RE–REGISTRATION | | | |

Please ring appropriate code number

A	B		A	B	
01		RADIOACTIVE IODINE (RAI) FOR HYPERTHYROIDISM	09		SPONTANEOUS HYPOTHYROIDISM + REPLACEMENT THERAPY following an episode of hyperthyroidism
	01	RAI for recurrent hyperthyroidism			
	05	Euthyroid – No Change		10	Euthyroid – No Change
	06	Thyroxine replacement for hypothyroidism		11	Hypothyroid – Replacement dose corrected
	21	Euthyroid – No Change (Patient not recalled)		22	Hypothyroid – Irregular thyroxine therapy corrected
02		SURGERY FOR HYPERTHYROIDISM		23	Reassessed – Thyroxine dose reduced
				24	Euthyroid – No Change (Patient not recalled)
	03	RAI for recurrent hyperthyroidism			
	05	Euthyroid – No Change	15		AUTOIMMUNE THYROIDITIS
	07	Thyroxine replacement for hypothyroidism			+ REPLACEMENT THERAPY
	21	Euthyroid – No Change (Patient not recalled)			Euthyroid before treatment
03		SURGERY + RAI FOR HYPERTHYROIDISM			

FIGURE 15.2   Part of the registration form for patients with thyroid disease, illustrating initial (first) registration (column A) and re-registration (column B) categories

history of the disease and the activities of the health care facilities which are responsible for patients. However, unless extremely large numbers of patients are observed over a long period of time very little useful information will accrue in these small subgroups. Furthermore there is a penalty, which includes greater complexity for the user (and an increasing number of errors) more complex and time consuming programming, processing of files and secretarial activities. This is not a finite problem; it would be possible to continuously refine and extend the definitions of clinical status and follow-up events. This inevitably outstrips the ability of most users to comply with the extensive criteria for registration, while the information 'feed-back' exceeds their needs in the routine management of patients. If professional health workers cannot see the point of information collection in a procedure such as this they are unlikely to do it either willingly or well. The enthusiasm for and ability to record detail is unlikely to extend beyond a small group of specialists and innovators.

DATA CAPTURE

The best conditions for data capture, including the completion of the registration documents will be met when the data-base is explicit and accompanied by clear definitions and operational criteria. The data base should be designed to fulfil clearly defined functions and answer specific questions. How is the data base to be completed? The options here include medical staff; trained interviewers, who may be para-

'People do not want computers. They want systems. Systems that will perform useful functions for the minimum possible cost . . . (and) meet the objectives specified by the user.'

There is a great danger that the advocates of computer technology in the design of registers will over-emphasize the possible gains and take insufficient account of many organizational problems. Certainly, unless the objectives of establishing the register are well thought out and the proposed system is capable of meeting them, an efficient computer-assisted register will only be a mirage. What gains will accrue from the use of computers in this situation? The possible advantages of using a computerized system can be summarized as follows:

1. The need to create a system, which is compatible with computing techniques, exerts an important discipline on the designers and may be responsible for several beneficial changes in methods of working.

2. The use of computing techniques may be a crucial and unavoidable step if large cumulative files holding information on many clinical and social variables are required either for continuing patient management or to evaluate the long-term outcome of disease or treatment.

3. If the need for a high level of transactions on a daily or weekly basis must be met, then computing techniques may be the only means of providing rapid, accurate information flow on a large scale for all essential register procedures.

4. Computing, used as an alternative to other forms of work organization (e.g. by permitting centralization and sharing of facilities), may lead to improved efficiency and cost-effectiveness, unattainable by other methods.

Those potential gains should form the basis of any study which is mounted to assess the need for computing in the design of a register. It should be appreciated, however, that although the techniques of systems analysis are used to study the clinical and organizational problems, the register and its mode of operation which results from this work will not necessarily be dependent on computing facilities.

The use of computing in the establishment and development of a register will highlight deficiencies in the organization and logic of the system if they remain at the time of implementation. The creation of a viable and adaptable computerized register which provides, in addition to patient identification, a cumulative file of clinical and biochemical variables, requires a lengthy and thorough trial and developmental stage using largely non-automated techniques. Those workers who intend to mount pilot studies on the establishment and use of registers, may be attracted to the principle of punched feature cards as a flexible and versatile manual approach which is also compatible with computer methods.[26] Premature conversion to an automated system or deficiencies in the computer-register interface could lead to chaos, or at least disrepute, particularly amongst occasional users or those with a limited interest in and knowledge of its working. The optimum point at which to convert the system to a computer-assisted operation must be a matter of judgement. However, the decision should be based on objective evidence of its efficiency and an estimate of the probable need for further modifications in design and the resources which will be required to meet them. It is of course inevitable that the demands of users will change and it is unreasonable to expect the originators' design to continue to meet all requirements 10 years from its inception. However, it is important that the original objectives of the system are not lost sight of; they will have determined the format and content of the programmes and any marked deviation from this plan may be disruptive, and require considerable consultation and reprinting of standard documents. The costs of re-programming may be high, especially if frequent amendments and changes are required.

COMPUTING TECHNIQUES IN THE USE OF EXISTING RECORDS

Newcombe's[27] studies of congenital abnormalities in Nova Scotia, largely based on pooled data from three separate sources, are of interest. He illustrates the value of automated or computer-assisted information sources and the relative ease with which they can be integrated. Similarly, the disadvantages of manual systems which are not compatible with mechanized methods are discussed. The study demonstrates the problems of achieving patient identification on data from different sources. In this exercise matching of patient records was achieved using nominal identifying data. Three main objectives for a system of notification and registration for congenital anomalies are cited:

1. To detect increasing incidence of an anomaly.

2. To identify risk factors such as prenatal exposure of mothers to injurious factors.

3. Follow-up of the children affected to provide information on the need for services.

Wagner and Newcombe's bibliography on record linkage, including computer methods is a useful guide to the literature up to 1970.[28]

FACILITIES AND MODE OF OPERATION

The type of equipment used, the capacity of the system and the mode of operation in a computer-assisted register will depend on the objectives of the project, the predicted size of the population to be covered and the size of the data-base held on each patient. Additional considerations will include the type of service required, such as the maximum acceptable time-lag between input of patient data and reporting of processed results or the period required to access a patient record from a peripheral clinic. The DVLC computing system and those operated by the banks, credit card companies and the police national computer are based on daily batch-processing, virtually all the information is recorded and processed using magnetic tape. This demonstrates that current technology allows the construction and operation of extremely large registers. New developments in mass storage techniques will both provide further scope in this field and simplify hardware configurations. One study of medical computer development[29] stressed the problems of using real-time processing techniques in some health care projects. Although it is likely that, in the future, many successful applications will be based on real-time processing, it is doubtful whether the cost and complexity of such a system will be justified in the development of the type of register being discussed here.

CONFIDENTIALITY: SOCIAL AND POLITICAL ISSUES

There have been several recent discussions in the medical press and elsewhere on the subject of confidentiality and privacy. In 1971, a review of health service computing contained advice on security measures.[30] More recently the issue has been stimulated by the Younger Report on privacy,[31] the government White Paper on Computers and Privacy 1974[32] and the Supplementary Report (1975).[33] In the area of health care there are several unanswered questions which are raised or emphasized by the growth of computing methods. One in particular concerns the use of medical records by non-medical professions, for example, social workers who are responsible for some aspects of continuing patient care in the community.[34] The Hippocratic Oath and the International Code of Medical Ethics state, in effect, that doctors will not divulge information about their patients to a third party. There is an on-going debate about who constitutes a third party. In a register for patients with inborn errors of metabolism there could be a large number of workers providing advice and care and directly contributing to the completion and maintenance of information in the data base. Kenny[34] cites a cynic's view that, 'the best safeguard we have against unwarranted intrusion into our medical records is the inefficiency of the present system'.

In the future it is clear that we will have to demonstrate very adequate safeguards for personal information in health care information systems. This is not simply a technological problem because, as Lackey[35] points out, ordinary carelessness in day to day operation may provide many accessible trails open for fraudulent acquisition of sensitive information. We can be certain that in any future proposals for national registers all these aspects will receive detailed attention. A recent statement by Dr David Owen,[36] replying in the House of Commons to a parliamentary question, underlines the socio-political implications of using computers in this type of health care activity: 'I am satisfied that the confidentiality of the information held on computer systems . . . is adequately safeguarded and I can assure the Hon. Member that no proposal for linking health information on a national basis would proceed without full public discussion. We would not want to waken up and find that it has suddenly occurred.'

Summary

There is much evidence which demonstrates the current lack of appropriate organization in collecting, collating and analysing information which is needed to provide and evaluate patient care. The register is one method of extending the expertise and facilities of special centres to the communities they serve. The establishment of a register requires extensive and careful preparatory work by a multidisciplinary team. Pilot studies, employing non-automated methods of handling information are essential. The concept of a central processing facility serving several centres is an attractive one, but in practice it may create several problems, particularly in the standardization of criteria for diagnosis, in ensuring the accuracy and completeness of information collected and the maintenance of follow-up records. Our experience would suggest that although computing facilities, if they are employed in a large scale register, may be centralized, responsibility for the maintenance of files should remain with each individual centre participating in the project. If the original objectives, criteria and operational procedures are complied with by all the participants then it will be possible to merge the files for the purpose of analysis and clinical research.

I am grateful to Mr A. F. Damodaran, Director, Grampian Health Board Computing Network Project, and to my colleagues in the Department of Community Medicine, University of Aberdeen, for their help and advice in the preparation of this paper. The information on SAFUR is derived from work carried out by the multicentre steering committee and in particular by Mr Edwin Alexander, Senior Systems Analyst, Grampian Health Services Information Unit

REFERENCES

1. MOORE, R. F. O. (1916). The retinitis of arteriosclerosis, and its relation to renal retinitis and to cerebral vascular disease. *Q.J. Med.*, **10**, 29
2. BROOKE, E. M. (1974). The current and future use of registers in health information systems. *WHO Offset Print No. 8.* (Geneva: World Health Organization)
3. World Health Organization Expert Committee on Health Statistics. (1967). *Epidemiological Methods in the Study of Chronic Diseases.* WHO Tech. Rep. Ser. No. 365
4. HEDLEY, A. J., SCOTT, A. M. and DEBENHAM, G. (1969). A computer assisted follow-up register. *Meth. Inform. Med.*, **8**, 67
5. HEDLEY, A. J. (1973). Long-term aftercare for patients treated for thyrotoxicosis. *Br. J. Surg.*, **60**, 771
6. BONNAR, J., GOLDBERG, A. and SMITH, J. A. (1969). Do pregnant women take their iron? *Lancet*, **i**, 457
7. DIXON, W. M., STRADLING, P. and WOOTON, I. D. P. (1957). Outpatient P.A.S. therapy. *Lancet*, **ii**, 871
8. JOYCE, C. R. B. (1962). Patient co-operation and the sensitivity of clinical trials. *J. Chron. Dis.*, **15**, 1025
9. PORTER, A. M. W. (1969). Drug defaulting in general practice. *Br. Med. J*, **1**, 218
10. HEDLEY, A. J., FLEMMING, C., CHESTERS, M. I., MICHIE, W. and CROOKS, J. (1970). The surgical treatment of thyrotoxicosis. *Br. Med. J.*, **1**, 519
11. SMALL, W. P. (1967). Lost to follow-up. *Lancet*, **i**, 997
12. CROOKS, J., CLARK, C. G., AMAR, S. S. and COULL, D. C. (1965). Preventive medicine and the gastrectomised patient. *Lancet*, **ii**, 943
13. HEDLEY, A. J. (1972). M.D. Thesis, University of Aberdeen
14. Department of Health and Social Security. (1974). Proceedings of the conference on psychiatric case registers, University of Aberdeen 1973. D. J. Hall, N. C. Robertson, and R. G. Eason (eds.). Statistical and Research Report Series No. 7.
15. GIBBINS, J. (1976). Personal communication
16. ACHESON, E. D. (1967). Medical Record Linkage. Nuffield Provincial Hospitals Trust. (Oxford University Press)

17. HOGBEN, L. and CROSS, K. W. (1948). The statistical specificity of a code personnel cypher sequence. *Br. J. Soc. Med.*, **2**, 149
18. PAGE, E. S. and WILSON, L. B. (1973). *Information Representation and Manipulation in a Computer.* Cambridge Computer Science Books 2. (Cambridge University Press)
19. HEDLEY, A. J., ALEXANDER, E. A. and INNES, G. (1976). Patient identification and documentation of deaths in a follow-up register. (In preparation)
20. THOMAS, G. E. (1968). The registration of children at risk of handicap. *Med. Off.* **120**, 162, 177, 191, 208
21. RICHARDS, I. D. G. and ROBERTS, C. J. (1967). The 'At-Risk' infant. *Lancet*, **ii**, 711
22. LOCKWOOD, E. (1971). Accuracy of Scottish hospital morbidity data. *Br. J. Prevent. Soc. Med.*, **25**, 76
23. INNES, G. and WEIR, R. D. (1968). Patient identification on a regional basis. In G. McLachlan and R. A. Shegog (eds.), *Computers in the Service of Medicine.* Nuffield Provincial Hospitals Trust. Oxford University Press.
24. HUNTER, D. (1976). Personal communication
25. ASHCROFT, L. (1974). Systems—not computers. *Systems*, **2**, 26
26. HARDEN, R.McG., HARDEN, K. A., JOLLEY, J. L. and WILKIN, T. J. (1975). Punched feature card retrieval systems in clinical research. *Br. J. Hosp. Med.*, **13**, 195
27. NEWCOMBE, H. B. (1969). Pooled records from multiple sources for monitoring congenital anomalies. *Br. J. Prevent. Soc. Med.*, **23**, 226
28. WAGNER, G. and NEWCOMBE, H. B. (1970). Record Linkage: Its methodology and application in medical data processing.
29. OCKENDEN, J. M. and BODENHAM, K. E. (1970). Focus on medical computer development. Nuffield Provincial Hospitals Trust. Oxford University Press
30. Department of Health and Social Security. (1971). *Using Computers to Improve Health Services—a Review for the National Health Service*
31. Home Office (1972). Report of the committee on privacy (the Younger Committee). HMSO, Command 5012
32. Home Office, (1975). *Computers and Privacy.* HMSO, Command 6353
33. Home Office. (1975). *Computers: Safeguards for Privacy.* HMSO, Command 6354
34. KENNY, D. J. (1975). Confidentiality and the growth of computers. *Hosp. Hlth. Serv. Rev.*, **71**, 6
35. LACKEY, R. D. (1974). Penetration of computer systems: an overview. *Honeywell Computer J.*, **8**, 90
36. OWEN, D. (1975). *Weekly Hansard.* House of Commons Parliamentary Debate, 16th May–23rd May 1975, pp. 1577–88

16

Mechanized storage and retrieval of information

Joan S. Emmerson and D. N. Raine

The inherited metabolic diseases present special problems of management: their rarity means that if the approximately 2000 cases likely to occur each year in the United Kingdom were evenly distributed among its 360 paediatricians, each would see only eight cases annually, and even if all cases in a given teaching area were attended by a single specialist, he would still have less than 100 cases each year, half of which would have cystic fibrosis, and the rest would be examples of 500 or more possible diseases. Since all, so far, are inherited by recessive and X-linked mechanisms and are associated with specific enzyme deficiencies, it is gratifying that the rate of recognition of new diseases has perceptibly declined whilst the number of known enzyme deficiencies continues to increase (Table 16.1).

The clinical manifestations of this group of diseases are quite diverse and their description is distributed through a wide range of general and specialist medical publications, and details of diagnostic tests and

Table 16.1   The number of recessive and X-linked disorders and the number of known enzyme deficiencies identified as their primary cause in the four editions of McKusick's *Mendelian Inheritance in Man*

Edition and year	Recessive	X-linked	Total	Known enzyme defects
1st 1966	531	119	650	—
2nd 1968	629	123	752	—
3rd 1971	789	149	938	103
4th 1975	947	174	1121	141

enzyme studies occur in a further range of scientific publications. McKusick has indicated (Table 16.2) those cited more than 80 times in compiling his catalogue[1] and while not all relate to inherited metabolic disease few can afford to disregard the long list of publications containing 79 or fewer citations relevant to this group of disorders.

In 1974, *Index Medicus* listed 225 papers under the general heading 'Metabolism, inborn errors' a figure which does *not* include those cita-

Table 16.2   Journals cited more than 80 times in the compilation of McKusick's *Mendelian Inheritance in Man*

New England Journal of Medicine
Lancet
Journal of Pediatrics
American Journal of Human Genetics
American Journal of Diseases of Children
Science
Nature (including *Nature New Biology*)
Pediatrics
Journal of Clinical Investigation
American Journal of Medicine
Archives of Disease in Children
Archives of Dermatology
Annals of Human Genetics (and *Annals of Eugenics*)
Journal of Medical Genetics
Journal of the American Medical Association
Archives of Neurology
Journal of Heredity
Blood
British Medical Journal
Neurology
Humangenetik
Annals of Internal Medicine
American Journal of Ophthalmology
Archives of Ophthalmology
Brain
Journal of Bone and Joint Surgery (U.S. and U.K.)
Proceedings of the National Academy of Sciences (U.S.)

tions listed under the headings for individual diseases. In 1975 *Medical Subject Headings* contained 70 main index terms relating to inborn metabolic disorders, including the general heading (Table 16.3). These differ somewhat from McKusick's disease headings and in some ways are less satisfactory. Thus, it is probably not useful to distinguish ochronosis from alkaptonuria; lactose intolerance is not accompanied by the equally specific sucrose and isomaltose intolerances, the list of mucopolysaccharidoses includes one term (the first) that is not widely used and omits types 2 and 4; the six enzyme defects contrast with the 141 that are known and include three that occur elsewhere in the list of headings; lipid disorders include deficiency of β- but not of α- lipoprotein—and so on. The treatment adopts a style appropriate to many other aspects of medical indexing but is not appropriate to the large number of quite specific inherited metabolic diseases.

Table 16.3   Medical   Subject   Headings   (MESH)   relating   to inherited metabolic disease

Metabolism, inborn errors	*Metabolism, inborn errors*
Amino acid metabolism, inborn errors	Glycogenosis 3
Albinism	Glycogenosis 4
Alkaptonuria	Glycogenosis 5
Ochronosis	Glycogenosis 6
Homocystinuria	Glycogenosis 7
Maple syrup urine disease	Glycogenosis 8
Phenylketonuria	Lactose intolerance
Amyloidosis	Mucopolysaccharidosis
Carbohydrate metabolism, inborn errors	Eccentro osteochondrodysplasia
	Lipochondrodystrophy
Fructose intolerance	Mucopolysaccharidosis 3
Galactosemia	Mucopolysaccharidosis 5
Glycogenosis	Mucopolysaccharidosis 6
Glucosephosphatase deficiency	
Glycogenosis 2	Glucosephosphatase deficiency
	Glucosephosphate dehydrogenase deficiency

Metabolism, inborn errors	*Metabolism, inborn errors*

Hypophosphatasia
Lactose intolerance
Lesch–Nyhan syndrome

Hyperbilirubinemia, hereditary

Crigler–Najjar syndrome
Gilbert's disease

Jaundice, chronic idiopathic

Lipid metabolism, inborn errors

Abetalipoproteinemia
Hyperlipemia, essential familial
lipoidosis
Lipoidproteinosis
Refsum's syndrome
Sphingolipidosis
Amaurotic familial idiocy
Angiokeratoma corporis
diffusum
Gangliosidosis
Gaucher's disease
Leukodystrophy, meta-
chromatic
Niemann–Pick disease

Metal metabolism, inborn errors

Fanconi syndrome
Hemochromatosis
Hepatolenticular degeneration
Hypophosphatasia
Hypophosphatemia, familial
Paralysis, familial periodic
Pseudohypoparathyroidism
Porphyria
Purine-pyrimidine metabolism,
inborn errors
Gout
Lesch–Nyhan syndrome
Renal tubular transport, inborn
errors
Acidosis, renal tubular
Aminoaciduria, renal
Hartnup disease
Cystinosis
Cystinuria
Fanconi syndrome
Glycosuria, renal
Hypophosphatemia, familial

It is obvious, therefore, that the single specialist cannot hope to be fully acquainted with or even easily obtain the best statements on more than a few diseases, and from a list of references offered by an efficient librarian he has little reason to select some and not others for special attention. There is no reason, however, why a specially designed information system should not be constructed by several workers involved in the field of inherited metabolic disease. If such a system were made widely available the benefit to patients, paediatricians and medical scientists would be both immediate and very great. The present discussion is concerned with the feasibility and possible structure of such a system.

Input of information

SOURCES OF CITATIONS: THE PRESENT SYSTEM

For the several years in which one of us has been engaged in work on inherited metabolic disease, a file of published literature has been formed by collecting offprints, photocopies and reference cards after surveying current issues of some 20 medical and scientific journals; the lists of references in those papers that have needed to be consulted further; from abstracting journals such as *International Abstracts of Biological Science* and from lists of titles, (The Royal Postgraduate Medical School *Library Bulletin* was used, but Life Sciences and Clinical Practice issues of *Current Contents* cover similar ground); and papers referred to in secondary review sources.

This *ad hoc* system—with all its human errors and imperfections—has resulted in 250 files on specific diseases, each containing between 1 and 100 citations. The files occupy six standard filing cabinet drawers and are arranged alphabetically (with minor modifications) using the standard names in the latest edition of McKusick *Mendelian Inheritance in Man*,[1] and the related scientific data on the enzymes and metabolic pathways involved are filed with the associated disease. With this system, to which much time has been devoted, information is available on only 23% of the recessive and X-linked diseases listed by McKusick, and whole areas of information (such as that published in neuropathology journals which are not regularly surveyed) are missing.

QUANTITATIVE ADVANTAGES OF MEDLARS

It was decided as a first step to examine the extent to which MED-LARS (MEDical Literature Analysis and Retrieval System), though in some ways imperfect, could improve on the *ad hoc* system so far adopted. A MEDLARS search covering the period January 1973–March 1975 was formulated. The search requested the retrieval of citations listed under the category 'Metabolism, inborn errors', including all the specific terms available. It was limited to 1000 references, on the grounds of cost, and because it was felt that this would be a reasonable number in the circumstances on which to judge the value of the material in terms of relevance. (It is not known how many more references there might have been in that period.)

Of the 1000 citations listed the first 300 were rated as important or otherwise and the language of the publication noted. The content of the papers was judged from the title only and assessment of their probable value and importance was influenced by any previous knowledge of the authors, the language, and experience of the quality of other publications in the journal cited. This very subjective assessment, which in the case of language can amount to frank prejudice, can be criticized from several viewpoints, but it differs little from the way in which an individual selects certain journals for regular reading, and departs from the way in which the *ad hoc* files were prepared only in that, for them, the full text rather than just the title was more often available. Papers rated as 'important' were those which anyone seriously concerned with a disease could hardly do without. Those rated 'not important' included those confirming facts already established, papers in obscure journals or languages, and papers reviewing several diseases from one particular aspect or in general. Thus, while these publications might have been important for the education of inexperienced workers or those of a particular nationality or clinical discipline, they were unlikely to contain additional vital information necessary for a sophisticated health care system in the Western World.

With these specifications, then, the analysis (Table 16.4) showed that one-third of the citations from the MEDLARS search were important. One-fifth of these were in languages other than English, but only one-tenth were in languages other than English, French or German. The *ad hoc* files, when compared with this analysis, contained only one-quarter of the citations rated as 'important' and very few indeed of those rated 'not important'. There would therefore be an immediate and substantial (fourfold) benefit from basing a special information system

Table 16.4 Analysis by language and 'importance' of a sample of 300 consecutive citations from a MEDLARS search on inborn errors of metabolism

	English	French and German	Other languages	Total
'Important'	93	16	10	119
'Not important'	102	30	49	181

on MEDLARS, and the level of redundancy would not be great, making the task of winnowing the grain from the chaff neither tedious nor excessive.

QUALITATIVE REPRESENTATION BY MEDLARS

While work continues on some disorders over years, it is not uncommon for other diseases to become fashionable for a few years and then, when the basic facts have been established, to disappear from the current literature. The MEDLARS search was, therefore, examined for evidence of this (Table 16.5). In fact, while such current vogues as the mucopolysaccharidoses and the sphingolipidoses dominate the list, classic diseases like galactosaemia and cystinosis are still represented by two or three citations each. In all, more than 40 diseases and groups of diseases are represented.

Table 16.5   Distribution according to subject of 119 MEDLARS citations concerned with a single disorder or group taken from a sample of 300 citations in a search on inborn errors of metabolism

Disorder	No. of citations	
Mucopolysaccharidoses	15	2 each:
Sphingolipidoses	14	Renal tubular acidosis
Lipidaemia	9	Histidinaemia
α_1-antitrypsin deficiency	7	Cystinosis
Phenylketonuria	5	Hypophosphatasia
Screening	5	Cystinuria
Porphyria	5	Lesch–Nyhan syndrome
Fabry's disease	5	Lactose intolerance
Glycogen storage disease	4	Lecithin-CAT deficiency
Wilson's disease	4	
Organic acidaemia	4	1 each:
G6PD deficiency	3	17 other diseases
Urea cycle defects	3	
Galactosaemia	3	

Retrieval of information

Since the use of MEDLARS can at once produce better results than the laborious manual method of collecting data, we may now consider ways of refining this to produce a quickly accessible, central, relevant list of references which can be tapped by a variety of workers who might have an immediate need to have information on one or more aspects of a given disease.

The first step would be to set up a MEDLARS search on the lines of the trial run already described, and this would be updated every month. The citations from the MEDLARS listing would be screened by workers experienced in the subject, and they would select, on the basis of their experience, and aided by the index terms applied to each citation, items to be included in the new system. The full text of these chosen citations would then be acquired. At some stage the full text of a sample of all citations should be examined and the value of selecting from this instead of the title only should be weighed against the additional burden in cost, time and the complexity of reading several languages. It is quite possible that review of the full text in some form will indeed prove to be the most satisfactory initial step in the system.

The form in which the full texts would be obtained, whether as an initial or second step, and subsequently filed, would be a matter for discussion. The possibilities are to obtain from a central source (in Britain the British Library, Lending Division, Boston Spa) a photocopy or microfiche of each paper. The former is easy to read directly but can be less satisfactory if (as in pathological studies or photographs of clinically important features) half-tone illustrations form an important part of the text. However, one photocopier, the Xerox 4000, has greatly improved this form of reproduction of half-tone plates.

Microfiche, of course, is not readily readable but its great advantage is that it can be stored in much less space than photocopies. Improved methods of making microfiche and of reconverting these to hard copy are constantly being investigated. There are on the market several different types of microfiche reader, some of which are relatively inexpensive.

The problem of copyright must be borne in mind, especially if full texts are to be stored in different centres or if there were any question of offering or reproducing numbers of copies from the original copy.[4-6] While many publishers are searching for a reasonable resolution of the problem of copyright in relation to photocopying, this is not yet in sight and meanwhile they remain very sensitive to infringements. Most journals publish a statement of their rights and policy in this regard. While it would be possible for the main centre for this special information system to retain the full texts of the citations it would be a logical step to transmit those required by a peripheral station as hard copy or when future developments permit, by wire, and acceptable conditions for this would need to be agreed.

Having acquired the full text of each citation in whatever form, the next step is to index it with appropriate descriptive terms (index terms, subject headings) by which it can be retrieved from a file. It is proposed that instead of MEDLARS indexing terms, the disease entities used in the latest edition of McKusick's *Mendelian Inheritance in Man* should be used. The fact that some new diseases or syndromes may not appear in the current edition of McKusick is outweighed by the often less precise descriptions used in *Index Medicus*, for example, lipochondro-dystrophy includes Hurler's disease, and gangliosidosis GM1 is in-cluded in amaurotic family idiocy. In addition to the main disease heading, each citation would be assessed using the pro-forma (Figure 16.1) for its contribution with regard to clinical description (CLIN), diagnosis (DIAG), treatment (TREAT), pathology (PATH), heterozy-gote detection (HET) prenatal detection (PREN), data relating to the enzyme defect and its assay (ENZ) and finally some papers would be designated because they were considered of such primary importance

Author(s) :

Title   :

Journal   :

Disorder (McKusick no.)	CLIN	DIAG	TREAT	PATH	HET	PREN	ENZ	KEY	Assessor
									FINAL

FIGURE 16.1   Pro-forma for the assessment of publications prior to entry into the information system

for the disease with which they are concerned that they should always be listed even after several years and the appearance of many more recent publications (KEY). Each citation would be assessed by two individuals (with clinical and laboratory orientations respectively) giving a double check on the input. Space is allowed in the pro-forma for a final decision after discussion of differences in assessment by the two primary surveyors. The original texts may be filed either alphabetically by the name of the first author or numbered sequentially and filed accordingly.

The information coded on the indexing form would constitute the data base for an on-line computerized system similar to MEDLARS but with obviously restricted range. The main centre would house a computer, which need not be large, with enough storage capacity to hold the data base. Storage would be on magnetic disc and subject specialists would need to decide how many years' information should be retained. In addition, computer terminals would be installed in as many centres as considered necessary in the overall plan. It has been suggested that in the United Kingdom about five centres could deal with all aspects of inborn errors of metabolism.[2,3]

A qualified computer programmer would work in conjunction with the subject experts. He would programme the data from the index forms for storage in the computer and would draw up instructions for its retrieval on-line. In effect this would be a mini-MEDLARS with a restricted data-base.

USE OF THE SYSTEM

The system would be available not only to workers located in a particular centre but also, through the nearest specialist centre, to paediatricians, family doctors, genetic counsellors, medical scientists and social workers with a specific problem. These would be workers without ready access to any general information source and for whom a specialized centre able to give a quick response to requests for literature on diagnosis or treatment, for example, would be invaluable. The centre would be able to produce references for a simple request combining a named disease and one of the sub-classifications (e.g. Refsums disease—prenatal detection) when the peripheral terminal would receive the most important (KEY) and some of the most recent references on its screen. Those available in that reference laboratory or local medical library would then be examined from the original or photostat copy. Copies of more obscure references would be requested from the central data bank and in the future it may be that microfiche images will be transmissible immediately by wire.

With technical instructions for using the terminal provided by computer staff it is not difficult to operate an on-line system. Provided that the user knows clearly what he needs and can select the appropriate index terms to describe the various aspects of his subject he needs only to be able to type (even with one finger) and to follow the instructions given.

Once the system is devised, the chosen references coded and stored in the central computer and the instructions for their retrieval specified, it can be used in different ways by individual centres according to their needs. It is assumed that the data bank will be regularly up-dated by the main centre on receipt of the monthly MEDLARS list and it is probable that the peripheral centres, since they will all be expert in this field, will contribute to this part of the system.

Most medical scientists are already familiar with MEDLARS and with MEDLINE, its development to on-line searching, and for this reason a detailed description of the workings of the system has been omitted. Many papers have been published on its applications and potentialities and for those who wish to investigate more closely the techniques of computerized literature searching and evaluate the effectiveness of these methods the recently published *Medlars Handbook*[7] gives an introduction to the system, a brief history of its development and examples of search methods. Among many other useful papers, McCarn and Leiter[8] and Rogers[9] evaluate such systems and Barber and colleagues[10] write specifically on the MEDUSA experiment carried out in Newcastle upon Tyne.

Costing

The system described is a very simple one to organize in computer programming terms. The software required would be relatively unsophisticated and the programmer effort and storage space comparatively small. The greatest effort will go into the reading and classification of the literature but since the specialists already do this to some extent they would now pool their efforts and gain a much greater return.

Capital equipment might cost £15 000 for the central computer unit with a further £5000 for each terminal, together with £1000 per annum for the rental of GPO facilities. In addition two programmer-clerks might be needed for operation and filing at a combined annual salary of about £6000. There would also be the comparatively low cost of the MEDLARS search. One would assume that the subject specialists would be employed in any case and that once the system was set up the amount of time they would need to select references from each monthly MEDLARS printout and to code them would be quite small.

REFERENCES

1. McKusick, V. A. 1975. *Mendelian Inheritance in Man*, 4th ed. (Baltimore: Johns Hopkins Press)
2. Raine, D. N. (1972). Management of inherited metabolic disease. *Br. Med. J.*, **2**, 329
3. Raine, D. N. (1974). The need for a national policy for the management of inherited metabolic disease. In D. N. Raine (ed.), *Molecular Variants in Disease. J. Clin. Pathol.* **8** (27 Suppl.) (Roy. Coll. Pathologists) 156 and chapter 1 of this volume
4. Henry, N. L. (1974). Copyright, public policy and information technology. *Science (N.Y.)*, **183**, 384
5. Walsh, J. (1974). Journals: photocopying is not the only problem. *Science (N.Y.)*, **183**, 1274
6. Henry, N. L. (1974). Copyright: its adequacy in technological societies. *Science (N.Y.)*, **186**, 993
7. Frankland, J. G. B. (1975). *U.K. Medlars: A Handbook for Users*. British Library Lending Division, Boston Spa, West Yorks
8. McCarn, D. B. and Leiter, J. (1973). On-line services in medicine and beyond. *Science (N.Y.)*, **181**, 318
9. Rogers, F. B. (1974). Computerized bibliographic retrieval services. *Lib. Trends*, **23**, 73
10. Barber, S. A. *et al.* (1973). On-line information retrieval as a scientist's tool. *Inf. Stor. Retr.*, **9**, 429

17

Computer-aided diagnosis of inherited metabolic disease

D. N. Raine, Nansi G. Rees and Susan H. Terry

The now very large number of inherited metabolic diseases, none of which occur in a given centre with sufficient frequency to allow the accumulation of useful experience in diagnosis, let alone management, poses a special problem in medical practice. There are already listed in the latest edition[1] of McKusick's *Mendelian Inheritance in Man* 141 recessive or X-linked disorders associated with a known enzyme deficiency, and there are altogether nearly 1200 diseases inherited by these mechanisms. It is beyond even the specialist to remember all that may be relevant in a given clinical situation, and for some time we have been exploring the extent to which the administrative role of the computer can be adapted to reducing this burden by selecting and reminding the clinician of those diseases that should be considered first.

The basis of the diagnostic system

The first attempt to deal with the problem, albeit without hardware, is worth mentioning because it provided the conceptual basis for the system subsequently developed. It was published[2] in the form of a table in which the clinical features of each disease were reduced to four terms in which the presence of mental subnormality was designated M; active neurological degeneration as N; the presence of eye abnormalities as E followed by the nature of the eye defect (such as cataracts, retinitis, macular spot); and the presence of other prominent features as O, which again were specified (for example, vomiting, hepatomegaly, skeletal, hair). In this way, each of nearly 200 diseases, named and numbered according to the most recent McKusick classification, were followed by a very concise clinical statement in standard form, and it was possible when presented with, for example, a patient with cataracts and abnormal hair to scan the 'clinical features' column of the table for

'E-cataracts' and to pick those entries in which this was accompanied by 'O-hair'.

This simple device, the compilation of which involved many hours of work by a number of people, contained some inherent defects and the user was warned when it was published[2] that it could be neither complete nor wholly accurate and did not contain sufficient information for diagnosis. However, while it remains a useful check list it proved too crude to be of value in directing or reminding the clinician to more than a small number of diseases with fairly specific characteristics. When faced with a mentally subnormal child it was little help to know that M occurred in more than 80 different clinical descriptions.

It can be seen that the underlying concept of this system is to scan the patient's clinical features against a matrix of typical descriptions of each disorder and to recognize those with which the patient matches most closely. This contrasts with the 'dichotomous key' adopted in, for example, elementary systems for the identification of flowers and animals. Since at the outset it was not known whether the *clinical* manifestations of inherited metabolic diseases would be sufficiently specific to allow either system to succeed without incorporating the definitive and specialized tests, it was decided that the matrix matching system made less demands and was more adaptable to successive modification and that it should be examined first.

DEVELOPMENT OF THE BASIC CONCEPT

Since a clinical classification based on four major features with an *ad hoc* extension of two of them, provided an inadequate basis for a diagnostic scheme, it was necessary to consider ways in which this should be extended. Theoretically, there was no reason why the matrix should not be open-ended in both directions allowing new diseases to be added vertically and the horizontal component to be extended indefinitely with new symptoms or signs. Since any new edition of the McKusick catalogue would provide a standard basis for the former it was only necessary to agree on a set of standard clinical terms for the latter. It was rather surprising to discover that, despite several years of international activity on medical classification and computer-aided diagnosis in other fields, no such standard list had been compiled—much less agreed.

It was therefore decided to explore this problem by seeking to devise a set of terms that would cover a limited group of disorders, and the mucopolysaccharidoses were chosen for this purpose. Many literature reports of patients with one of the several varieties of mucopolysaccharidosis were read and the clinical terms used were noted. Only English and French language reports were used but these were drawn from several countries. The definition of these terms as they appeared in English language medical dictionaries of English and American origin were then compared and those terms which did not appear in one, or whose definitions in both were not closely similar, were rejected. Similarly, indefinite terms and those calling for subjective judgement were also rejected. Some consideration was also given to the extent to which the terms selected could be translated unequivocally into several European languages, but the examination of this aspect of the problem received only limited attention due to the lack of a large polyglot medical dictionary.

Examples of terms that can be used include kyphosis, lordosis, gingival hypertrophy, hernia and skin nodules, but others have quite different meanings in Britain and America or are indefinite or peculiar to one or other nation: gibbus (humpback in UK, an X-ray change in USA), thin enamel on teeth, diastasis recti, night blindness, sagittal ridge and coronary occlusion.

A final selection of 43 terms was assembled into a proforma, and the clinical descriptions of mucopolysaccharidosis patients in the literature re-examined. Two things were concluded from this exercise:

1. To extend this approach to all other inherited metabolic diseases would involve more work than would be justified without further indication that a useful diagnostic system would result, and

2. Many individual case reports in the literature are astonishingly incomplete making them of limited value as the basis of a diagnostic programme.

This latter problem will be overcome, once the list of terms has been devised, if this is then used in a binary manner (yes or no, or + or −) to describe future patients or to review retrospectively with the clinician concerned those already described in the literature. Accurate and systematic individual case reports will ultimately be required since a typical description of a particular inherited metabolic disease is not always possible. Since many of these disorders develop during childhood all the features of a given condition rarely occur simultaneously. The more detailed the set of descriptive terms used the less certainly will a particular pattern of positive and negative features emerge. Moreover, since all of the diseases are rare, several years may elapse before sufficient cases can be accumulated from which a truly typical clinical description can be derived. Indeed, the means whereby these two problems can be overcome in a computer-aided diagnostic system has yet to be devised and again it was considered that, before spending time on this, more indication of the practical validity of the basic concept should be sought.

The first pilot study

Since four clinical features were too few and an indefinite number presents too great a task to begin with, it was decided to select about 20 major features covering most parts of the body affected by these diseases and including any features that were likely to be especially discriminating. This number was chosen for no better reason than it was greater than four and was likely to be manageable in compiling a data bank. In the event the 22 features included in Figure 17.1 were chosen.

The next task was to compile a data bank in terms of these 22 features and a pilot survey of 83 diseases was begun. The diseases were chosen because they were fairly definite in presentation, clinically or therapeutically relatively important, covered a wide spectrum of symptoms, and a useful file of literature was immediately available. In three instances, α_1-antitrypsin deficiency, Crigler–Najjar syndrome and galactosaemia, the clinical presentation at different ages was considered to be so different that entry of a single clinical picture could be misleading. The first two of these were therefore entered as both 'childhood' and 'adult' forms, and galactosaemia as 'infantile' and 'childhood' forms separately, making 86 entries for the 83 diseases (Table 17.1).

The data bank was compiled by two of us (S.M.T. and N.G.R.) using a number of reference books and special monographs as well as the literature files which varied greatly in the completeness of their coverage. In the light of experience of a number of differences of interpretation by the two compilers some of the clinical features were annotated by listing certain clinical abnormalities included by the term, making the proforma (Figure 17.1) to be completed by the clinician for his patient more helpful.

All of the diseases were assessed by the two surveyors independently and all differences were discussed by the three authors and a final

DIAGNOSIS OF INHERITED METABOLIC DISORDER

PATIENT:

D.O.B.   SEX [M][F]

N.H.S. NO:

HOSPITAL:

Reg. No:

Terms include symptoms listed below: Mark box present (+)
                                                        or absent (−)

Terms / abnormalities	Symptom	Mark box
	Onset before 8/12	
	Onset after 8/12	
Abnormal amount, form, texture, brittleness or pigmentation	Distinctive odour	
	Hair abnormality	
Abnormal pigmentation, rashes, infiltrations, tumours, ichthyosis, eczema, sun sensitivity	Skin abnormality	
	Jaundice	
	Cyanosis	
	Goitre	
Diarrhoea Constipation Steatorrhoea	Vomiting	
	Bowel abnormality	
	Hepato(spleno)megaly	
Virilization; abnormal external genitalia	Genital abnormality	
	Neurol./mental degeneration	
Ptosis, epilepsy, deafness. Abnlty of movement/tone; nystagmus, delayed motor development	Other functional neurolog. abnlty	
	Mental retardation	
Abnormal height for age	Skeletal abnormality	
<3rd or >97th%	Renal calculi	
Abnormal joints, Scoliosis, rickets	Anaemia	
Abnormal X-ray density	Acidosis	
	Lens corneal defect	
Ward testing only—sugar, protein, change on standing, stain in nappie	Retinal abnormality	
	Urine abnormality	
	Specify Other	

Further comment:

Medical Officer: Date:

FIGURE 17.1 Proforma to be completed for patients for whom computer-aided diagnosis is required, detailing the 22 clinical features and some of the abnormalities they include

Table 17.1   The 86 entries for 83 diseases used in the first pilot study of a system for computer aided diagnosis of inherited metabolic disease

Acrodermatitis enteropathica	(20110)
Adenylate kinase deficiency, anaemia due to	(20160)
α_1-Antitrypsin deficiency, (1) infant, (2) adult	(20740)
Angiokeratoma, diffuse (Fabry's)	(30150)
Argininaemia	(20780)
Argininosuccinic aciduria	(20790)
Aspartyl-glycosaminuria	(20840)
Carnosinaemia	(21220)
Cerebral cholesterinosis	(21370)
Cerebro-hepato-renal syndrome	(21410)
Ceroid storage disease	(21420)
Citrullinuria	(21570)
Corneal dystrophy (Groenouw type 2)	(21780)
Crigler–Najjar syndrome, (1) childhood, (2) adult	(21880)
Cystinosis, type 1	(21980)
Cystinosis, type 2	(21990)
Cystinuria	(22010)
Diphosphoglycerate mutase deficiency of erythrocyte, anaemia due to	(22280)
Farber lipogranulomatosis	(22800)
Formiminotransferase deficiency	(22910)
Fructose -1,6, diphosphatase deficiency	(22970)
Fucosidosis	(23000)
Galactokinase deficiency	(23020)
Galactosaemia, (1) infantile, (2) childhood	(23040)
Gangliosidosis, generalized GM1, type 1	(23050)
Glutathione peroxidase deficiency, haemolytic anaemia due to	(23170)
Glutathione reductase, haemolytic anaemia due to deficiency of, in red cells	(23180)
Glutathione synthetase deficiency of erythrocytes, haemolytic anaemia due to	(23190)
Glycinaemia; propionic acidaemia	(23200)
Glycogen storage disease, type 1	(23220)

Glycogen storage disease, type 2	(23230)
Glycogen storage disease, type 3	(23240)
Glycogen storage disease, type 4	(23250)
Glycogen storage disease, type 5	(23260)
Glycogen storage disease, type 6	(23270)
Glycogen storage disease, type 7	(23280)
Glycoprotein storage disease	(23290)
Hartnup disease	(23450)
Hepatolenticular degeneration	(27790)
Hexokinase deficiency, haemolytic anaemia	(23570)
Histidinaemia	(23580)
Homocystinuria	(23620)
β-Hydroxyisovaleric aciduria and β-methylcrotonyl glycinuria	(21020)
Hydroxykynureninuria	(23680)
Hypophosphatasia	(24150)
Hypoxanthine-guanine phosphoribosyl transferase deficiency (Lesch–Nyhan)	(30800)
Isovaleric acidaemia	(24350)
Krabbe disease	(24520)
Lactosyl ceramidosis	(24550)
Lecithin-cholesterol acyl-transferase deficiency	(24590)
Lipase, congenital absence of pancreatic	(24660)
a-β-Lipoproteinaemia	(20010)
Lowe oculocerebrorenal syndrome	(30900)
Mannosidosis	(24850)
Maple syrup urine disease	(24860)
Menke's syndrome	(30940)
Metachromatic leukodystrophy, juvenile	(25020)
Methionine malabsorption syndrome	(25090)
Methylmalonic aciduria, type 1	(25100)
Methylmalonic aciduria, type 2	(25110)
Mucopolysaccharidosis, type 1 (Hurler)	(25280)
Mucopolysaccharidosis, type 3 (A and B, Sanfilippo)	(25290, 25292)
Mucopolysaccharidosis, type 7	(25322)
Myeloperoxidase deficiency	(25460)
Nervous system disorder resembling Refsum's and Hurler disease	(25640)
Niemann–Pick disease	(25720)

Orotic aciduria, types 1 and 2	(25890, 25892)
Oxalosis, type 1	(25990)
Oxalosis, type 2	(26000)
Phenylketonuria	(26160)
Phosphohexose isomerase	(17240)
Pyroglutamic aciduria	(26613)
Pyruvate kinase deficiency of erythrocyte	(26620)
Refsum syndrome	(26650)
Sea-blue histiocyte disease	(26960)
Sulphocysteinuria	(27230)
Trypsinogen deficiency	(27600)
Valinaemia	(27710)
Wolman disease	(27800)
Xanthinuria	(27830)
Xeroderma pigmentosum	(27870)
Xerodermic idiocy of de Sanctis and Cacchione	(27880)
Xylosidase deficiency	(27890)

description agreed. The extent to which the two primary surveyors disagreed gives some indication of the extent to which more remote users of the system, when compiled, might misinterpret the 22 features and give a 'wrong' description of their patient. The frequency of disagreement on specific features also identifies the more ambiguous terms which perhaps should be replaced as the system is developed. The differences that did occur (Table 17.2) reflects the different clinical experience of the two surveyors, one of whom had a general medical and surgical background, and the other a more specialist knowledge of child psychiatry and mental subnormality.

Once the data bank on the 86 entries was agreed its value in diagnosis could be tested. This was done by issuing the enquiry proforma (Figure 17.1) to clinicians in charge of patients, past and present, with an already diagnosed inherited metabolic disease. After explaining the structure of the form, the clinician was asked to complete it for the clinical state of the patient at the time of presentation and not to indicate any symptoms or signs that developed subsequently. At this stage data was obtained on 28 patients representing 18 diseases.

Much of the preliminary work was done by scanning the patient's data against the matrix by hand, but the results presented here are those

Table 17.2 The number of differences between initial statements and that finally agreed for each of 22 terms by the two primary surveyors compiling the data bank for 86 entries on 83 diseases

Term	'Errors' out of 86		
	Surveyor A	*Surveyor B*	*Total*
Onset before 8/12	4	3	7
Onset after 8/12	4	3	7
Distinctive odour	0	0	0
Hair abnormality	4	2	6
Skin abnormality	4	5	9
Jaundice	3	4	7
Cyanosis	0	1	1
Goitre	0	0	0
Vomiting	1	6	7
Bowel abnormality	3	2	5
Hepato(spleno)megaly	5	5	10
Genital abnormality	0	2	2
Neurol./mental degeneration	1	19	20
Other functional neurol. abnlty.	11	6	17
Mental retardation	9	4	13
Skeletal abnormality	2	6	8
Renal calculi	0	0	0
Anaemia	5	3	8
Acidosis	3	1	4
Lens corneal defect	6	0	6
Retinal abnormality	4	4	8
Urine abnormality	17	3	20

obtained subsequently after the process had been mechanized using a programme devised by Mr K. D. Griffiths of the Department of Clinical Chemistry, Birmingham Children's Hospital, using a Wang 2200B computer to which we later had access through the courtesy of Mr P. Scott at the Department of Clinical Chemistry, Selly Oak Hospital, Birmingham.

THE NATURE OF THE SCANNING PROCESS

When the patient's data is matched against the data bank all, or as many as possible, of the patient's clinical features, as recorded on the proforma, are used. When matched against the characteristics of a particular disease two things are of interest. The first is the number of characteristics coinciding between patient and data bank: the more that coincide the more probable that disorder represented the correct diagnosis, and the second is the proportion of this number of coincidences to the number of characteristics of the particular disease: the greater the proportion the more probable that disorder will represent the correct diagnosis.

This may be made more clear by considering the examples in Figure 17.2 which includes a data bank in which five diseases A–E are described in terms of five clinical features 1–5. Patients X, Y and Z with the clinical features given will be matched against the data bank in turn.

Data Bank

	1	2	3	4	5
A				+	
B		+	+	+	
C	+	+	+		+
D	+			+	
E		+			+

Patients

	1	2	3	4	5
X	+	+	+		+
Y			+		+
Z	+	+	+	+	

Results

	X		Y		Z	
	Corr.	%	Corr.	%	Corr.	%
A	0	—	0	—	1	100
B	2	66	1	33	3	100
C	4	100	2	50	3	75
D	1	50	0	—	2	100
E	2	100	2	100	1	50

Diagnosis in order of probability

X	Y	Z
C*	E*	B*
E	C*	C*
B	B	D
D	(A D)	A
A		E

FIGURE 17.2   Model system to illustrate the matching processes and expression of results. The asterisk denotes maximal number of correlations. For further explanation see text

Patient X who has four features does not match with any characteristics of disease A but two of his features coincide with two of the characteristics of disease B. Thus, there are two correlations with disease B, but since the latter contains three characteristics the maximum amount of coincidence possible between this patient and the disease represents only 66% of the full clinical picture of the latter. This process is repeated with the results shown for each patient in Figure 17.2. Thus, for patient X the maximum correlation achieved is four, using all of the patients clinical features, and this represents a complete match with one disease only, disease C. It would be reasonable to conclude that patient X is more likely to have disease C than any other disease in the data bank. (It must always be recognized that for undiagnosed patients the correct diagnosis may not be in the data bank at all.)

For patient Y, again, all the clinical features are used but there is maximal correlation with two diseases, C and E. However, the matching features represent only half of the characteristics of the former, whereas the match in the latter is complete. This, therefore, gives the advantage to E over C. In patient Z none of the diseases correlate on all four clinical features presented by the patient. However, two diseases, B and C, match on three out of the four and again there is a difference in the percentage match giving B the advantage over C.

With the real data bank this process is performed mechanically and the diseases are printed out in blocks of equal number of correlations starting with the greatest. Within each block of diseases each with the same number of correlations the diseases are further sorted into descending order of percentage correlation.

TESTING THE SYSTEM

Using the data available at presentation on patients with known diagnoses, print-outs were obtained and the position of the correct diagnosis in the list determined: the higher this occurred, the more successful the system is decreed to be. With a new, undiagnosed patient the clinician will be anxious to know how far down the list he should go, checking each diagnostic possibility by further clinical observation or by a specific laboratory investigation, before he might reasonably expect to reach the correct diagnosis.

The results obtained are shown in Table 17.3 and Figure 17.3. Table 17.3 shows the wide variety of metabolic diseases used to test the

Table 17.3   The position of the correct diagnosis in 28 patients subjected to preferential ordering by the pilot system of computer-aided diagnosis comprising 86 entries on 22 clinical features

Angiokeratoma, diffuse	3
α_1-Antitrypsin deficiency	3
Argininosuccinic aciduria	2
Cerebro-hepato-renal syndrome	3, 7
Cystinosis type 1	1
Galactosaemia	3
Hepatolenticular degeneration	2, >23
Homocystinuria	7, 3
Hypophosphatasia	1, 1
Lesch–Nyhan syndrome	5
Lowes syndrome	4, 4
Maple syrup urine disease	1, 15, 1
Menke's kinky hair syndrome	1, 3
Metachromatic leukodystrophy	1, 8, 1
Methylmalonic aciduria	3
Mucopolysaccharidosis type 1H	2
Phenylketonuria	2
Propionic acidaemia	11

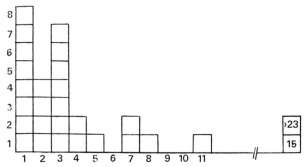

FIGURE 17.3   Frequency with which the correct diagnosis of 28 patients with an inherited metabolic disease occurred in various positions in the print-out from the first pilot study of a system for computer-aided diagnosis

system so far. The position of the correct diagnosis in the list for the few examples of each disease that are available shows that while none so far seem to come out consistently badly, several, like hepatolenticular degeneration and maple syrup urine disease, are occasionally too low in the list for the system to have been of use. However, Figure 17.3 gives a remarkably encouraging picture, for out of 28 patients the correct diagnosis appears at the top of the list in eight, while 79% are within the first five and 89% within the first 10.

Conclusion

It is clear from these results that the diagnosis of the inherited metabolic diseases can be greatly facilitated by a system of preferential ordering on the basis of their clinical presentation. It is also clear in this model system where the weaknesses lie. It may be necessary to add to the 22 clinical features used in the present study, and certainly, great benefit can be anticipated from replacing the terms relating to mental and neurological abnormalities by others more specific. Now that such a system has been shown to be feasible, the additional effort to improve and perfect it can be justified. It is proposed to increase the data bank to include about twice the present number of diseases and it will then be of interest to apply the system to patients in whom the correct diagnosis is not yet known.

Postscript

The system now has 157 diseases in the data bank based on the same 22 clinical features. A test of this with 36 patients with a known diagnosis has recently been reported.[3] In seven instances the correct diagnosis came at the top of the list, 66% were within the first five and 83% within the first 10.

REFERENCES

1. McKusick, V. A. (1975). *Mendelian Inheritance in Man*, 4th ed. (Baltimore: Johns Hopkins University Press)
2. Raine, D. N. (1972). Management of inherited metabolic disease. *Br. Med. J.*, **2**, 329
3. Raine, D. N., Rees, N. G., Terry, S. M. and Griffiths, K. (1976). Computer-aided diagnosis of inherited metabolic disease. *Arch. Dis. Child.*, **51**, (In Press)

THE FOURTH MILNER
LECTURE

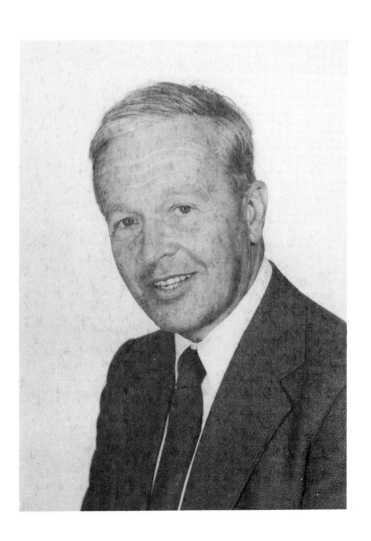

18

The biochemical autopsy: a tool for studies of genetically-determined brain disorders

The Milner Lecture delivered at the 1975 annual meeting of the Society for the Study of Inborn Errors of Metabolism

Thomas L. Perry

Your invitation to deliver the Milner lecture to the 1975 annual meeting of the Society is an honour which gives me great pleasure. I am also very happy to visit Britain again, and to renew friendships that commenced when I attended your annual meetings in Belfast and Leeds in 1970 and 1971. The papers and discussion of the past two days devoted to systematic detection of inherited metabolic diseases, and to their efficient and humane management in the community, have been interesting and important. I wish to use this opportunity, however, to emphasize the need for continuing scientific research on the biochemical complexities of inherited metabolic disorders. For health care to be really excellent, one must blend humanitarian intentions and good organization with unsatisfied scientific curiosity.

Much attention has been given in the published symposia of the Society, and indeed in this meeting, to inherited diseases affecting children. I feel it is time for physicians and other scientists interested in inborn errors of metabolism to pay much more attention to inherited diseases affecting adults, and, although I am a paediatrician by training, I intend to present several recent examples where some progress has been achieved on the biochemical basis of such diseases in adults. I wish to use this lecture also to challenge the often-repeated dictum that one should not hope to discover biochemical errors in diseases inherited in autosomal dominant fashion. Finally, since many serious inherited disorders affect the brain, causing mental retardation in childhood, or psychoses and mental deterioration in adult life, I wish to use this occasion to make a plea for more frequent serious biochemical studies of the brain itself, and of the cerebrospinal fluid (CSF), the physiological fluid which bathes the brain. I hope I will not be thought immodest if I use examples from our own laboratory in Vancouver to make these points, since I have greatest familiarity with them.

Glycine encephalopathy

Infants with hyperglycinaemia are found not infrequently in systematic screening programmes where amino acids are examined in the plasma or urine of newborns. Other cases come to attention when infants with severe neurological symptoms are investigated biochemically. The hyperglycinaemias have been classified up to now as ketotic when symptoms and laboratory signs of ketoacidosis have been present, and as nonketotic when lowered blood pH and ketonuria have not been demonstrable.

Hyperglycinaemia often accompanies propionic acidaemia[1] and methylmalonic acidaemia,[2] and has also been observed in some patients with isovaleric acidaemia[3] and β-ketothiolase deficiency.[4] In these disorders of organic acid metabolism, diagnoses are based on the detection of abnormal amounts of organic acids in urine and plasma, and on appropriate enzyme assays carried out on cultured fibroblasts or on biopsy or autopsy specimens of liver. Presumably the elevation of plasma glycine concentrations in these patients, and the demonstrated *in vivo* impairment of glycine cleavage,[5] are secondary to the accumulation of the abnormal organic acids in liver and possibly other tissues. When these organic acidaemias are promptly recognized and effectively treated, either with a low-protein diet or, in the vitamin B_{12}-responsive forms of methylmalonic acidaemia, with supplemental vitamin B_{12}, infants often do well and may suffer no permanent neurological damage.

The majority of infants with hyperglycinaemia, however, have no recognizable abnormality in organic acid metabolism. In these nonketotic hyperglycinaemic patients, abnormal organic acids are not detectable in plasma and urine, and ketoacidosis is absent, yet many develop an overwhelming neurological illness early in infancy. This is characterized by intractable seizures, spasticity, early death, or severe mental retardation in those patients who survive infancy.[6] Baumgartner and his colleagues[7] have recently demonstrated with sophisticated enzyme assay techniques that propionate and methylmalonate metabolism are entirely normal in infants with true nonketotic hyperglycinaemia. Various treatments of non-ketotic hyperglycinemia have all proved ineffective.

We have asked ourselves why there is such a profound difference in the clinical symptoms of infants with different forms of hyperglycinaemias, even though all may show comparable elevation of glycine concentrations in their fasting plasma. In particular, it is puzzling that some patients with hyperglycinaemia unassociated with organic acidosis may have no evidence at all of neurological disease,[8] while others are desperately ill. The answers to these questions became more clear when we measured glycine concentrations in the CSF of hyperglycinaemia patients, and particularly when we measured the glycine content of autopsied brain in three of these patients.[8]

GLYCINE IN PLASMA AND CSF

Table 18.1 shows the concentrations of glycine in these fluids in three infants with non-ketotic hyperglycinaemia whom we studied, and in two other children who had hyperglycinaemias of undetermined type (but *not* ketotic). The latter two patients had 2–4-fold elevations of glycine in plasma, but essentially normal concentrations of glycine in their CSF. By contrast, while plasma glycine was either normal or elevated only 3- or 4-fold in the three infants with true non-ketotic hyperglycinaemia, glycine concentrations were increased to levels 15–30 times above normal in their CSF. The enormous elevation of glycine in their CSF suggested that they might have an unusual accumulation of glycine in their brains.

BRAIN GLYCINE

Two of our non-ketotic hyperglycinaemic patients, and one of the patients with hyperglycinaemia of undetermined type, died and were autopsied. Amino acid analyses of various regions of their brains, using techniques developed in our laboratory[9-11] demonstrated a marked accumulation of glycine in the brains of the two non-ketotic hyperglycinaemic infants (Table 18.2, Cases 4 and 5), but not in the brain of the hyperglycinaemic infant of undetermined type (Table 18.2, Case 1).

GLYCINE CLEAVAGE ENZYME ACTIVITY

My colleague, Dr Nadine Urquhart, then measured the *in vitro* activities of the glycine cleavage enzyme in specimens of brain and liver

Table 18.1   Glycine concentrations in fasting plasma and cerebrospinal fluid

Subjects	Fasting plasma glycine ($\mu mol/l$)	CSF glycine ($\mu mol/l$)	CSF/ plasma ratio
Adult controls*	219 ± 54 (77)	6.4 ± 1.7 (43)	0.03
Infant controls*	209 ± 46 (12)	5.2 ± 2.0 (34)	0.02
Patient 1, hyperglycinaemia,? type	556†	9.8	0.02
Patient 2, hyperglycinaemia,? type	734†	5.5	0.01
Patient 3, non-ketotic hyper-glycinaemia	810†	159.1†	0.20
Patient 4, non-ketotic hyper-glycinaemia	631†	142.2†	0.23
Patient 5, non-ketotic hyper-glycinaemia	266†	87.6†	0.33

* Mean $\pm$ SD are shown for control groups, with numbers of subjects in parentheses
† Mean glycine values of repeated specimens
(Taken from Perry *et al.*,[8] with permission)

from these three autopsied hyperglycinaemic infants. The glycine cleavage enzyme system splits glycine into carbon dioxide, ammonia, and a one-carbon fragment derived from the number 2 carbon atom of glycine. This fragment is attached to tetrahydrofolic acid to form N^5, N^{10}-methylene tetrahydrofolic acid. This is illustrated in the diagram in Figure 18.1. The glycine cleavage reaction is apparently the main degradative pathway for glycine in mammalian brain.[12] The one-carbon units produced by the glycine cleavage system can then be further utilized by a second enzyme, serine hydroxymethyltransferase, to convert intact molecules of glycine into serine (Figure 18.1). Thus absence of activity of the glycine cleavage enzyme system in brain would not only prevent splitting of glycine, but would also result in a deficiency of methylene units for conversion of other glycine molecules into serine.

Table 18.2 Glycine content of several regions of central nervous system*

Subjects	Frontal cortex	Occipital cortex	Cerebellar cortex	Caudate nucleus	Putamen-globus pallidus	Spinal cord
14 Neurologically normal adults	1.24 ± 0.44	1.57 ± 0.64	1.81 ± 0.64	1.70 ± 0.36	2.01 ± 0.67	
Neurologically normal infant, age 8 m	2.09	2.01	2.61	2.44	2.36	2.22
Patient 1, age 14 m, hyperglycinaemia,? type	2.04	1.97	2.02		2.18	
Patient 4, age 10 m, nonketotic hyperglycinaemia	4.51	3.55	10.05	6.40	7.43	8.90
Patient 5, age 8 m, nonketotic hyperglycinaemia	4.84	4.24	8.13	6.62	8.40	8.33

* Values expressed in μmol/g wet weight; mean ± SD are shown for adult control group (Taken from Perry et al.,[8] with permission)

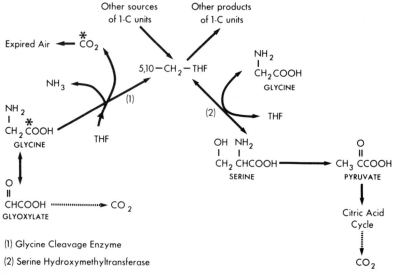

FIGURE 18.1   Metabolism of glycine and interconversion of glycine and serine. THF denotes tetrahydrofolic acid; 5,10–CH$_2$–THF denotes N^5,N^{10}-methylene tetrahydrofolic acid; and 1-C unit denotes single-carbon unit. The two relevant enzymes, the glycine cleavage enzyme and serine hydroxymethyltransferase, are indicated by numbers in parentheses. The asterisk marks the radioactive carbon atom followed in both in vivo studies and in vitro enzyme assays (Taken from Perry *et al.*,[8] with permission)

Table 18.3 shows that activity of the glycine cleavage enzyme was undetectable in the brains of the two infants with non-ketotic hyperglycinaemia, while appreciable activity was present in the brain of the infant who died with hyperglycinaemia of undetermined type. Considerable *in vitro* activity of the glycine cleavage system was nevertheless present in liver tissue of both non-ketotic hyperglycinaemics.

COMMENT

These observations suggest that 'true nonketotic hyperglycinaemia', as Baumgartner and his colleagues[7] term the disorder, or glycine encephalopathy as we prefer to call it, differs from all the other hyperglycinaemias in that it involves a profound accumulation of glycine in brain, which can easily be predicted by amino acid analysis of the CSF in living patients. Although many infants with this disorder must have died and come to autopsy, it is surprising that only one previous measurement of glycine in brain has been reported.[13] There too brain glycine content was greatly elevated.

Table 18.3   Glycine cleavage enzyme activity in brain and liver*

Subject†	Frontal cortex	Cerebellar cortex	Liver
Control 1			
(52 y, 10 h)	92	456	2859
Control 2			
(8 m, 5 h)	145	227	3622
Patient 1			
(14 m, 4 h)	59	125	165
Patient 4			
(10 m, 3 h)	0	0	993
Patient 5			
(8 m, 9 h)	0	0	1087

* nmol $^{14}CO_2$ formed/h/g protein
† Figures in parentheses indicate age at death, and interval from death until tissue was frozen at $-80°C$
(Taken from Perry et al.,[8] with permission)

How does one explain finding complete absence of glycine cleavage enzyme activity in the brain in glycine encephalopathy, but appreciable activity in the liver? One possibility is that the enzymes in the two organs are not identical, and that the brain isozyme is defective in glycine encephalopathy. But if this were the case, it is difficult to explain why most of the affected infants who have been studied appear to have developed normally *in utero*, and then to have become ill somewhere between the first few days to few months after birth. Elevated plasma glycine levels are apparently harmless, while elevated brain glycine content can be lethal. One can readily understand how the placental circulation could keep plasma glycine levels within normal limits in the fetus, but it is more difficult to conceive that this could prevent glycine accumulation in brain, if the glycine cleavage enzyme system were inactive in fetal brain.

Another possibility is that an inhibitor of the glycine cleavage enzyme accumulates, especially in brain, in glycine encephalopathy. Such an inhibitor might cross the placenta and be metabolized by the mother until the infant was born, thus explaining why hyperglycinaemic infants appear normal at birth. We found no evidence for the presence of such an enzyme inhibitor in the brains of the first two infants we studied with glycine encephalopathy. However, we have recently received the brain of a third baby who died of a rapidly progressive form of the disease early in infancy, and we intend to search further for a possible inhibitor. A third possibility is that some small molecule serves as an activator of the glycine cleavage enzyme in brain, and that this activator is supplied by the mother during pregnancy, but cannot be synthesized by the infant on its own.

The mechanisms for the profound neurological disturbance in glycine encephalopathy need further study. There is substantial evidence[14] that glycine may function as an inhibitory synaptic transmitter in the spinal cord, and possibly at certain synapses in the brain as well. Thus, a massive accumulation of this putative inhibitory compound might seriously impair function of the brain. Another possibility that should be explored is the effect of a profound shortage of one-carbon fragments might have on various synthetic biochemical pathways in the rapidly growing infant brain.

If it is true that high plasma glycine levels are innocuous, while high brain glycine levels are severely damaging, it is easy to see why the various therapeutic measures that have so far been tried in glycine encephalopathy have proved ineffective. I do not think this is the sort of metabolic disorder which can be benefited by special diets low in one or more amino acids. Unfortunately, the humanistic inventiveness of people like Mr Jerome Milner cannot solve all of our problems for us. Likewise, pouring benzoic acid into such an infant, and hoping that this will mop up the excessive glycine by converting it to hippuric acid, can hardly be expected to work, since there is no evidence that the enzyme glycine-N-acylase is present in brain.

At the moment, we have no available therapy for glycine encephalopathy. We cannot yet detect the disorder prenatally by amniocentesis, and all we can presently do is to provide prompt genetic counselling to parents, when a case is detected, as to the 1 in 4 risk that their next baby will have the same disorder. If, however, we knew that an inhibitor was poisoning an otherwise normal glycine cleavage enzyme in brain, or that a small molecular enzyme activator was missing in glycine encephalopathy, or even that the neurological damage was due largely to lack of one-carbon fragments, we might yet be able to devise an effective therapy for this disorder. This example, I feel, emphasizes the need for closer alliances between research laboratories and broad community efforts in the provision of effective medical care.

Disorders inherited as autosomal dominants

HUNTINGTON'S CHOREA

I had been interested in Huntington's chorea for some time when I was told by a prominent medical geneticist that I was absolutely wasting my time to look for a biochemical abnormality in this disorder, since it was inherited as an autosomal dominant. Fortunately, a mixture of common sense and nonconformism led me to continue my efforts.

To both the scientist and the humanist, Huntington's chorea is a most interesting disease. Heterozygotes for the mutant gene develop the disorder if they live to mid-adult life, when the symptoms commence. These include loss of previously normal intelligence, personality changes, development of a wide variety of psychotic symptoms, commission of minor crimes, and choreiform and athetoid involuntary movements. Typically, symptoms appear in the 4th decade of life after previous excellent health, and pursue a relentless progressive course until death 12–15 years later. At autopsy, marked atrophy is found in the striatum, and to a lesser extent throughout the cerebral cortex. In North America, approximately 1 in every 10 000 persons is heterozygous for the Huntington's chorea gene and can be expected to develop the disorder if he or she survives long enough. About 1% of the population chronically confined to institutions for the mentally ill consists of patients with Huntington's chorea. Most patients have already produced their children by the time they are recognized to be ill, and these children must in turn endure years of anxiety worrying about the 50% chance that they too will develop the disorder.

Huntington's chorea has also an interesting history. Many of the patients now suffering from the disorder in French Canada are descendants of a woman who emigrated from Brittany to Montreal in 1645.[15] Three persons carrying the mutant gene for Huntington's chorea came by ship to the American Colonies from the village of Bures in East Anglia in 1630. Their affected descendants not only account for many of the present cases in the United States, but some of them were tried for witchcraft and hanged in the late 17th century by the religious bigots in New England.[16,17] It is a sobering thought to find oneself 200 years later investigating the biochemical basis of witchcraft!

Since many fruitless efforts had been made to discover biochemical abnormalities peculiar to Huntington's chorea in the urine and blood of affected patients, we elected to examine biochemically the brains of patients dying of this disorder. Fortunately, a biochemical technique with which we were familiar, automated amino acid analysis, paid off handsomely. We discovered[18] that γ-aminobutyric acid (GABA), and its histidyl dipeptide, homocarnosine, were considerably reduced in content in the caudate nucleus, putamen-globus pallidus, and substantia nigra, in autopsied brain from choreic patients, as compared to values found in the same regions of autopsied brain from persons dying without neurological or psychiatric disease. Glycerophosphoethanolamine was significantly increased in content in the same regions of choreic brain. Table 18.4 presents our latest mean values for GABA and homocarnosine content, representing six regions of autopsied brain for 11 patients dying with Huntington's chorea, and 16 control adult subjects. One can see that there are highly significant reductions of GABA in the caudate nucleus, putamen-globus pallidus, substantia nigra, and occipital cortex in choreic brain, and highly significant reductions of homocarnosine in the putamen-globus pallidus and the cerebellar cortex.

A large body of evidence suggests that GABA is an important inhibitory synaptic transmitter in mammalian brain. This has been reviewed recently by Krnjevic.[14] Thus it is tempting to speculate that a deficiency of GABA might account for the movement disorders characteristic of Huntington's chorea, and perhaps for the disordered mentation as well. Figure 18.2 summarizes the synthetic and degradative pathways of GABA metabolism in mammalian brain, and shows the relation between it and other compounds occurring in brain. Glutamic acid decarboxylase (GAD) is the enzyme which synthesizes GABA from glutamic acid, and GABA transaminase (GABA-T) is the first enzyme in the degradative pathway of GABA.

When we reported the deficiency in GABA in brain in Huntington's chorea, a number of investigators, led by the group at Cambridge University, studied the activity of the enzyme GAD in autopsied choreic brain. All of them[19-23] have found GAD activity reduced in those areas of choreic brain that are pathologically most affected. However, GAD activity has also been found to be decreased in the brains of patients dying with Parkinson's disease[24] and with senile dementia.[25] Our group[23] found GAD enzyme activity reduced in choreic brain, but to our surprise we found equally low GAD activity in the brains of two control adults who died suddenly without neurological or psychiatric

Table 18.4 GABA and homocarnosine content of autopsied brain of Huntington's chorea patients and control subjects

Amino compound		Frontal cortex	Occipital cortex	Cerebellar cortex	Caudate nucleus	Putamen-globus pallidus	Substantia nigra
GABA	Controls (16)	1.79 ± 0.13	2.01 ± 0.14	1.76 ± 0.12	2.94 ± 0.22	4.55 ± 0.29	5.75 ± 0.25
	Choreics (11)	1.59 ± 0.14	1.38 ± 0.12†	1.61 ± 0.11	1.57 ± 0.26*	1.76 ± 0.24*	2.18 ± 0.22*
Homocarnosine	Controls (16)	0.34 ± 0.05	0.57 ± 0.09	0.72 ± 0.07	0.29 ± 0.05	0.87 ± 0.09	0.95 ± 0.08
	Choreics (11)	0.20 ± 0.04	0.31 ± 0.06	0.37 ± 0.07†	0.23 ± 0.05	0.35 ± 0.06*	0.66 ± 0.08‡

Results are expressed in μmol/g wet wt., and represent mean ± S.E.
Figures in brackets indicate number of brains analysed
* $P < 0.001$ (as compared with normal subjects)
† $P < 0.005$
‡ $P < 0.02$

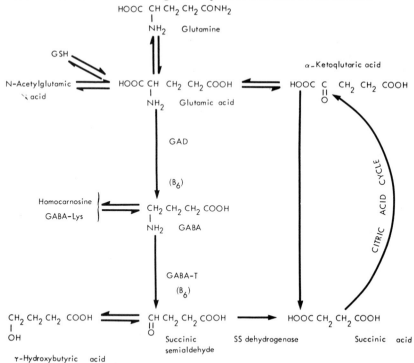

FIGURE 18.2   Metabolism of γ-aminobutyric acid in mammalian brain. GAD represents glutamic acid decarboxylase; GABA, γ-aminobutyric acid; GABA-T, γ-aminobutyric acid transaminase; SS dehydrogenase, succinic semialdehyde dehydrogenase; GSH, reduced glutathione; and GABA-Lys, γ-aminobutyryllysine

disease of any sort. Although these two control subjects had very low *in vitro* activity of the synthetic enzyme, their brain GABA content was normal and in this latter respect they differed markedly from the choreic patients.

If one considers the possible explanations for the low GABA content of the basal ganglia in Huntington's chorea, three mechanisms come to mind (Figure 18.2). First, the mutant gene may have caused a deficiency of GAD activity, perhaps starting in mid-adult life. We searched for a possible inhibitor of GAD, by carrying out mixing experiments of homogenates of choreic and control brain in our enzyme assays,[23] but found none. A second possibility is that the mutant gene might produce excessive activity of the degradative enzyme, GABA-T (Figure 18.2). We measured GABA-T activity in choreic brain and found it no greater than in control brain.[23] A third possible explanation for the low GABA content of brain in Huntington's chorea, one which might also account for the observed deficiency of GAD activity, is that a population of neurones which utilize GABA as a synaptic transmitter, and which therefore contain large amounts of GAD for synthesizing GABA, has been lost, for reasons as yet unknown. We think this third possibility is very likely. It will probably be necessary to search carefully for a potential toxic substance that accumulates in certain brain regions in Huntington's chorea, or for absence of some key nutrient substance, that in turn causes progressive death of GABAergic neurones.

Meanwhile, one urgently wants to do something therapeutically for patients with Huntington's chorea that will relieve their symptoms and prolong their lives, and offer some hope to their children who are at risk for the disease. We have shown in rats[11] and in squirrel monkeys[26] that one can produce sustained elevation of GABA content in brain through inhibition of the degradative enzyme, GABA-T, by continued administration of either amino-oxyacetic acid or isonicotinic acid hydrazide (isoniazid). Recently we have been administering isoniazid, in doses considerably higher than those used in treating tuberculosis, to a limited number of patients with Huntington's chorea. The results are not very promising, even though we have laboratory evidence to suggest that we are indeed elevating these patients' brain GABA contents. If those neurones that normally release GABA at their synapses are dying or dead, supplying extra brain GABA by a pharmacological manoeuvre as we have done might well be ineffective.

HEREDITARY MENTAL DEPRESSION WITH TAURINE DEFICIENCY

Having been successful in finding a distinct biochemical abnormality, although not necessarily the primary one, in Huntington's chorea, we have more recently examined brain in two other degenerative neurological diseases that are inherited in autosomal dominant fashion. Again nonconformist curiosity has been rewarded!

A family in British Columbia has been afflicted with a severe neuropsychiatric disease characterized throughout by mental depression and late in the illness by parkinsonian symptoms. The pedigree of this family is shown in Figure 18.3. Patients of both sexes in three successive generations have been affected. Each of the seven family members with the disorder had enjoyed good physical and mental health until reaching the age of 45 to 50. The affected patients then developed mental depression, fatiguability and lethargy, sleep disturbances, and progressive

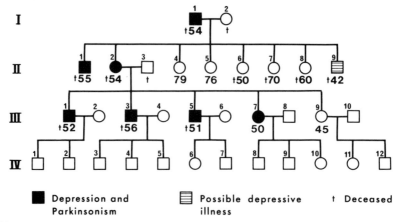

| ■ Depression and | ▤ Possible depressive | † Deceased |
| Parkinsonism | illness | |

FIGURE 18.3   Pedigree of a family with hereditary mental depression and parkinsonism. Numbers under symbols indicate present age or age at death

weight loss. Patients III-1,3 and 5 also had an unusual impairment of depth perception. During the latter half of their illnesses, the patients all developed certain features of parkinsonism, such as an impassive facial expression, a tendency to hold the trunk stiffly, and tremor of the hands. They also had difficulties in speech, swallowing, and breathing in the last years of their illnesses, and died suddenly and unexpectedly of apparent central respiratory failure. The duration of the illness from first symptoms to death has varied between 4 and 6 years in the six affected family members who have died. Mental depression in these patients failed to respond to tricyclic antidepressants, monoamine oxidase inhibitors, and to electroconvulsive therapy. The parkinsonian symptoms were not alleviated by administration of L-dopa or amantadine.

We were fortunate to obtain fasting plasma and CSF from patient III-3 shortly before his death, and specimens of several regions of his brain at autopsy. Amino acid analyses of these specimens were performed and showed a deficiency of taurine in plasma, CSF, and brain,[27] but no other abnormalities. Patient III-3's fasting plasma taurine concentration was 23 μmol/l, whereas our mean for 67 normal adults is 56 $\pm$ 13 μmol/l. His CSF taurine concentration was 1.0 μmol/l, while our mean value for 53 adults with various neurological diseases is 6.5 $\pm$ 1.7 μmol/l.

Table 18.5 presents the content of taurine in several regions of patient III-3's brain, as compared with the taurine content of the same regions

Table 18.5 Taurine content of several regions of autopsied brain from patient III-3 and control subjects

Subjects	Substantia nigra	Putamen-globus pallidus	Caudate nucleus	Frontal cortex	Occipital cortex	Cerebellum
Neurologically normal (16)	1.18 (± 0.31)	1.52 (± 0.45)	1.38 (± 0.46)	1.13 (± 0.31)	1.14 (± 0.35)	2.97 (± 0.73)
Huntington's chorea (11)	1.60 (± 0.58)	1.90 (± 0.68)	1.93 (± 1.01)	1.58 (± 0.77)	1.31 (± 0.44)	3.53 (± 0.94)
Parkinsonism (3)	1.25 (± 0.15)	1.45 (± 0.28)	1.28 (± 0.29)	1.40 (± 0.77)	0.90 (± 0.13)	2.29 (± 0.42)
Patient III-3	0.97	0.80	0.71	0.64	0.54	1.06

Results are expressed in μmol/g wet weight and represent mean and S.D.

of autopsied brain in 16 neurologically normal adults, 11 patients dying with Huntington's chorea, and three patients dying with parkinsonism. The patient's taurine content is considerably lower than that of these various control subjects in all the examined brain regions, with taurine deficiency being most marked in the cerebellar cortex. The contents of other sulphur-containing amino compounds, such as methionine, cystathionine, cystine, and oxidized and reduced glutathione were normal in III-3's brain. No traces could be found of *S*-adenosylhomocysteine, homocystine, cysteinesulphinic acid, cysteic acid, or hypotaurine, other easily-measurable sulphur amino acids which are metabolic intermediates between methionine and taurine.

At about the time that patient III-3 died, his sister, III-7, developed symptoms of the same disorder. She has been getting slowly worse for $2\frac{3}{4}$ years, and we have had the opportunity of exploring certain aspects of taurine metabolism in her that were not studied in her brother. In the first place, her fasting plasma and CSF taurine concentrations, although low, have remained within normal limits during the first 2 years of her illness. She absorbs taurine normally from her gastrointestinal tract, does not excrete excessive amounts of taurine in her urine, and has normal taurine content in her platelets. If she has the same brain taurine deficiency that her brother exhibited at death, it does not seem likely that the deficiency arises from failure to absorb dietary taurine or from leakage of taurine from the body.

Figure 18.4 shows the relevant pathways of taurine metabolism in man, and those known to occur in human brain are indicated by heavy arrows. The probable main pathway in human brain involves oxidation of cysteine to cysteinesulphinic acid, decarboxylation of the latter to hypotaurine (with pyridoxal phosphate a necessary cofactor), and then further oxidation of hypotaurine to taurine.[28] A small fraction of taurine in rat brain is further metabolized to isethionic acid,[29] and isethionic acid presumably also occurs normally in human brain. Since no traces of hypotaurine were detectable in the brain specimens of patient III-3, it is unlikely that his taurine deficiency was due to an enzymatic failure at the level of hypotaurine oxidation. Cysteinesulphinic acid is a relatively unstable compound, however, and failure to detect it in brain obtained at autopsy 12 hours after death (as was the case with patient III-3) does not rule out the possibility of a deficiency of activity of the enzyme cysteinesulphinic acid decarboxylase in III-3's brain during life. Measurements of cysteine or cystine content in autopsied brain speci-

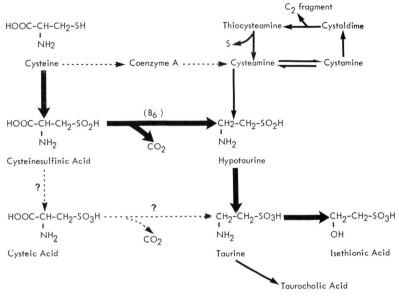

FIGURE 18.4 Taurine metabolism in man. Heavy arrows indicate metabolic steps known to occur in human brain (Taken from Perry *et al.*,[27] with permission)

mens are valueless, since both compounds accumulate rapidly after brain death, as a result of the hydrolysis of glutathione. Therefore, determination of the amount of cysteine and cystine in patient III-3's brain neither provided evidence for, nor ruled out an enzymatic block between cysteine and cysteinesulphinic acid. If and when further patients are found whose brain taurine content is reduced at autopsy, *in vitro* enzymatic studies of brain obtained as quickly as possible after death may provide the answer as to the site of the metabolic failure.

It is tempting to speculate as to how a deficiency of taurine might cause the symptoms that were seen in affected patients in this pedigree. Taurine is one of the major free amino compounds present in human brain, its content being much higher in the cerebellar cortex than in other brain regions that have been studied.[10] Taurine inhibits the firing of central neurones in brain, as does GABA,[30] and there is some evidence that taurine may serve as an inhibitory synaptic transmitter or modulator in the central nervous system[31–33] and in the retina.[34] Thus a widespread deficiency of this amino acid might produce a variety of neurological and psychiatric symptoms, and possibly even the abnormalities in visual depth perception experienced by three of our patients.

Meanwhile, on the assumption that our new patient, III-7's, symptoms are due to a gradually decreasing taurine content in her brain, we have fed her large amounts of taurine by mouth in an effort to increase the content of taurine in her brain. We were able to show that when ^{35}S-labelled taurine is administered to rats and to squirrel monkeys, some of the radioactive taurine can later be recovered from brain cells.[35] Patient III-7 has taken taurine orally in the very high dosage of 0.25 mmol/kg every 4 hours five times daily for a period of 6 months. This dosage has been sufficient to keep her plasma taurine concentrations continuously elevated to levels 8–10 times the normal fasting taurine concentration. She has had no observed toxic effects from these large doses of taurine, but unfortunately she has also shown no sustained improvement, and her symptoms of apathy, depression, inability to make simple decisions, and disordered sleep are slowly increasing. It is possible that even though we demonstrated some passage of radioactive taurine into brain in laboratory mammals, the actual amount that enters human brain when plasma taurine levels are elevated 10-fold is too little to be beneficial. If this is the case, administration of large amounts of L-cystine to our patient, or of massive amounts of pyridoxine (in case her cysteinesulphinic acid decarboxylase fails to bind normally to its cofactor, pyridoxal phosphate), might be helpful. We intend to try both of these manoeuvres on her. Another possibility, of course, is that the taurine deficiency which we found in the autopsied brain of patient III-3 was unrelated causally to the hereditary disorder that killed him. If this is the case, we may be barking up the wrong tree in attempting to raise patient III-7's brain taurine content.

HEREDITARY CEREBELLAR ATROPHY

Cerebellar atrophy inherited in autosomal dominant fashion is the latest hereditary disorder in which systematic amino acid analysis of autopsied brain specimens has rewarded us with an interesting biochemical finding. Through the initiative of our collaborator, Dr Robert D. Currier, at the University of Mississippi, we were provided with the rapidly-frozen brains of two adults who died of a progressive cerebellar disorder. This disease has occurred in at least five successive generations of a large kindred in the southern United States.[36] The patients in this pedigree have been classified as probably having olivopontocerebellar atrophy, Type IV,[37] a dominant disorder possibly involving the climbing fibres, whose cell bodies are located in the inferior olivary nucleus, and which rise to synapse with the Purkinje cells in the molecular layer of the cerebellar cortex. We have also examined brain obtained at autopsy from a patient in an unrelated Canadian family in which a degenerative cerebellar disorder has occurred in at least five members, of at least two successive generations.

Each of these three patients, from two different families with degenerative cerebellar disorders, showed a new amino acid disorder. Aspartic acid, a possible candidate for an excitatory synaptic transmitter in the brain,[14] was markedly reduced in content in the cerebellar cortex, although its content was normal in the cerebral cortex, the caudate nucleus, the putamen-globus pallidus, and the substantia nigra. Table 18.6 shows the differences in aspartic acid content between control subjects and our three cerebellar atrophy patients in the cerebellar cortex, the inferior olivary nucleus, the pons, and the dentate nucleus. The reduction of aspartic acid in the cerebellar cortex is quite striking when one views amino acid analyser chromatograms, as illustrated in Figure 18.5.

We are a long way from being able to explain the significance of an aspartate deficiency localized in the olivopontocerebellar system, to relate the biochemical abnormality to the symptoms, or even to propose

Table 18.6 Aspartate content of autopsied brain in hereditary cerebellar ataxia and controls

Subjects	Cerebellar cortex	Pons	Inferior olivary nucleus	Dentate nucleus
Neurologically normal (16)	1.98 ± 0.74			
Adult controls (3)		1.46 ± 0.06	0.72 ± 0.22	1.02 ± 0.19
OPCA IV	0.42	0.96	0.34	0.26
OPCA IV	0.68	0.72	0.43	0.27
Hereditary cerebellar ataxia, type?	0.58	0.76	0.49	0.52

Results are expressed in μmol/g wet weight, and represent mean and S.D.

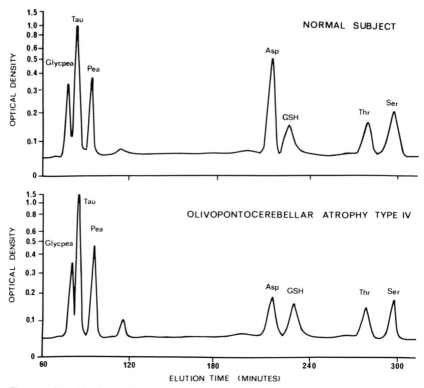

FIGURE 18.5   Tracings of chromatograms of free amino compounds in deproteinized extracts of human cerebellar cortex. In each case, approximately 100 mg wet weight of autopsied brain has been chromatographed, and only the first part of each chromatogram is shown. Aspartic acid (Asp) is greatly reduced in the cerebellum of the patient with olivopontocerebellar atrophy

any rational therapy for the disorder. We have explored the possibility that a deficiency of N-acetylaspartate in the cerebellar cortex has in turn caused the deficiency of aspartate. N-acetylaspartate occurs in large quantities in brain. Its physiological function is unknown, although it has recently been suggested that it plays a role in neuronal protein synthesis.[38],[39] Preliminary analyses suggest that the N-acetylaspartate content of the cerebellar cortex is normal in our patients with hereditary cerebellar atrophy.

HOMOCARNOSINOSIS

That there may well be further neurological disorders inherited in autosomal dominant fashion, and involving abnormalities in amino acid metabolism in brain, is suggested by a recent report by Gjessing and Sjaastad[40] from Norway. These investigators have discovered three adult siblings with mental retardation and progressive spastic paresis who have greatly increased levels of homocarnosine in their CSF. The normal mean concentration of homocarnosine found in the CSF of a large miscellaneous group of adult neurological patients was 1.8 ($\pm$ 1.8) μmol/l.[41] The three Norwegian siblings, *and their mother as well*, have CSF homocarnosine levels 25–40 times higher than this normal level. This is again an example of the potential value of applying amino acid analysis to CSF in neurological and mental diseases, and it suggests that biochemical examination of the brain in homocarnosinosis may eventually disclose interesting new findings.

Conclusions

The experiences we have had with interesting genetically determined disorders in our laboratory in Vancouver have helped clarify for me several ideas that I would like to stress in closing.

1. Applying relatively sophisticated laboratory techniques to CSF can really pay off when one studies neurological or mental diseases of unknown aetiology. I think we should probably obtain CSF more often than we usually do, and we should carry out some newer and more imaginative laboratory tests than just protein, sugar, and colloidal gold determinations on this valuable fluid. Sometimes one can get information about what is going on chemically in the brain that cannot be obtained from plasma or urine. The greatly elevated CSF glycine concentration in glycine encephalopathy, as contrasted to the normal or barely elevated CSF glycine levels of all the other hyperglycinaemias, is a good example of this.

2. The decreasing frequency of autopsies ought to be of concern to every health professional who hopes to improve the quality of medical care. It may be that traditional morphological examinations of tissues obtained at autopsy are now often unrewarding when it comes to providing new knowledge about unsolved diseases. But certainly the use of new methods such as electron microscopy, sophisticated virological studies, and especially biochemical techniques on autopsy tissues can help us to understand the causes of unexplained illnesses, and should eventually lead to successful treatments for some of them.

In my view, it is a tragic waste of human suffering to fail to arrange for well-planned autopsy studies when a child or adult dies of a mysterious hereditary disorder. When such disorders involve the brain, as they often do, the brain should be subjected to a variety of modern biochemical analyses. These should *not* be limited to amino acid analyses. This technique, with which we have some expertise in our laboratory, is only one of many which ought to be carried out. Therefore, it would be desirable to enlist the aid of different groups of investigators, each group having different laboratory skills.

Autopsies should be done as rapidly as possible after the death of a patient with an insufficiently understood hereditary disorder, and specimens of brain, liver, and other organs should be frozen at −70 °C or lower, if possible within 1 or 2 hours of death. This may make it possible for sophisticated enzyme studies to be carried out months or years later, whenever a biochemical abnormality has been found.

3. Modern biochemical investigations on brain should not be limited to children, but need to be carried out more often in adults with neurological or mental disease. Huntington's chorea, which primarily affects adults, is as common as phenylketonuria, and in terms of human misery it probably wreaks much more havoc than phenylketonuria. Some genetically-determined diseases of adults, such as the schizophrenias and the depressive psychoses, are much more frequent than the hereditary 'rare-butterfly' conditions of children to which many of us have devoted our attention. I recommend the work of Grote and colleagues[42] as a good example of an important and well-conceived experiment. This group of scientists, located in a department of psychiatry, carried out studies of the activities of four enzymes involved in catecholamine metabolism in autopsied brain of depressed patients who committed suicide, and in brain from appropriate control subjects who died suddenly.

4. Our experiences in biochemical studies of brain in Huntington's chorea, hereditary depression with taurine deficiency, and hereditary cerebellar atrophy have certainly convinced me that it is well worth while devoting more attention to the possible biochemical basis of disorders inherited as autosomal dominants. Professor Harry Harris[43] has recently discussed some of the possible mechanisms by which clinical disease may occur in persons heterozygous for a mutant gene, and thus having disorders classified as inherited in dominant fashion.

In many inborn errors of metabolism, specific enzyme activity in the heterozygous state has been found to be generally intermediate between that present in normal individuals and that present in abnormal homozygotes. In the extreme case where the abnormal gene leads to complete loss of enzyme activity, the heterozygote usually shows about one half the average activity found in normal homozygotes. If, as is usually the case, enzyme activity in normal homozygotes is many times the minimum actually required for efficient metabolic function, the reduced enzyme activity in heterozygotes will have no clinical consequences. If, however, the enzyme catalyzes a rate-limiting step in a metabolic pathway, and enzyme activity in the normal homozygote is only slightly in excess of that required, the heterozygote with a 50% reduction in activity of this rate-limiting enzyme might well have troubles. This seems to be the case in acute intermittent porphyria, a disorder usually appearing in mid-adult life which is inherited as an autosomal dominant, and where heterozygotes have critically reduced activity of the rate-limiting enzyme uroporphyrinogen synthetase.[44] It would be interesting to learn, for instance, whether any one of the three enzymes required to convert cysteine into taurine in brain (Figure 18.4) might in normal individuals have only just sufficient activity, so that reduced activity in heterozygotes could lead eventually to brain taurine deficiency.

Sometimes a gene mutation may result in increased activity of a specific enzyme, and the resulting disturbance of a metabolic pathway may give rise to overt pathological consequences. This is the case in an unusual type of gout where it has been shown[45,46] that heterozygotes for the mutant gene possess a phosphoribosylpyrophosphate synthetase with specific enzyme activity per molecule of enzyme about 2.5–3.0 times greater than normal. Thus it was reasonable for us to explore the possibility that an abnormally great GABA-T enzyme activity (Figure 18.2) might result in excessively rapid degradation of GABA in the brain in Huntington's chorea.

Another possibility in diseases inherited as autosomal dominants is that the absence of one normal allele in the affected heterozygotes results in insufficient production of key structural (i.e. non-enzymic) proteins which must be formed in substantial quantities for optimal cell functioning. If only one-half the usual amount of such structural proteins were formed, certain cells might function poorly, or gradually die off. This might be the case, for instance, with the GABA-utilizing neurones in Huntington's chorea, or with one particular type of neurone in the cerebellum in hereditary cerebellar atrophy. However, loss of a population of neurones in the brain might well be accompanied by dramatic secondary biochemical changes which could be detected by appropriate biochemical analyses, and which might account for important symptoms occurring in the affected patients.

5. Finally, I believe that the kinds of studies which I have described today demonstrate the intimate relationship that ought to exist between the research laboratory on the one hand, and practising physicians, nurses, nutritionists, and social workers on the other, if people are to get the highest possible quality of health care. Government agencies in these days of inflation and rapidly-rising health care costs tend sometimes to consider further medical research an expensive luxury or 'elitist', and to suggest that all we need is a more equitable and economic distribution of health care. I believe that our desire to relieve human suffering, just as much as our intellectual curiosity, demands continued vigorous research into the unsolved areas of inherited disease.

The studies from our laboratory referred to in this paper were supported by grants from the Medical Research Council of Canada, and from the Huntington's Chorea Foundation. I am grateful to my colleagues Mrs Shirley Hansen, Mrs Janet MacLean, and Dr Nadine Urquhart who have contributed greatly to the research described here

REFERENCES

1. ANDO, T. and NYHAN, W. L. (1974). Propionic acidemia and the ketotic hyperglycinemia syndrome. In W. L. Nyhan (ed.), *Heritable Disorders of Amino Acid Metabolism*, pp. 37–60. (New York; John Wiley & Sons)
2. MORROW, G. (1974). Methylmalonic acidemia. In W. L. Nyhan (ed.), *Heritable Disorders of Amino Acid Metabolism*, pp. 61–80. (New York: John Wiley & Sons)
3. ANDO, T. KLINGBERG, W. G., WARD, A. N., RASMUSSEN, K. and NYHAN, W. L. (1971). Isovaleric acidemia presenting with altered metabolism of glycine. *Pediatr. Res.*, **5**, 478
4. HILLMAN, R. E. and KEATING, J. P. (1974). Beta-ketothiolase deficiency as a cause of the ketotic hyperglycinemia syndrome, *Pediatrics*, **53**, 221
5. ANDO, T., NYHAN, W. L., CONNOR, J. D., RASMUSSEN, K., DONNELL, G. N., BARNES, N. D., COTTOM, D. and HULL, D. (1972). The oxidation of glycine and propionic acid in propionic acidemia with ketotic hyperglycinemia. *Pediatr. Res.*, **6**, 576
6. NYHAN, W. L. (1974). Nonketotic hyperglycinemia. In W. L. Nyhan (ed.), *Heritable Disorders of Amino Acid Metabolism*, pp. 309–23. (New York; John Wiley & Sons)
7. BAUMGARTNER, E. R., BACHMANN, C., BRECHTBÜHLER, T. and WICK, H. (1975). Acute neonatal nonketotic hyperglycinemia: normal propionate and methylmalonate metabolism. *Pediatr. Res.*, **9**, 559
8. PERRY, T. L., URQUHART, N., MACLEAN, J., EVANS, M. E., HANSEN, S., DAVIDSON, A. G. F., APPLEGARTH, D. A., MACLEOD, P. J. and LOCK, J. E. (1975). Nonketotic hyperglycinemia: glycine accumulation due to absence of glycine cleavage in brain. *N. Engl. J. Med.*, **292**, 1269
9. PERRY, T. L., STEDMAN, D. and HANSEN, S. (1968). A versatile lithium buffer elution system for single column automatic amino acid chromatography. *J. Chromatogr.*, **38**, 460

10. PERRY, T. L., BERRY, K., HANSEN, S., DIAMOND, S. and MOK, C. (1971). Regional distribution of amino acids in human brain obtained at autopsy. *J. Neurochem.*, **18**, 513

11. PERRY, T. L. and HANSEN, S. (1973). Sustained drug-induced elevation of brain GABA in the rat. *J. Neurochem.*, **21**, 1167

12. BRUIN, W. J., FRANTZ, B. M. and SALLACH, H. J. (1973). The occurrence of a glycine cleavage system in mammalian brain. *J. Neurochem.*, **20**, 1649

13. BACHMANN, C., MIHATSCH, M. J., BAUMGARTNER, R. E., BRECHBÜHLER, T., BÜHLER, U. K., OLAFSSON, A., OHNACKER, H. and WICK, H. (1971). Nicht-ketotische Hyperglyzinämie: perakuter Verlauf im Neugeborenenalter. *Helv. Paediatr. Acta*, **26**, 228

14. KRNJEVIC, K. (1974). Chemical nature of synaptic transmission in vertebrates. *Physiol. Rev.*, **54**, 418

15. BARBEAU, A., COITEUX, C., TRUDEAU, J.-G. and FULLUM, G. (1964). La chorée de Huntington chez les Canadiens français: étude préliminaire. *Union Méd. Can.*, **93**, 1178

16. VESSIE, P. R. (1939). Hereditary chorea: St. Anthony's dance and witchcraft in colonial Connecticut. *J. Conn. State Med. Soc.*, **3**, 596

17. CRITCHLEY, M. (1973). Great Britain and the early history of Huntington's chorea. In A. Barbeau, T. N. Chase and G. W. Paulson, (eds.), *Huntington's Chorea 1872–1972, Advances in Neurology*. Vol. 1, pp. 13–17. (New York: Raven Press)

18. PERRY, T. L., HANSEN, S. and KLOSTER, M. (1973). Huntington's chorea: deficiency of γ-aminobutyric acid in brain. *N. Engl. J. Med.*, **288**, 337

19. BIRD, E. D., MACKAY, A. V. P., RAYNER, C. N. and IVERSEN, L. L. (1973). Reduced glutamic-acid-decarboxylase activity in post-mortem brain in Huntington's chorea. *Lancet*, **i**, 1090

20. BIRD, E. D. and IVERSEN, L. L. (1974). Rigidity in Huntington's chorea. *Lancet*, **i**, 463

21. MCGEER, P. L., MCGEER, E. G. and FIBIGER, H. C. (1973). Choline acetylase and glutamic acid decarboxylase in Huntington's chorea. *Neurology*, **23**, 912

22. STAHL, W. L. and SWANSON, P. D. (1974). Biochemical abnormalities in Huntington's chorea brains. *Neurology*, **24**, 813

23. URQUHART, N., PERRY, T. L., HANSEN, S. and KENNEDY, J. (1975). GABA content and glutamic acid decarboxylase activity in brain of Huntington's chorea patients and control subjects. *J. Neurochem.*, **24**, 1071

24. LLOYD, K. G. and HORNYKIEWICZ, O. (1973). L-Glutamic acid decarboxylase in Parkinson's disease: effect of L-dopa therapy. *Nature (London)*, **243**, 521

25. BOWEN, D. M., WHITE, P., FLACK, R. H. A., SMITH, C. and DAVISON, A. N. (1974). Brain-decarboxylase activities as indices of pathological change in senile dementia. *Lancet*, **i**, 1247

26. PERRY, T. L., URQUHART, N., HANSEN, S. and KENNEDY, J. (1974). γ-Aminobutyric acid: drug-induced elevation in monkey brain. *J. Neurochem.*, **23**, 443

27. PERRY, T. L., BRATTY, P. J. A., HANSEN, S., KENNEDY, J., URQUHART, N. and DOLMAN, C. L. (1975). Hereditary mental depression and parkinsonism with taurine deficiency. *Arch. Neurol.*, **32**, 108

28. JACOBSEN, J. G. and SMITH, L. H. Jr. (1968). Biochemistry and physiology of taurine and taurine derivatives. *Physiol. Rev.*, **48**, 424

29. PECK, E. J. Jr. and AWAPARA, J. (1967). Formation of taurine and isethionic acid in rat brain. *Biochim. Biophys. Acta*, **141**, 499

30. CURTIS, D. R. and WATKINS, J. C. (1965). The pharmacology of amino acids related to gamma-aminobutyric acid. *Pharmacol. Rev.*, **17**, 347

31. JASPER, H. and KOYAMA, I. (1969). Rate of release of amino acids from the cerebral cortex in the cat as affected by brain-stem and thalamic stimulation. *Can. J. Physiol. Pharmacol.*, **47**, 889

32. KACZMAREK, L. K. and DAVISON, A. N. (1972). Uptake and release of taurine from rat brain slices. *J. Neurochem.*, **19**, 2355

33. LÄHDESMÄKI, P. and OJA, S. S. (1972). Neurotransmitter or modulator: Does taurine qualify? *Scand. J. Clin. Lab. Invest.*, **29** (Suppl. 122), 71

34. PASANTES-MORALES, H., URBAN, P. F., KLETHI, J. and MANDEL, P. (1973). Light-stimulated release of (^{35}S) taurine from chicken retina. *Brain Res.*, **51**, 375

35. URQUHART, N., PERRY, T. L., HANSEN, S. and KENNEDY, J. (1974). Passage of taurine into adult mammalian brain. *J. Neurochem.*, **22**, 871

36. CURRIER, R. D., GLOVER, G., JACKSON, J. F. and TIPTON, A. C. (1972). Spino-cerebellar ataxia: study of a large kindred. I. General information and genetics. *Neurology*, **22**, 1040
37. KONIGSMARK, B. W. and WEINER, L. P. (1970). The olivopontocerebellar atrophies: a review. *Medicine*, **49**, 227
38. ROUX, H., MURTHY, M. R. V. and BERLINGUET, L. (1974). Role of N-acetylamino acids in cerebral protein synthesis. I. Incorporation of radioactivity from labelled acetyl and aminoacyl moieties into protein. *Brain Res.*, **79**, 235
39. CLARKE, D. D., GREENFIELD, S., DICKER, E., TIRRI, L. J. and RONAN, E. J. (1975). A relationship of N-acetylaspartate biosynthesis to neuronal protein synthesis. *J. Neurochem.*, **24**, 479
40. GJESSING, L. R. and SJAASTAD, O. (1974). Homocarnosinosis: a new metabolic disorder associated with spasticity and mental retardation. *Lancet*, **ii**, 1028
41. PERRY, T. L., HANSEN, S. and KENNEDY, J. (1975). CSF amino acids and plasma-CSF amino acid ratios in adults. *J. Neurochem.*, **24**, 587
42. GROTE, S. S., MOSES, S. G., ROBINS, E., HUDGENS, R. W. and CRONINGER, A. B. (1974). A study of selected catecholamine metabolizing enzymes: a comparison of depressive suicides and alcholic suicides with controls. *J. Neurochem.*, **23**, 791
43. HARRIS, H. (1975). *The Principles of Human Biochemical Genetics*. 2nd ed. (Amsterdam: North-Holland Publishing Co.)
44. MEYER, U. A., STRAND, J., DOSS, M., REES, A. C., and MARVER, H. S. (1972). Intermittent acute porphyria: demonstration of a genetic defect in porphobilinogen metabolism. *N. Engl. J Med.*, **286**, 1277
45. BECKER, M. A., KOSTEL, P. J., MEYER, L. J. and SEEGMILLER, J. E. (1973). Human phosphoribosylpyrophosphate synthetase: increased enzyme specific activity in a family with gout and excessive purine synthesis. *Proc. Nat. Acad. Sci. U.S.A.*, **70**, 2749
46. BECKER, M. A., MEYER, L. J., WOOD, A. W. and SEEGMILLER, J. E. (1973). Purine overproduction in man associated with increased phosphoribosylpyrophosphate synthetase activity. *Science (N.Y.)*, **179**, 1123

Index